ANESTHESIA
FOR
OBSTETRICS

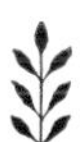

ANESTHESIA FOR OBSTETRICS

Labor — Delivery — Infant Care

ROBERT A. HINGSON

Professor of Anesthesia, Western Reserve University; Director of Anesthesia, University Hospitals of Cleveland

LOUIS M. HELLMAN

Professor of Obstetrics & Gynecology, State University of New York, College of Medicine at New York; Director of Obstetrics & Gynecology, Kings County Hospital

J. B. LIPPINCOTT COMPANY

PHILADELPHIA

MONTREAL

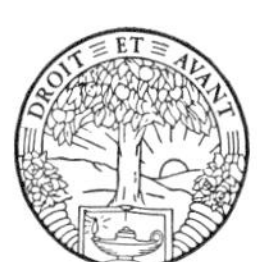

Certain portions of this book appeared in *Control of Pain in Childbirth,* edition 3, by Clifford B. Lull and Robert A. Hingson, copyright, 1948, by J. B. Lippincott Company.

Distributed in Great Britain by
Pitman Medical Publishing Co., Limited, London

Library of Congress Catalog Card No. 55-9914

Printed in the United States of America

Dedication

To those obstetricians and anesthesiologists whose singleness of purpose, mutual respect for problems held in common and co-operative endeavors lead women through childbirth in comfort and safety.

Dedication

To those obstetricians and anesthesiologists whose singleness of purpose, mutual respect for problems held in common and co-operative endeavors lead women through childbirth in comfort and safety.

Preface

There comes a time in the development of two interlocking medical disciplines when each reaches such a stage of complexity that a definitive text on problems and relationships of each to the other becomes obligatory. The authors believe that such a time is at hand in the specialties of obstetrics and anesthesia. In America, obstetrics has solved what may be termed its public health problem. Prenatal care, hospital delivery and safe deliverance are taken for granted. In an age when we turn with more and more interest to the patient's reaction to life's experiences, safe deliverance with optimal comfort and the prevention of psychic trauma are of increasing importance and demand considered evaluation of the available methods of management. Not only is freedom from pain an added nicety to delivery, but technics properly chosen and administered often can tip the balance between tragedy and success.

Anesthesia and analgesia have developed from rather simple technical skills to an increasingly complex specialty involving not only some of the most complicated and least understood aspects of human physiology but also the related sciences of chemistry and physics. With greater knowledge has come greater safety, but only in the hands of knowledgeable and trained personnel. As these two disciplines interlock, depending more and more each upon the other, it is only out of their mutual respect and understanding of each other's problems that safe and comfortable childbirth can be obtained.

The historical section of this volume has been given a place of importance, for it is believed that man's comprehension of the present and his ability to evaluate the future depend upon his understanding of the past. Man should feel himself not as an isolated seeker of scientific truth but as a part of a continuing stream of human enlightenment. This is particularly true when one deals with the process of human reproduction where not only a mechanical procedure is involved but also the mores, the religious beliefs and the prejudices of society play their part. Without some intelligent knowledge of what has gone before no firmly founded progress will be achieved.

Our society permits the physician special privileges granted to no other human being. Of these the obstetrician perhaps shares most. Thus he bears to the patient a closeness of relationship and a feeling of responsibility not found in the other branches of medicine. This special relationship has made him difficult to deal with and has given him a reputation for un-co-operativeness. When the anesthetist is projected into this situation as a third responsible party, he often finds it confusing and not to his liking. In this text we have tried to delineate fields of individual responsibility and areas where mutual co-operation might be beneficial.

In every section the authors have tried to present as briefly as possible the obstetric problems involved so that the anesthetic and analgesic technics may have some comprehensible reason for being. In presenting the obstetric problem it has been necessary to be somewhat didactic. The solutions of the various complications are chosen because the authors believe that they are effective. However, neither they nor the readers should regard these solutions as sole answers to the problems involved.

Finally, neither the anesthesiologists nor the obstetricians should be beguiled by the complexities or the brilliance of their skills. Always it is well, although somewhat humiliating, to remember that nature can perform the process involved quite safely and frequently unaided. The extra niceties of pain relief are added for a variety of reasons, but the *sine qua non* ever should be safety for mother and child.

THE AUTHORS

Introduction

A broad survey of the progress of relief of pain in childbirth from the time of the first delivery under anesthesia on January 19, 1847, until the present reveals definite periods of discovery, custom and enthusiasm. Commencing with chloroform, we have progressed through the morphine and scopolamine era; embarked with anticipation upon the battle of the barbiturates; entered hopefully the field of block anesthesia with continuous caudal and low dosage spinal; and, finally, completed the circle with markedly reduced drug therapy and natural childbirth.

It is worthy of note that Simpson's primary aim was the saving of the mother's life. The humanitarian aspects of obstetric pain relief, although important to him, were secondary. It is quite impossible now to realize the horrors of obstetrics in his day. Long, long labors were carried out frequently against impossibly contracted pelves, and when, finally, physically and mentally exhausted, the mother was subjected to a most painful and difficult operative delivery without anesthesia, it is a wonder that she survived.

Simpson proved to his own satisfaction that the prospects of survival were better if the patient was anesthetized during difficult surgical procedures.

Mortality Accompanying Amputations of the Thigh

Name of Reporter	*Number of Cases*	*Number of Deaths*	*Percentage of Deaths*
Malgaigne, Paris . . .	201	126	62 in 100
Peacock, Edinburgh .	43	21	50 in 100
Phillips' Collection . .	660	263	40 in 100
Lawrie, Glasgow	184	73	40 in 100
Total	1088	483	44 in 100
Anesthetized Patients	135	33	24 in 100

He felt that it must be so also with midwifery. Time has proven this concept to be correct so far as complicated delivery is concerned. With present-day methods it is of less import in the normal delivery.

Carl Gauss remarked continually on the well-being of his postpartum *Dämmerschlaf* cases. This, too, has been a frequent and a correct observation of all interested in this subject.

It remained for Frederick C. Irving to transfer the idea of the lifesaving properties of anesthesia, as conceived by Simpson, to the thesis that the abolition of maternal pain, permitting slower, gentler and more timely deliveries, would save infant lives as well. Through the initiation of a very large program at the Boston Lying-in Hospital, where all mothers were relieved of the pains and the memories of their labors, he attempted to prove his point.

Up to this point concepts concerning obstetric anesthesia and analgesia remained simple and straightforward. Subsequently, a marked improvement occurred in the safety factors of all surgical procedures. The conquest of hemorrhage through blood banks and of infection by means of antibiotics changed not only surgery but the practice of obstetrics, the statistical results of which became immeasurably better. The possible lifesaving properties of obstetric pain relief then were subject to closer scrutiny. The entire problem of perinatal loss—and it is one of some magnitude—came into focus. The transplacental narcotic effect of previously employed drugs began to seem somewhat undesirable, and thus block anesthesia appeared to be attractive. The technics involved do reduce to a minimum the fetal effect of drugs, but they are complicated, and their sequelae require increased training and skill. The perfection of methods for block anesthesia made deliveries free from pain possible in conscious women. This experience added visible knowledge to the influence of the methods of seminarcosis and general anesthesia that childbirth could be accomplished in a very pleasant and satisfying fashion. The fact that today some several million women have been delivered comfortably and completely awake under the conduction block methods has made possible a more complete acceptance of the principles re-enunciated by Grantly Dick Read which conclude that pain is reduced and in the normal patient is negligible if fear and tension are controlled. Public acceptance of this concept would have been inconceivable 20 years ago. It is only through the fact that over 4 generations of women have had the pains of labor relieved to some degree since Simpson first practiced his art that the fear and the trepidation regarding childbirth have been so allayed as to make the naturalness of the phenomena acceptable. Furthermore, there has been an increasing awareness and interest in psychological phenomena by both physician and layman. Now it is generally admitted that the awareness of the birth process and the actual physical and mental co-operation with it are advantageous to the psychological growth of women. Facts relating to the problems of childbirth are actually being taught and understood in an increasing number of high schools and colleges and through the facilities of an informed press which reaches nearly every person. We have emerged from the era in which both physician and patient believed that childbirth was so unnatural and the pain so indescribable that it was necessary to eliminate consciousness of the event by various combinations of pharmacologic agents. Following this education and better understanding of body physiology, we have a new generation of mothers who actually are curious concerning all the phenomena relating to childbirth, and many of them are anxious to participate consciously in all or a considerable part of this experience. This new attitude has reduced definitely the total amount and the duration of systemic narcosis in early labor and has held to a minimum its use in terminal labor; and yet, in indicated cases under competent management of the obstetrician and the anesthetist team, it has made more acceptable the use of both systemic narcosis and anesthesia of all types. Against this historical background and with full realization of the psychological importance of reproduction, the authors set forth the following basic principles for the use of analgesia and anesthesia as valuable adjuvants to the mother and the obstetrician without danger to the baby during labor and delivery:

BASIC PRINCIPLE 1

Complete and safe anesthesia of both the encephalic and the anatomic varieties with 100 per cent intensity in obliterating pain should be available instantaneously in every maternity for any patient who needs it. This holds true for spontaneous delivery, operative delivery or cesarean section. Should one type prove to be inadequate through technical or pharmacologic failure, another can be instituted immediately.

BASIC PRINCIPLE 2

No single agent or method of pain relief in the hands of every obstetrician-anesthetist team is acceptable universally. Since the requirements of multiparous and primiparous normal patients and of those presenting complicated abnormalities of physical structure and metabolic efficiency vary considerably, different methods of pain relief are recommended.

Unfortunately, maternity hospitals all over the world have not yet worked out satisfactory programs whereby obstetric anesthesia is administered by competent personnel on a 24-hour basis on a level commensurate with present-day knowledge.

NEGLECT OF OBSTETRIC ANESTHESIA CAN HARM OUR RELATIONS WITH PATIENTS, HOSPITALS

Leading anesthesiologists have emphasized the important added margin of safety possible in childbirth through professional anesthesia services. On the other hand, this phase of anesthesiology is often neglected in the rush of more complicated procedures, and administration of obstetric anesthesia is left to technicians. Failure to develop this phase of our specialty in more and more institutions may be a serious disservice to the patient and to the hospital, from both a medical and human relations standpoint.

WHAT THE PATIENT EXPECTS

Newspapers from time to time publish articles on deaths occurring under anesthesia during the simplest operations. It is possible that many of these could not be avoided. It is equally true that a qualified anesthesiologist can often prevent shock or other conditions responsible for death under anesthesia. The importance of having a trained physician at the head of the operating table during any surgical procedure, no matter how large or how small, is constantly emphasized by the Society. More and more patients realize the importance of professional anesthesia. Death for any reason during elective surgery simply cannot be tolerated. The patient knows that better anesthesia care is available than ever before, and expects it.

OPPORTUNITY FOR CONFUSION

Probably no one is more confused about anesthesia than an expectant mother going to the hospital for the first time. For weeks she has been reading popular articles about new drugs, hypnosis, natural childbirth, spinals, saddle block, and similar subjects. She has discussed the subject of anesthesia with her friends. And she is hopelessly confused on the subject. Then she arrives at the hospital in pain, usually at a time when her obstetrician is not present. She may get too much analgesic, not enough analgesic, or the wrong kind of anesthetic for her condition.

A mother having her third child recently had her baby held back until the obstetrician arrived, then had it without benefit of anesthesia whatsoever. The baby suffered a brain injury in childbirth. And this happened at a maternity hospital that supposedly is one of the finest in America.

24-HOUR SERVICE ESSENTIAL

It is worth pointing out that if professional anesthesia is desirable at 8 o'clock in the morning, it is equally desirable at midnight. A hospital with a qualified anesthesia staff has the right to expect service on a round-the-clock basis for its patients. More and more hospitals are certain to demand such service, and to take steps to obtain it if their staff physicians do not meet the challenge.

A great many anesthesiologists are recognizing this problem and meeting the need, one result being that a qualified physician is usually on hand. This can be particularly important to obstetric patients, who obviously cannot schedule their exact hour of arrival at the hospital in advance.

THE MEASURING STICK

Most obstetric patients recall the anesthesia care they receive or the lack of it as the most vivid impression of the type of medical care accorded them. A mother who has an unpleasant experience in childbirth is going to have a sorry opinion of the quality of anesthesia care at your hospital for the rest of her life, no matter whether you had anything to do with her care or not.

How much better would it be if she received some information about anesthesia from you in advance of her confinement, and knew that a physician anesthesiologist would be on hand to greet her and provide her with the finest care available before her obstetrician arrived and during the period of childbirth.

PRACTICAL PROBLEMS

Naturally, there are practical problems in many institutions where the supply of physician anesthesiologists is small and the number of maternity cases is substantial. On the other hand, who is to tell the public that professional anesthesia is vital in every surgical procedure, yet is not to be provided in obstetric cases where the well-being of both mother and child is at stake?

It may be a long time before practical problems can be removed and professional anesthesia services can be provided for every obstetric patient in your hospital. But planning towards this end is essential in our specialty. It is important from a sound medical viewpoint. And it is equally vital in terms of the sound human relationships needed for the orderly growth and development of our specialty.*

The authors are indebted for a full decade of collaboration and support to the pharmaceutical companies of America: Abbott Laboratories; Astra Pharmaceutical Company; Ciba Pharmaceutical Products; Eli Lilly and Company; Merck and Co., Inc.; Parke, Davis and Company; Sharp and Dohme, Inc.; E. R. Squibb and Sons; Winthrop-Stearns, Inc.; and Becton, Dickinson and Company. We are also indebted to the Johns Hopkins University and Hospital and Sinai Hospital, of Baltimore; Western Reserve University and University Hospitals, of Cleveland; the State University of New York, College of Medicine at New York and the Kings County Hospital; and the United States Public Health Service.

We owe much to Nicholson J. Eastman, Allen F. Guttmacher, Thomas Parran, Leonard Scheele, Ralph Chester Williams and Selwyn D. Collins in their high administrative capacities; without their co-operation and active consultation this work would have been impossible.

* By the American Society of Anesthesiologists on Professional Relations Policies and Ideas, February, 1955.

Of singular significance was the statistical *Arbeit* of Ruth Phillips and her associates of the Division of Public Health Methods in the correlation of our data.

We also thank the following personnel of the Baltimore Pain Study: Physicians Erin Griffin, of Wellington, New Zealand, Nellie Knottenbelt, of Leiden University, Holland, Lawrence Cheng-Chung, of Shanghai, China, Ruth Merrill, Andy Bowdon, Jack Riley, Harold Davidson and the late Whedon Johnson; nurses Ruth Blevin, Patricia Doolin, Katie Sue Floyd, Mary Hoffman, Ruth Montgomery, Dorothy Plummer and Martha Stern; coding clerks and statisticians Omer L. Heusman and Agnes Shriver; secretaries Lalla Nelson, Julianna Duffy, Rosemary Deckel, Leona Peck and Jacqueline Hartenstein.

For reading and correcting proof we are indebted to Dr. William A. Cull, Assistant Professor of Anesthesia in charge of the Division in the MacDonald House (Obstetrics & Gynecology), Western Reserve University, Cleveland, Ohio, and to Mary Jane Fitzpatrick.

Finally, we acknowledge the help of all our colleagues and nurses on the attending and hospital staffs of the Departments of Obstetrics of the Johns Hopkins and Sinai Hospitals, of Baltimore.

Contents

1 Obstetric Amnesia, Analgesia and Anesthesia in Broad Perspective

During the decade 1945 to 1955, progress in the understanding and the utilization of the principles of obstetric analgesia and anesthesia during childbirth has exceeded the accomplishments of the previous century so dramatically and effectively introduced by the lifework of Sir James Y. Simpson, of Edinburgh.

Maternal mortality in the United States, which was greater than 1 per cent at the beginning of the century, has been reduced from 9.1 per thousand in 1919 to the all-time low of about 1.5 per thousand live births (Fig. 1).

Perinatal infant mortality has been reduced from the staggering losses of more than 10 per cent near the turn of the century to about 3.5 per cent (Fig. 2). This figure includes the previable prematures, the intra-uterine deaths due to nonpreventable anoxia and hypoxia of mechanical origin and the 0.5 per cent of infants with congenital anomalies incompatible with life. Many of the intra-uterine deaths stem from interference with placental circulation in such conditions as premature separation, placenta previa and toxemia. Obviously, obstetric anal-

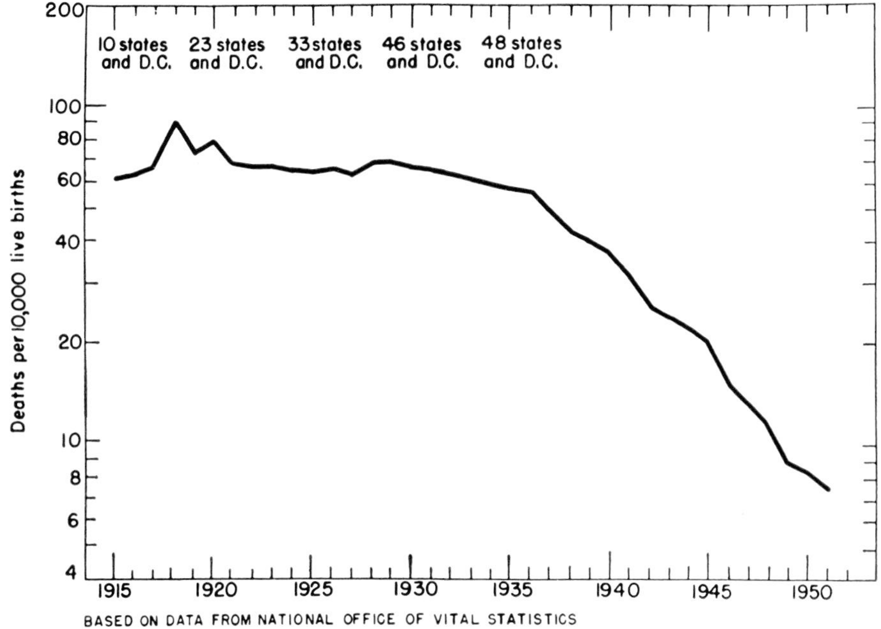

FIG. 1. Undoubtedly emphasis upon and the institution of better obstetric anesthesia have combined, with improved prenatal care, antibiotics and improved operating-room and delivery-room safeguards, in reducing the 20-year plateau of maternal mortality almost tenfold since 1936.

gesia and anesthesia cannot influence this fetal wastage; however, it must be employed with increased vigilance and skill to protect these handicapped mothers.

Likewise, maternal and fetal morbidity have been lowered strikingly. As in 1849, Simpson produced evidence emphasizing that anesthesia produced reductions in surgical mortality from amputations, so do we document evidence in the following chapters that much of the salvage of mother and baby life in this era is due to intelligent use of analgesia and anesthesia and the related supervision of respiration and infant resuscitation.

The afferent pathways of labor and delivery pain identified through the works of Head, in 1894, and Cleland, in 1933, were understood and appreciated by the obstetrician and the anesthetist only in the past decade.

The obstetric textbooks of the past 2 centuries, at most, devoted only a few pages to quoted and poorly defined technics on the management of obstetric anesthesia. The character and the intensity of the birth outcry became a gauge of progress in labor in estimating cervical dilatation and degree of pelvic descent of the presenting part. The historical manuscripts from all the early civilizations describing the pains concomitant with childbirth were read but unheeded. The 61 Biblical references to the agony of travail, the picturesque *Poena Magna* in ancient Roman writings, and the dissatisfactions of the feminine maternal half of our population were not enough to bring proper scientific emphasis and *opus* into the birth rooms of the world. Textbooks on anesthesia, which presented in well-organized chapters the minutiae of pharmacology and technic in all types of surgical anesthetics, presented only a few scattered paragraphs on this vital subject. Neither did authors of obstetrics or of anesthesia take cognizance of the fundamental differences of depth, duration and induction or the altered anatomic, endo-

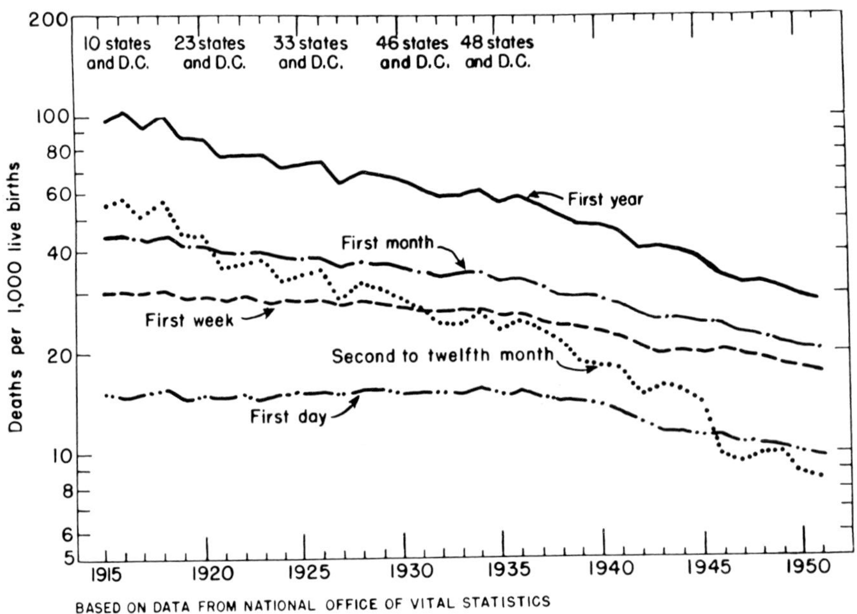

FIG. 2. Thirty-five year graph showing decline in infant mortality particularly evident since 1935. Described in text.

crinologic and physiologic differences between the obstetric and the surgical patient. Of greater significance was the fact that no attempt was made until recently to determine the temporal factors and the hemodynamics of transplacental narcosis with the resultant effect on perinatal physiology.

The late Clifford Lull, together with Robert A. Hingson, presented the first complete text covering the knowledge of the subject in *Control of Pain in Childbirth,* in 1944,* almost a century after the first obstetric anesthetic. Since this time, 3 editions of this work and 3 complete texts by other American authors (obstetricians), 2 by British authors and monographs by French, Spanish and Portuguese authors in Europe and South America on the subject, together with more than 800 scientific papers in the medical literature, bear evidence of the increasing significance of this field. Finally, it is being recognized that surgical and obstetric anesthesia are as different as surgery and obstetrics. It is essential for the obstetrician to understand the principles of anesthesia and for the anesthetist to understand the obstetric principles of labor and delivery. *The basic theme of this text is the development of teamwork between obstetrician and anesthetist in the management of maternal and infant comfort and safety.*

The mere mention of the approximate 4,000,000 births per year in the United States, with use of some forms of pain-relieving drugs in more than 75 per cent of them, indicates the importance of the subject. It is interesting to reflect on the fact that this represents 24,000,000 woman-hours in labor if the conservative figure of 6 hours of active labor per average case is standard. By way of comparison, the 535 members of both Houses of Congress spend approximately 200 8-hour days in each session for a total of 800,000 congressman man-hours or approximately 3 per cent of the time deliberating the nation's present as the maternal population spends in actual labor producing the population foundation of the nation's future.

Furthermore, the last decade has seen the number of American hospital deliveries rise to 85 per cent of the births. The movement of the patient from the bedroom to the hospital not only makes available better anesthesia and analgesia but also increases the demand for more and better pain relief.

The decade has seen a major focus of attention on the quantitative assay of obstetric pain, as well as the qualitative assay of the efficiency of the analgesic and anesthetic drugs.

These drugs include the widespread use of Demerol and related synthetic analgesics. Studies now are being undertaken on n-allyl-normorphine, the antagonistic drugs to morphine and Demerol. The British have reintroduced trichloroethylene. Also in this group are the muscle relaxant drugs curare and succinylcholine, whose place in obstetrics now is understood better. The recent introduction of the steroid Viadril into obstetric anesthesia merits consideration. Finally, and of no less significance, has been the relatively recent development of the vast field of conduction anesthesia. This is through the continuous caudal, peridural, spinal, saddle block and pudendal block. It is by this latter group that at least one fourth of the nation's obstetric anesthetics are managed.

The development of the psychosomatic approach to obstetric pain relief parallels the general development and interest in this phenomenon in all of medicine. Such an approach would have been untenable a generation ago when fear of obstetric pain was universal and

* Lull, C. B., and Hingson, R. A.: Control of Pain in Childbirth, Philadelphia, Lippincott.

relief could be expected only through obliteration of memory and consciousness. The vast difference in the attitude of the well-educated young matron today is so great as to be scarcely recognizable. To her to whom no traditional fear of pain or danger to life remains, the verbalization of relief of pain, tension and fear makes good sense. Parturition becomes a natural life experience in which she desires to partake actively.

Regardless of how one feels about Read's and Nikolaev's ideas concerning childbirth, it must be admitted that their emphasis on the proper mental and physical preparation of pregnant women for delivery is a distinct contribution. However, there is inconclusive evidence that the prescribed exercises serve in any way to accelerate or ease labor. As with the other Read technics of muscle relaxation and concentration on the child, they can be considered as unwitting hypnotic shortcuts to a psychological lobotomy.

This is not meant to deprecate any such technics, for they are used instinctively by any good physician, but it is said merely to place them in proper perspective. Such approaches appeal to the educated private patient and even to those who read and understand popular journalism. If the psychological lobotomy fails to some degree, at least the use of drugs will have been cut down. However, natural delivery is not the goal for every woman nor need it be considered as the ideal for American obstetrics. As a matter of fact, Grantly Dick Read makes little sense to the mother of the slums or her sister from Tobacco Road or to the Southern Negress in the "Help me, Jesus" stage of labor. As Klein and Potter so aptly point out, her fears and superstitions are so much more primitive and basic that she cannot and does not comprehend the psychological approach to pain. To her, reality is found in the encephalic obliteration or dulling of consciousness. Nerve block is barely acceptable.

One should be as careful with the psychological scalpel as with the surgeon's scalpel and should be no less trained in its use. The great danger in the total acceptance of the Read philosophy is not patient harm but a deterioration of the quality of anesthesia available so that when needed, it is neither expertly given nor wisely chosen.

The principles of better maternal anesthesia have been built on firm foundations. The 10-year Chicago study of infant mortality and the 3-year Baltimore obstetric anesthesia study have contributed much to this end. There is a current focus of attention on the salvage of the premature infant and efforts to avoid the tragic and unnecessary mortalities associated with cesarean section.

In the last decade, this mass of knowlelge developing from discoveries and new critical analyses in both the specialties of anesthesia and obstetrics has become so extensive and of such vital significance to the comfort and the safety of mothers and newborn babies. It also has become so confusing and controversial that the authors feel obliged as a combined endeavor to compile, organize, epitomize and present these data. The effort of this book will be to do so in concise technics that will be readily available and utilizable by practitioners and students of each specialty.

The authors recognize that the best application of pain relief in obstetrics needs constant revision, most careful records and analysis of factual data, not the least of which is a fair and open mind to compare the new with the old in forming opinions. Also, we have found of advantage the unbiased appraisal of the individual parturient and the mass of parturients concerning the degree of comfort and security experienced by them during labor and delivery with the various methods. It is quite certain that no single method or technic yet designed is satisfactory for all cases. Yet most of the standard forms of management of labor and delivery will provide the same relative efficiency and safety for the majority of normal parturients having full-term normal babies provided that those technics are administered properly.

The character of labor, its intensity and duration and the pain threshold of the patient, her emotional stability and previous anesthetic and obstetric experiences are factors that sometimes call for the skilled execution of one technic when another would be otherwise satisfactory.

Unquestionably, the accumulation of medical knowledge concerning the safe conduct of labor and delivery and of the management of pain relief during this period has far surpassed its clinical application. In reviewing the progress that has been made during the first century of control of pain in childbirth, the authors are convinced that there should be closer correlation between the use of knowledge derived from the basic sciences of anatomy, physiology and pharmacology and the clinical application of medical technics in obstetrics and anesthesiology. While the transplacental narcosis, a by-product of obstetric amnesia, analgesia and general anesthesia, is a deplorable condition, its dangers can be offset to some degree by the maintenance of adequate transplacental oxygenation of the fetus during the period of labor. The more vigorous and prolonged the contractions during labor, the more necessary is the saturation of the maternal oxyhemoglobin transport system in order that hypoxia of the infant may be relieved between contractions. Certainly the 50 per cent nitrous oxide and 50 per cent air analgesia technics of Britain and the Continent would be most disadvantageous to the baby in such situations, since this reduces the available alveolar oxygen to the dangerous level of 10 per cent. The partial pressure of oxygen under these circumstances approaches

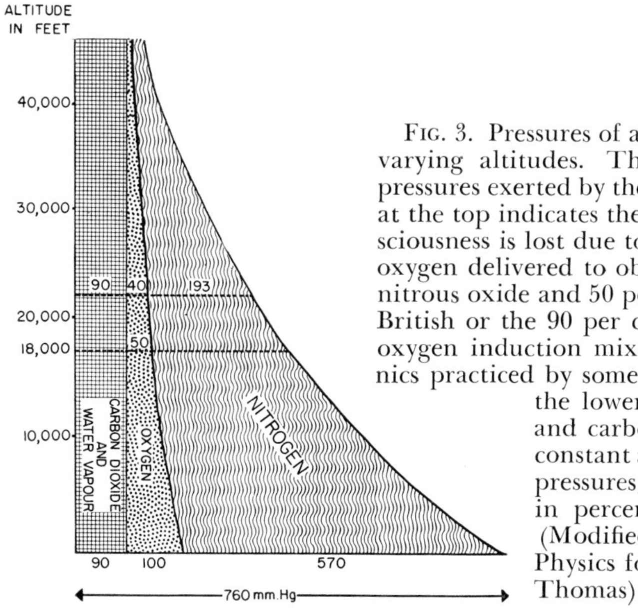

Fig. 3. Pressures of alveolar gases when breathing air at varying altitudes. The shaded areas show the partial pressures exerted by the component gases. The dotted line at the top indicates the approximate height at which consciousness is lost due to hypoxia. The partial pressure of oxygen delivered to obstetric patients by the 50 per cent nitrous oxide and 50 per cent air analgesic technics of the British or the 90 per cent nitrous oxide and 10 per cent oxygen induction mixtures in critically dangerous technics practiced by some hospitals in America is shown by the lower dotted line. Note: Water vapor and carbon dioxide in the alveolus remain constant at 90 mm. Hg and combined partial pressures, regardless of altitude or variations in percentage of anesthesia gas mixtures. (Modified from MacIntosh & Mushin: Physics for the Anesthetist, Springfield, Ill., Thomas)

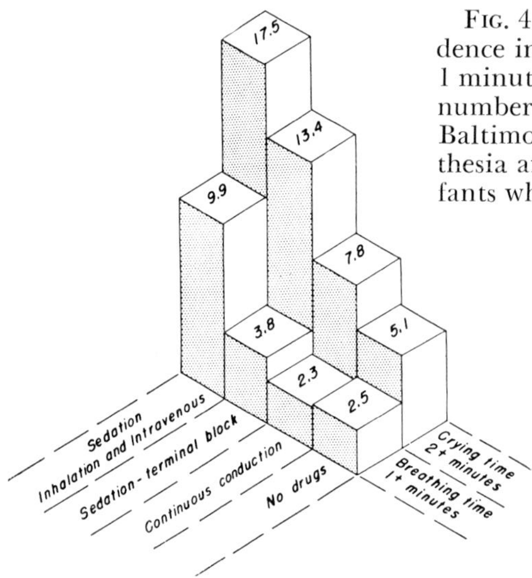

FIG. 4. This 3-dimensional graph illustrates the incidence in percentage of delay in breathing time beyond 1 minute, and of crying time beyond 2 minutes, of total number of infants born to 7,704 mothers in a 3-year Baltimore obstetric anesthesia study by method of anesthesia and analgesia used. Twins, cesarean sections, infants who died before onset of labor and analgesia, and infants with congenital malformations incompatible with life were excluded.

the hazardous conditions found at altitudes of 20,000 feet above sea level—only a few feet below the critical altitude where the normal nonpregnant individual loses consciousness from anoxia! (Fig. 3.) Happily, in this decade, there are many technics, including all of the conduction anesthesia methods, which permit 100 per cent oxygen inhalation by the mother.

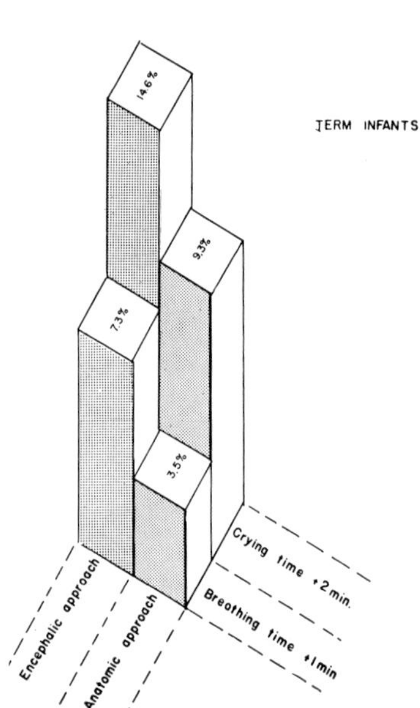

FIG. 5. This summarizes the information in Figure 4 relating to full-term infants in this study. The encephalic approach methods include systemic narcosis during labor and all inhalation and intravenous anesthesia methods. The anatomic approach methods include all local, spinal, caudal and extradural anesthesia methods.

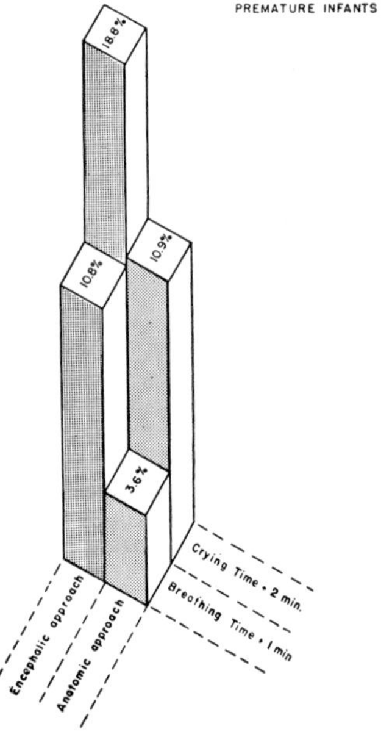

FIG. 6. This summarizes the information in Figure 4 relating to the 988 premature infants in this study. Undoubtedly, the premature infant is jeopardized far less when spared the transplacental narcotic effect of inhalation and intravenous anesthesia.

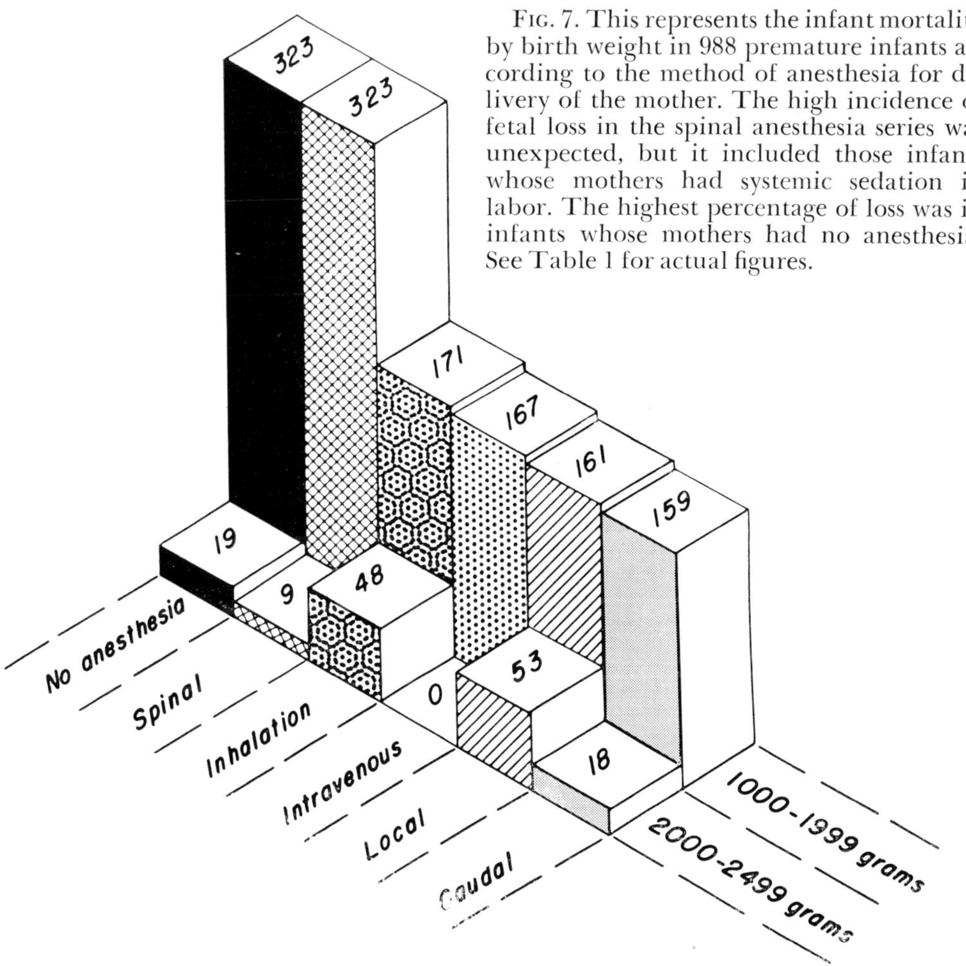

FIG. 7. This represents the infant mortality by birth weight in 988 premature infants according to the method of anesthesia for delivery of the mother. The high incidence of fetal loss in the spinal anesthesia series was unexpected, but it included those infants whose mothers had systemic sedation in labor. The highest percentage of loss was in infants whose mothers had no anesthesia. See Table 1 for actual figures.

In modern obstetrics, in maintaining optimum comfort during childbirth it is necessary to develop the maximum co-operation between obstetricians and anesthetists in the correlation of the principles of both specialties. In surgical procedures, there is only one patient to consider, whereas in parturition, there are two—the mother and the baby. The respiratory center of the latter is especially vulnerable to sedative and anesthetic drugs, and, since these agents, if given systemically, regularly traverse the placenta, the probability of their obtunding the initiation of respiration at birth is apparent as shown by Figures 4 to 7 and Table 1.

Also, it is necessary to recognize that the degree of complete pain relief in labor and, to a lesser extent, during delivery, is of secondary importance to parturient progress during labor and delivery.

Again, in contrast with surgery, where complete anesthesia may be instituted with a rapid induction to the required depth for muscular relaxation, in obstetrics intensity of anesthesia must be balanced with physiologic uterine activity and progress in labor. Rarely, even in this decade, and much less frequently than in times past, all degrees of pain relief must await the diagnosis and the treatment of the factors of desultory

TABLE 1. STILLBIRTHS AND NEONATAL LOSS FOR PREMATURES[1] BY TWO BIRTHWEIGHT GROUPS ACCORDING TO METHODS OF ADMINISTERING DRUGS

METHOD	*Number of Cases*[2]			*Rate per 1,000 Total Births*		
	STILL-BIRTHS	NEONATAL DEATHS	TOTAL BIRTHS	STILL-BIRTHS	NEONATAL DEATHS	TOTAL DEATHS
			1,000 to 1,999 Gm.			
Total	*4*	*41*	*211*	*19.0*	*194.3*	*213.3*
No anesthesia	1	10	34	29.4	294.1	323.5
Intravenous		1	6		166.7	166.7
Inhalation		6	35		171.4	171.4
Conduction						
Caudal	3	8	69	43.5	115.9	159.4
Spinal		11	34		323.5	323.5
Local		5	31		161.3	161.3
Combination of methods			2			
			2,000 to 2,499 Gm.			
Total	*2*	*9*	*500*	*4.0*	*18.0*	*22.0*
No anesthesia		1	53		18.9	18.9
Intravenous			29			
Inhalation		5	104		48.1	48.1
Conduction						
Caudal	2	1	163	12.3	6.1	18.4
Spinal		1	115		8.7	8.7
Local		1	19		52.6	52.6
Combination of methods			17			

1 Prematures include all infants weighing 1,000 to 2,499 Gm.
2 Twins, cesarean sections, infants who died before onset of labor and analgesia and infants with congenital malformation incompatible with life are excluded.

labor. Happily for the comfort of the patient, sometimes the treatment is a complete rest with adequate sedation with barbiturates and morphine in desultory labor in the first stages of cervical dilatation, or it is the institution of continuous caudal analgesia in prolonged cases of uterine dysfunction with or without augmenting oxytocic intravenous drip therapy.

The optimal time for starting medicinal analgesia is the responsibility of the obstetrician and demands astute judgment that can be garnered only from experience. The most common error, often producing grave consequences, is to start it too soon! In retrospect, many of our worst cases of prolonged labor may be charged sometimes to the premature use of sedative drugs or to the premature employment of some form of vertebral conduction anesthesia. One rule should be absolute: *Such medication never should be started until positive proof exists that the cervix is showing progressive effacement and dilatation characteristic of labor in the acceleration phase.* Analgesia and anesthesia are too important to the patient in the last half of labor and delivery to waste and misuse them or to store them in the fatty depots of mother and fetus in false or desultory labor with 10- and 20-second contractions that occur every 5 to 10 minutes. If an error is to be made, it will be a less costly mistake if the medication is started too late rather than too early. In 1951, in an analysis of 202 instances of prolonged labor in the Boston Lying-in Hospital, it was believed that analgesic drugs were the major cause in 19 cases. Adriani has reported that saddle block anesthesia has a tendency to slow and even stop some labors notwithstanding the fact that it definitely accelerates others. The authors have reported the same experience with continuous caudal analgesia in continued warnings since 1942.

CHARACTERISTICS OF GOOD AND SAFE ANESTHESIA

1. It must be both predictable and controllable.

2. It must have a rapid and not unpleasant onset without a latent profound or summation of effect.

3. It must be reversible with prompt restoration of physiologic vital body or organ functions in both mother and baby.

4. It must be eliminated rapidly or destroyed promptly into harmless by-products that leave a minimum of sequellae from its use.

5. The effective antidote to counteract any sudden, inadvertent toxic effect of the drug, as well as the means of carrying on effective respiration and oxygenation, should be readily available.

CHARACTERISTICS OF GOOD AND SAFE ANALGESIA

1. If administered by inhalation, it should be weak enough to be employed continually for 4 to 5 minutes at delivery without taking the "average" patient into the excitement stage or into full anesthesia.

2. Inhalation analgesia should be produced within 15 seconds (the usual interval between the beginning of a uterine contraction and the development of pain).

3. Systemic or inhalation analgesia should be compatible with prolonged administration without significant toxic effect.

4. Transplacental effect on the infant must not exceed the limits of safety.

5. Ideally, the systemic effects should not require prolonged, continuous individual nursing attention or strait-jacket confinement.

VITAL SAFEGUARDS AND STANDARD EQUIPMENT FOR EACH DELIVERY ROOM

1. Assorted mechanical oral and nasal airways

2. Negative suction apparatus for the aspiration of mucus, vomitus or blood

3. Endotracheal tubes, connectors and adapters and laryngoscopes

4. Transparent, properly fitting face masks with workable pressure-limiting valves

5. Tables that readily assume the Trendelenburg position

6. Therapeutic oxygen readily available through properly working gas machines so that intermittent positive pressure can be administered promptly to mother and baby

7. Since most of the anesthetic, amnesic and analgesic drugs depress and interfere with the heat-regulating mechanisms, the temperature of the labor and delivery rooms should be maintained at about 80°F. For example, assuming a respiratory minute volume of 8 L. per minute, the heat lost by the patient when ether is given by the circle method is about 180 calories per minute. The parturient, especially in states of shock, fatigue or starvation after prolonged labor, should not be exposed to drafts or sudden changes in temperature. Likewise, drafts and low environmental temperatures are dangerous in parturients with respiratory diseases and following

the hypometabolism of prolonged semi-narcosis.

AMNESIA, ANALGESIA AND SOPORIFIC DEPRESSION DURING LABOR

The state of amnesia through depression of the frontal lobe cortex may be achieved by the specific pharmacologic action of scopolamine, one of the alkaloids of belladonna, or by obtunding frontal lobe cerebration with one or a combination of the barbiturates alone or with such analgesics as morphine or Demerol.

Scopolamine can be used alone to produce a pure amnesia; it can be used with a soporific to produce an amnesia plus sleep; it can be used with morphine or Demerol and Amidone or Nisentil to produce amnesia plus analgesia; or it can be used in combination with both a soporific and an analgesic. The pure pharmacologic action of the belladonna group will be considered first.

The Belladonna Group

The belladonna group of drugs includes scopolamine, hyoscyamine and atropine. They are considered to be parasympathetic depressant drugs with a diversant action on the central nervous system. Atropine produces a stimulation of the medulla and the higher cerebral centers when therapeutic doses are used. Later there is a central nervous system depression.

Scopolamine, on the other hand, is a primary depressant of the central nervous system in such a manner as to cause drowsiness, fatigue and dreamless sleep, and sometimes forgetfulness. It is this action which indicates the use of scopolamine as a preanesthetic medication and as an amnesic agent in the obstetric management of the first stage of labor.

Not infrequently, however, therapeutic doses of scopolamine cause excitement, restlessness, hallucinations and delirium. From our experience we cannot emphasize too strongly that in these instances during the first stage of labor, the use of the drug should be discontinued, and one of the other forms of management should be substituted. The limitations of the various combinations of "twilight sleep" should be recognized and remedied by the selection of a more satisfactory analgesic agent during labor.

Goodman and Gilman* state:

> Atropine and scopolamine differ quantitatively in their peripheral parasympatholytic actions. Scopolamine is the stronger blocking agent for the iris, ciliary body, and certain secre-

* Goodman, Louis, and Gilman, Alfred: Pharmacological Basis of Therapeutics, ed. 2, New York, Macmillan, 1955.

Atropine:

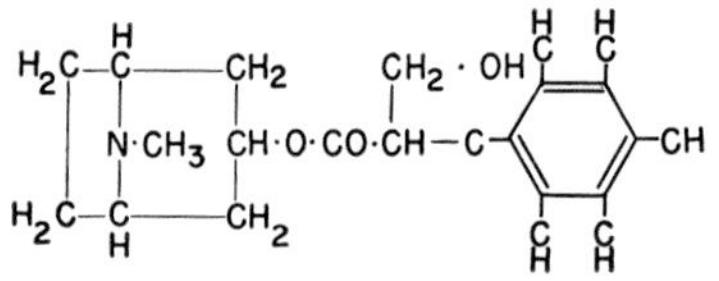

$C_{17}H_{23}O_3N$ — Mol. wt. 289.36

Scopolamine:

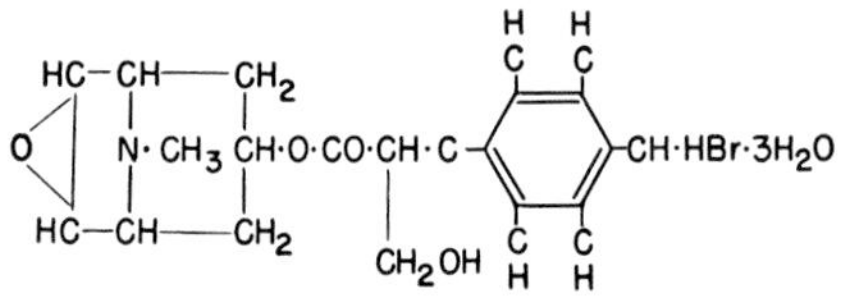

$C_{17}H_{21}NO_4 \cdot HBr \cdot 3H_2O$ — Mol. wt. 438.32

tory (salivary, bronchial, and sweat) glands. The action of atropine is more pronounced and more prolonged than that of scopolamine on the heart, intestine, and bronchiolar musculature. Atropine is more useful than scopolamine for peripheral autonomic blocking actions because in clinical doses it lacks any significant central sedative effect. Scopolamine is occasionally used for its ocular effects, but otherwise it is administered mainly for its central effects.

The following organs are moderately depressed under the action of the belladonna alkaloids: higher and motor cerebral centers, lacrimal glands, mucous and salivary glands, ocular ciliary muscle, heart, pancreas, stomach, intestines, uterus, bladder and the cerebral cortex of the baby. The respiratory, vasomotor and temperature-regulating centers and the respiratory mechanisms are stimulated under the action of these drugs.

The maximum effect after therapeutic doses of the drug is achieved in about 1½ hours. The duration of effect is usually from 3 to 5 hours, which in some instances is prolonged for 8 to 12 hours.

These drugs are eliminated through the kidneys. Adriani has found that one therapeutic dose was eliminated within 36 hours.

Reynolds has pointed out, with possible significance, that atropine exerts an inhibitory effect upon the hyperemia to which estrogen gives rise in the whole uterus. Likewise, fright and hypoxia cause a vasoconstriction in the endometrial vessels after a latent period of 17 seconds—which probably represents the circulation time after epinephrine release. These factors are included in this discussion in order that the obstetrician might consider the harmful effects of extreme belladonna dosages in extremely apprehensive patients who are laboring in a noisy maternity. The authors have observed profound bradycardia and fetal thrashing in utero after a vasopressor was used in these circumstances.

Demerol

Demerol (ethyl 1-methyl-4-phenylpiperidine 4-carboxylate hydrochloride) was introduced by Eisleb and Schaumann in Germany, in 1939, as Dolantin, Dolantol or D-140. It is a white crystalline substance slightly soluble in water and with a strong alkaline reaction. The hydrochloride is employed medicinally. It is readily soluble in water and has a neutral reaction with a slightly bitter taste. The solution is not decomposed by a short boiling period.

Batterman and Rovenstine were pioneers during its developmental period in America. Previously it had been investigated extensively on the European continent.

Pharmacologically, Demerol has a distinct relaxing action on the smooth muscles of the bowel, the uterus, the bronchial tree and the urinary bladder. This action as an antispasmodic has been attributable to a depression of the parasympathetic nerve endings and of smooth muscle directly. The former action resembled that of atropine but was not so marked, while the direct muscular depression was greater than that produced by papaverine. After careful experiments on animals and human subjects, Barlow, using the Hardy, Wolff and Goodell technic, concluded that in

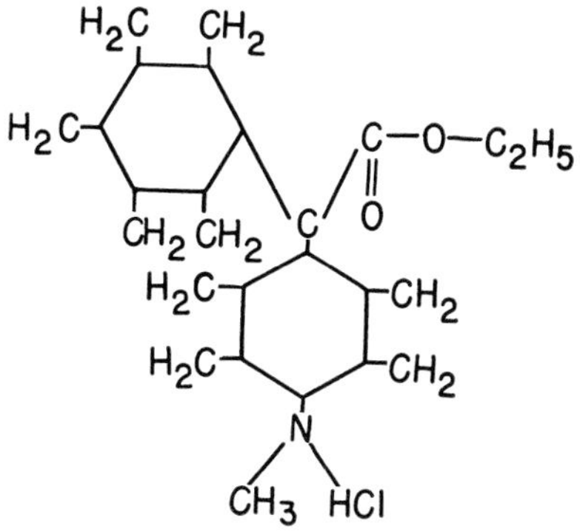

Demerol (Meperidine) (Pethidine)

analgesic potency Demerol was intermediate between codeine and morphine.

The preliminary consensus by those who have given it considerable trial is that Demerol is a safe analgesic approximating the effectiveness of morphine for the relief of pain. As compared with morphine, its structural formula is relatively simple.

The use of Demerol in obstetrics was first reported by Benthin in Germany; frequently, he observed mild uterine atony. In America it was first tested in obstetrics by Gilbert and Dixon in Baltimore. Later, it was used more thoroughly by Frederick C. Irving at the Boston Lying-in Hospital.

These investigators have confirmed that Demerol has analgesic properties approaching the efficiency of morphine in its action upon the higher centers. When used with scopolamine it takes the place of morphine as a supplementary amnesic agent in a large percentage of cases. Twenty per cent of cases receiving therapeutic doses of Demerol developed increased diaphoresis, and 36 per cent of ambulatory subjects developed mild reactions, such as dizziness, euphoria, intense thirst, nausea and occasional vomiting. The depression of the respiratory and the gastro-intestinal systems is definitely less than when morphine is used. Gilbert and Dixon state that the parturients slept occasionally between pains, but at no time were they narcotized to the point that they did not respond to questioning in conversational tone. There was no reaction upon the pupil, and the miosis of morphine was not seen.

The drug passes to the baby through the placenta. The use of any of the general anesthetics just before delivery significantly accentuates the depressive effect on the baby.

Our own observation in the use of Demerol leads us to believe that there is a moderate retardation of the baby's respiratory mechanism with a degree of central nervous system depression comparable with that present in the mother. We have seen one baby sleep for 6 minutes after the use of Demerol and scopolamine when only 2 minutes of nitrous oxide was used as terminal delivery anesthesia. This baby's respiration was fairly well established, but it did not respond to the usual forms of external stimulation for this period. However, premature babies definitely are not narcotized to a degree comparable with that often seen with morphine.

At present, Demerol is used in doses of 100 mg. each 3 to 4 hours during early labor; later, supplements of 0.4 mg. (1/150 gr.) of scopolamine or small doses of the barbiturates are added every 2 hours as needed. Irving first used Demerol intravenously but now recommends it as intramuscular injections.

With the exception of continuous caudal analgesia and the reintroduction of trichlorethylene, this method of obstetric pain relief is one of the newest to be added to our valuable agents. Sufficient evidence is now at hand to define it as one of the safer drugs. However, cases refractory to its use who indicate little degree of pain relief have been observed generally. Occasional shocklike reactions, with pallor, sweating, disturbed vasomotor mechanisms and hypotension, occur following its use. At least 2 maternal mortalities associated with immediate shock, hypotension and convulsions, have occurred following the use of 100 mg. intramuscularly and intravenously, respectively.

When used alone, Demerol is satisfactory in almost 60 per cent of cases. Its use as a supplement to scopolamine and the barbiturates as a preferred agent must await the recommendations and commendations of the parturients who, unfortunately, still bear the brunt of the pains of travail.

It is our recommendation that at the

present stage of clinical experience the dose of Demerol administered intravenously in conjunction with barbiturates or other depressant drugs or anesthetics should not exceed 25 mg., as a rule, in any one 15-minute period in order that due time can be given to observe its effect. Furthermore, Demerol should not be used intravenously as an analgesic in medicine, surgery or obstetrics or as an anesthetic unless facilities are available for adequate oxygenation, assisted respiration and controlled respiration. Nalorphine (Nalline) hydrochloride—a specific antidote—also should be available.

Antidote. Nalorphine (Nalline) hydrochloride has been reported to be a specific antidote against respiratory depression that may result from overdosage or unusual sensitivity to narcotics, including Demerol. In unconscious patients, it is given in intravenous doses of from 5 to 40 mg., depending upon the severity of the depression. Also, it has been given to the newborn in doses of from 0.1 to 0.2 mg. injected into the umbilical vein. We do not encourage its prophylactic use or its use in questionable indications.

Beck* states that Demerol "in conjunction with scopolamine . . . offers the best means of securing analgesia and amnesia in labor with the least risk to the mother and child." Later, he says that "local anesthesia combined with Demerol and scopolamine is the simplest, safest and most satisfactory method for the average woman in the hands of the average practitioner."

Demerol when used in control of labor pain has been shown to produce satisfactory analgesia, to shorten labor in the primipara and to be without significant effect upon the baby. With large doses of Demerol a moderate sedative effect is noted, and sleep frequently is induced between pains. In none of the obstetric patients so far observed was excitement, disorientation or irrationality encountered, such as may be seen frequently with the barbiturates and the other preparations used for the production of amnesia in addition to analgesia during labor.

Demerol alone produces analgesia but not amnesia. If amnesia also is desired, scopolamine or barbiturates also should be used. However, when barbiturates are used the fact that their action is potentiated by Demerol should be kept in mind.

Roby and Schumann, at the Harvard Medical School, and Schumann, independently, recorded and analyzed over 1,000 obstetric cases at the Boston Lying-in Hospital. All patients received identical medication at fixed intervals. The routine consisted of the following: Initial medication was 100 mg. Demerol and 0.6 mg. (1/100 gr.) scopolamine intramuscularly, followed by 0.4 mg. (1/150 gr.) scopolamine 45 minutes later. After 4 hours another dose of 100 mg. Demerol with 0.3 mg. (1/200 gr.) scopolamine was given. Thereafter, when necessary, 100 mg. Demerol was given every 4 hours and 0.3 mg. scopolamine every 2 hours. Newly admitted parturients expected to deliver within 2 hours received 100 mg. Demerol and 0.6 mg. scopolamine intravenously,* taking at least 2 minutes for this injection. The same amounts of Demerol and scopolamine, intravenously, were used as premedication for cesarean section 45 minutes prior to induction of anesthesia.*

Entirely satisfactory amnesia was obtained in 70.5 per cent of 847 patients; 16.9 per cent had analgesia but no amnesia, and 12.6 per cent constituted failure of amnesia. In examining the partial and the total failures it became apparent that a number of the patients had re-

* Beck, A. C.: Obstetrical Practice, ed. 6, pp. 979 and 984, Baltimore, Williams & Wilkins, 1955.

* Not recommended by the authors.

ceived medication too late to benefit materially from its effects.

With regard to the effect of Demerol-scopolamine on the length of labor, it appeared that a substantial shortening of the time of labor could be obtained in comparison with a series of 500 cases delivered under barbiturate-scopolamine analgesia. Thus, under the Demerol routine, the average primipara's labor apparently was reduced by 2.5 hours, and the multiparous labor by 1.2 hours, representing a 17 per cent and 14 per cent reduction, respectively.

In order to gain an approximate estimate of the effect of Demerol on the quantity of the anesthetic agent required, comparative studies were made on 18 uncomplicated pelvic deliveries treated with Demerol and 19 identical cases with patients receiving barbiturates and scopolamine. The results suggest that Demerol and the barbiturates are equivalent in preanesthetic value.

The analgesic effect of Demerol was evident from a group of 37 patients who precipitated without anesthesia; 29 of these were delivered with no recollection of pain whatever in spite of the fact that several patients sustained lacerations requiring repair. No depressant effect of the analgesia was apparent.

To investigate the effect on the newborn infant, a detailed analysis was made of 897 cases. Of these, 737 babies were active, 107 slightly slow (all of these were normal and required no further attention), 30 were slow, and there were 6 neonatal deaths and 17 stillbirths. Each of the stillbirths and neonatal deaths could be explained on the basis of congenital deformity or pathologic state, and there was an adequate obstetric explanation for the slowness of the newborn infants, all of whom were discharged as normal with the mother.

An analysis of 44 premature infants showed that 91 per cent were in satisfactory condition; 2 prematures were slow; and 2 were stillbirths. There is little to suggest a respiratory depressant effect in this group.

Demerol was used with satisfactory results as the premedication in 17 cesarean sections. The average length of medication was 30 minutes in 14 with active infants, 1 hour and 45 minutes in 2 with slightly slow babies, and 45 minutes in 1 patient with slow reaction.

Patients treated with Demerol and receiving general anesthesia have been relatively free from mucus and excitement during the induction.

Schumann concludes that in view of the satisfactory amnesia, the absence of pulmonary complications and the freedom from depressant effects upon the fetus, Demerol in conjunction with scopolamine is considered to be superior as an obstetric analgesic to other analgesics in common use.

The combined use of barbiturates and scopolamine has been compared with the use of Demerol and scopolamine by Irving (Harvard Medical School), who analyzed 14,676 cases receiving the former and 2,446 cases receiving the latter. The barbiturate-scopolamine medication produced complete and almost complete amnesia in 85 per cent of the patients, while the combination of Demerol and scopolamine resulted in only 75 per cent of complete or almost complete amnesia. However, there were 3 deaths associated with the use of pentobarbital, but no deaths were due to Demerol. The incidence of respiratory complications in mothers after Demerol was 2 in 2,446 cases, as compared with as many as 44 in 14,676 barbiturate cases. This bears out the claim that Demerol is rarely a respiratory depressant and, in spite of its lessened effectiveness as an adjuvant in producing amnesia, it is a safer drug for routine use in a large clinic. The second disadvantage of the barbiturates is the production of excitement which is caused distinctly less often by Demerol and scopolamine. Usually, excitement was controlled in those given barbiturates by 100 mg. Demerol or retention enemas of paraldehyde. Only 62 per cent of babies breathed spontaneously after barbiturates and general anesthesia as compared with 82 per cent of the Demerol group.

According to Beck, the combination of Demerol and scopolamine offers the best means of securing analgesia and amnesia in labor with the least risk to mother and child, while the manner in which the cervix "melts away" under this medication is surprising.

Hingson (in a paper read at the Nashville Postgraduate Assembly) has summarized his experiences with Demerol in more than 27,000 obstetric cases. In 8,000 women in labor who were delivered by nurses and midwives, a 100-mg. dose of Demerol was the sole analgesic and anesthetic agent. In 10,000 cases delivered under spinal anesthesia in private practice, the major analgesic consisted of from 100 to 200 mg. Demerol. In 9,000 women delivered in the Baltimore obstetric anesthesia study, Demerol was given during the course of labor to more than 40 per cent of the service patients and more than 60 per cent of the private patients with no maternal labor complications or fetal deaths attributable to the drug. The safety of Demerol has been so impressive that it is now routine to administer to all patients who enter the labor suite and operating rooms for labor, minor surgical procedures or examinations a blanket relaxing dose of 50 mg. Demerol between the hours of 7 A.M. and 7 P.M. At the onset of active labor, barbiturates and Demerol or Demerol and scopolamine are instituted, with a maximum dose of 200 mg. Demerol administered during any one labor.

In preference to barbiturates, Barnes (1950) administers Demerol combined with chloral to the mother as soon as the uterine contractions are strongly marked. Besides the analgesic action, this combination of drugs produces a sensation of well being.

Schade (Worthington, Minn.) considers the combined administration of Demerol and scopolamine the method of choice for obtaining analgesic and amnesic effects in obstetrics.

Bookstaver (Norwegian Hospital, Brooklyn) attests to the apparent harmlessness of Demerol analgesia in the conduct of premature labor. In 235 such cases in which 100 mg. Demerol was used, there were only 9 deaths (3.8%), which compares very favorably with 3 deaths (25%) in 11 cases in which morphine was the analgesic.

In Barnes' series (University College Hospital, London, 1947) of 500 patients to whom Demerol was given during labor no effect on uterine contractions could be observed in 67 per cent; in 23 per cent contractions appeared to increase; while in 9 per cent they appeared to diminish. However, there was no shortening of labor. In kymograph recordings taken before, during and after intravenous administration of Demerol and scopolamine, Roberts (Postgraduate Medical School, London, 1950) found that although the intervals between uterine contractions may be lengthened after the injection of Demerol, the delay appears in only 2 or 3 contractions following the onset of action of the drug, the rhythm soon becoming re-established. However, Demerol should not be given too early during labor as it may inhibit weak contractions and so delay labor. Demerol does not raise the incidence of postpartum hemorrhage (Josephine Barnes; Roberts, 1948).

Roberts reported (1948) that he gives Demerol at full dilatation or within 10 minutes of delivery without adverse effects upon the fetus. Patterson (Alleghany General Hospital, Pittsburgh) recommends that Demerol not be given near the time of delivery to minimize any possibility of depressing fetal respiration. On the other hand, Gottschalk (University of Colorado Medical School) noted that the administration of Demerol and hyoscine to the mother prior to delivery exerts little or no effect upon the respiration of the newborn baby, regardless of the time of administration of the drugs. He obtained 53 kymographic records on 31 newborns whose mothers had received from 100 to 300 mg. Demerol with from 0.6 to 1.5 mg. hyoscine during a 9-hour period before delivery, comparing these with 15 records obtained on 9 infants whose mothers had not received Demerol and hyoscine. The medication was given intravenously 10 minutes before delivery in 2 instances and 1 hour or less prior to delivery in 17 instances (31 records). The infants varied in age from 7 minutes to 1 hour. Ransom (London) has found that a dose of 150 mg. Demerol given intramuscularly to the mother in labor has its maximal effect upon the infant in from 1 to 1¼ hours and wears off in from 8 to 10 hours. A total of 250 mg. Demerol may be given during the last few hours before delivery. If more than this is to be given there should be an interval of 8 or 9 hours between doses. That Demerol has relatively little influence upon the fetus is borne out by Way and his co-workers (1949), who found that when 100 or 200 mg. Demerol was given during labor, less than 1 per cent of the total dose appeared in the urine of the infants.

Adanon

Another member of the Demerol series, Adanon (*dl*-6-dimethylamino-4,4-diphenyl-3-heptanone), has been studied by us in the control of pain in labor. Apparently the analgesic efficiency of this drug is between 10 and 20 times that of Demerol, with a toxicity about twice as great. Our experience with this agent indicates that, as an analgesic, its duration of action is more fleeting. Several patients have obtained relief for periods of from 30 to 45 minutes only following its administration. Most of them described the intensity of their pains as being from 50 to 75 per cent relieved following the prescribed dosage of 5 mg. by mouth. This newer member of the series is an indication that possibly more potent and less toxic examples of this same group will yet be developed and explored clinically.

The new agent just described is being prepared by Winthrop-Stearns, Inc. We have administered it both by mouth and intravenously, in doses ranging from 5 to 20 mg. per hour. In several cases we have noticed an oxytociclike action of this agent, which stimulated more vigorous and more frequent uterine contractions. In the German series this synthetic analgesic was A-4624.

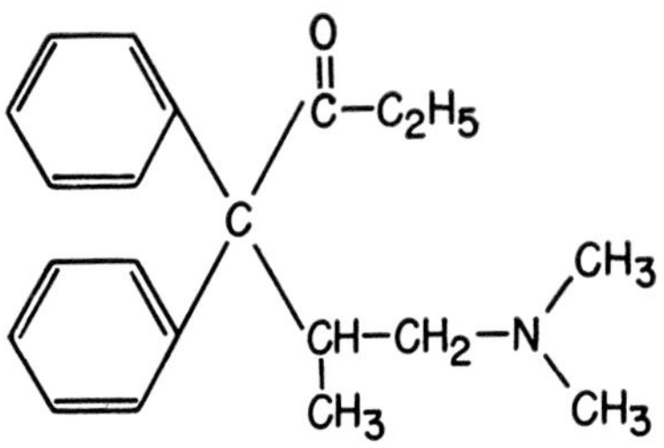

Adanon

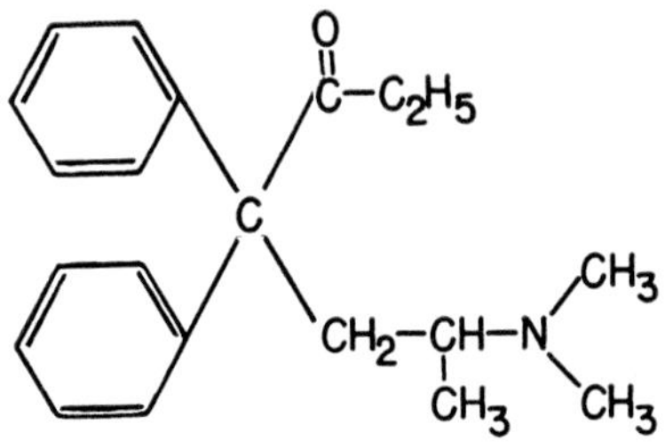

Dolophine

Dolophine

Eli Lilly and Company has developed another one of these systemic analgesics under the name of Dolophine. It can be seen from the accompanying structural formulas that these two components are practically identical. We have used both of them and have not been able to determine any great difference in their analgesic efficiency or in their side effects. We believe that they are both an improvement over Demerol, and both have produced mild fetal embarrassment.

Nisentil

The most careful evaluation of Nisentil to date is that of William M. Kane, of Margaret Hague Hospital, Jersey City, who came to the following conclusions on the basis of 1,000 obstetric cases:

1. Nisentil was found to give satisfactory analgesia in 98.1 per cent of the deliveries.
2. Nisentil (60 mg.) in combination with scopolamine ($\frac{1}{150}$ gr.) injected subcutaneously was found to give the best results. Nisentil may be repeated safely in proportion to subjective response.
3. There were no maternal side effects of Nisentil except in 8 patients (0.8%) who complained of being very dizzy. There was no vomiting.
4. Fetal respiratory depression was present in either a moderate or marked degree in 4.9 per cent of the cases.
5. The over-all fetal mortality was 1.7 per cent. None of these deaths was attributable to Nisentil.
6. Nisentil is a valuable drug in obstetric analgesia. Its rapid onset of action, relatively short period of maximum effect and its minimal depression of respiration in the infant make it an almost ideal drug in the obstetric field.

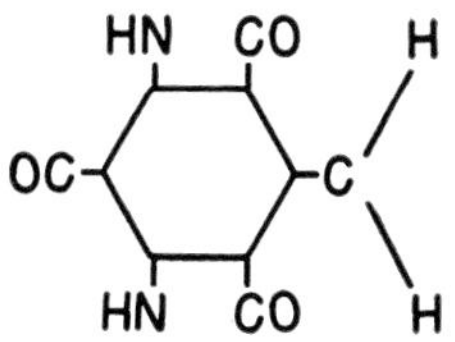

Barbituric acid
(malonyl urea)

Hypnotics (Barbiturates)

In 1933, Irving and his associates reported on a year's clinical research with various combinations of the barbiturates, either alone or with scopolamine, Pantopon, magnesium sulfate and rectal ether. Four of these methods, giving highest efficiency, were all based upon the use of Sodium Amytal or sodium pentobarbital. In the order of their efficiency, these were (1) sodium pentobarbital and scopolamine, (2) Sodium Amytal and rectal ether, (3) Sodium Amytal and scopolamine and (4) sodium pentobarbital and rectal ether. "Twilight sleep" was the least efficient, being more closely compared with Pantopon, magnesium sulfate and rectal ether.

Three of the conclusions of Irving and his associates are worthy of note. They found that all methods of analgesia delay the infant's respiration to some extent. In two control series (one without analgesia and one with nitrous oxide and oxygen only) they noted delayed respiration in 1.9 per cent and 20 per cent, respectively. They also concluded that opium and its derivatives should not be used during labor because of the effect upon the infant's respiration. Finally, they found sodium pentobarbital and scopolamine the most effective combination, the chief objection to it being restlessness of the patient and, in the occasional case, the manifestation of a hypotension with a shocklike reaction. They found that this hyperexcitability could

TABLE 2. EVALUATION OF AMNESIA SCOPOLAMINE WITH OTHER SPECIFIED DRUGS*

Drugs with Scopolamine	Mothers with Known Evaluation		Excellent		Good		Fair		Poor	
	Number	*Per Cent*	*Number*	*Per Cent*	*Number*	*Per Cent*	*Number*	*Per Cent*	*Number*	*Per Cent*
Nembutal	740	100	346	46.8	137	18.5	134	18.1	123	16.6
Nembutal and Demerol	432	100	271	62.7	78	18.1	36	8.3	47	10.9
Seconal	371	100	135	36.4	75	20.2	65	17.5	96	25.9
Seconal and Demerol	1,516	100	1,092	72.0	213	14.1	123	8.1	88	5.8
Seconal and Nembutal	111	100	80	72.1	14	12.6	7	6.3	10	9.0
Seconal, Nembutal and Demerol	194	100	156	80.4	23	11.9	9	4.6	6	3.1
Demerol	550	100	196	35.6	132	24.0	117	21.3	105	19.1
Scopolamine only	32	100	11	34.4	3	9.4	4	12.5	14	43.7
Morphine and barbiturates	15	100	2	13.3	1	6.7	4	26.7	8	53.3
Morphine, barbiturates and Demerol	8	100	4	50.0	1	12.5	1	12.5	2	25.0
Heroin and barbiturates	19	100	14	73.7	3	15.8	1	5.3	1	5.2
Seconal, Delvinal and Demerol	2	100	—	—	1	50.0	1	50.0	—	—

* Baltimore Obstetric Anesthesia Study, *quoted by* Bryce-Smith, Roger, and Hingson, R. A.: Anesthesiology **15**:351-352, 1954.

be controlled on occasions with rectal ether.

In 1921, Hamblen and Hamlin, of the University of Virginia, reported a series of 50 cases—the first 17 receiving an initial dose of 9 gr. and subsequent doses of 6 gr. of Sodium Amytal as needed. The remaining cases received an initial dose of 15 to 18 gr. and 1 or 2 additional doses of 6 gr. They stated that excellent results were not obtained with an additional dose of less than 15 gr. Constant nursing supervision was required. Their experience showed that postpartum quiet and sleep occurred from 8 to 12 hours with no fetal narcosis.

B. C. Hirst sent to many clinics a questionnaire regarding the technic of obstetric analgesia and anesthesia. The most widely used agents seemed to be the barbiturates. Pentobarbital sodium appeared to be chosen most frequently. The barbiturates are given by mouth. The use of them intravenously by Latin-American physicians has not spread to the United States with the exception of the clinics of Dr. Pierce Rucker, of Richmond, and Dr. Roy L. Grogan, of Fort Worth. Both these obstetricians report satisfactory obstetric analgesia and anesthesia with intravenous barbiturates.

During the period of the Baltimore obstetric anesthesia study we administered Seconal Sodium orally, intravenously and intramuscularly to more than 2,000 patients or Nembutal (pentobarbital) to more than 1,150 patients as the major soporific drug or as the sole agent during labor. When the patient arrived on the labor floor in rapid and advanced labor, intravenous administration of Seconal Sodium and scopolamine was frequently sufficient for the anesthesia for delivery as well. When indicated, terminal administration of nitrous oxide or terminal conduction nerve block provided the necessary supplement.

The intravenous dosage schedule was as follows: (1) 150 to 200 mg. of short-acting barbiturate intravenously when the patient arrived on the delivery floor if the cervix was dilated 6 cm. and contractions were regular and forceful; (2) 0.4 mg. of scopolamine intravenously at

TABLE 3. PERCENTAGE OF MOTHERS WITH COMPLICATIONS IMMEDIATELY FOLLOWING ADMINISTRATION OF SPECIFIED DRUGS DURING ANALGESIA*

Drugs	Per Cent				Number[1]			
	All Mothers	*No Complications*	*Minor*	*Major*	*Mothers*	*No Complications*	*Minor*[2]	*Major*[3]
No amnesic drugs	100	95.1	4.6	.3	3,103	2,950	142	11
Nembutal only	100	90.3	8.7	1.0	392	354	34	4
Nembutal and Demerol	100	92.7	7.3	—	55	51	4	—
Nembutal and scopolamine	100	97.2	2.7	.1	809	786	22	1
Nembutal, Demerol and scopolamine	100	97.6	2.2	.2	456	445	10	1
Seconal only	100	92.7	7.3	—	301	279	22	—
Seconal and Nembutal	100	95.7	4.3	—	23	22	1	—
Seconal and Demerol	100	95.4	4.6	—	218	208	10	—
Seconal and scopolamine	100	96.9	3.1	—	423	410	13	—
Seconal, Demerol and scopolamine	100	97.3	2.5	.2	1,612	1,569	40	3
Seconal, Nembutal and scopolamine	100	98.3	1.7	—	121	119	2	—
All barbiturates, Demerol and scopolamine	100	97.1	2.7	.2	2,276	2,211	61	4

1 Twins, cesarean sections, infants who died before onset of labor or analgesia and infants with congenital malformations incompatible with life are excluded.

2 Minor complications: delayed onset, nausea and vomiting.

3 Major complications: vomiting with aspiration, cyanosis, apnea, laryngospasm, shock, convulsions, chills. Mothers are counted only once; if she had a major and minor complication, she is counted for major complication only.

* Baltimore Obstetric Anesthesia Study, *quoted by* Bryce-Smith, Roger, and Hingson, R. A.: Anesthesiology **15**:351-352, 1954.

the same time and (3) 0.2 mg. of scopolamine by hypodermic injection.

The schedule for oral and intramuscular administration was as follows: (1) 200 to 300 mg. at the onset of established labor; (2) within 20 minutes, 0.4 to 0.6 mg. of scopolamine hypodermically; (3) supplementary scopolamine as required by the patient in intervals of 30 minutes to 2 hours, not to exceed a total dose of 1.5 mg., and (4) repeat doses of 100 to 200 mg. of barbiturate every 4 hours as needed.

As seen in Table 2, 371 of these patients received Seconal only; 1,516 received Seconal and 100 mg. of Demerol; 111 received Seconal as the first intramuscular injection and Nembutal intravenously 4 hours later, and 194 received Seconal intramuscularly, Nembutal intravenously and Demerol intramuscularly 4 hours later.

As seen in Table 3, no major complications were observed in any patient who received Seconal; this compared favorably with those complications observed in patients who had combinations with other barbiturates. The minor complications of delayed onset of adequate relief and some nausea with occasional vomiting were seen more frequently than with the other combinations.

Likewise, it was significant that 20.3

per cent of the patients who received Seconal only reported at the psychologists' examination, 24 hours after delivery, that there was no relief. This compared unfavorably with the 4.8 per cent of patients who reported no relief from comparable doses of Nembutal given intravenously. However, when used in combination with scopolamine, phenobarbital or Demerol, no significant difference was recorded in the "no relief" group.

We observed no serious complications that could be ascribed to the drug itself among the babies delivered to these patients. There was a delay in the breathing and crying time of the premature and the mature infants when compared with those born to mothers who did not have sedative drugs or anesthetics.

Summary and Conclusions

Short-acting barbiturates, both orally and parenterally, are useful sedatives with all forms of conduction analgesia, provided such analgesia is effective.

As a basal narcotic for obstetric and surgical patients who are to be anesthetized in their rooms before surgery, it may be administered simply and, because

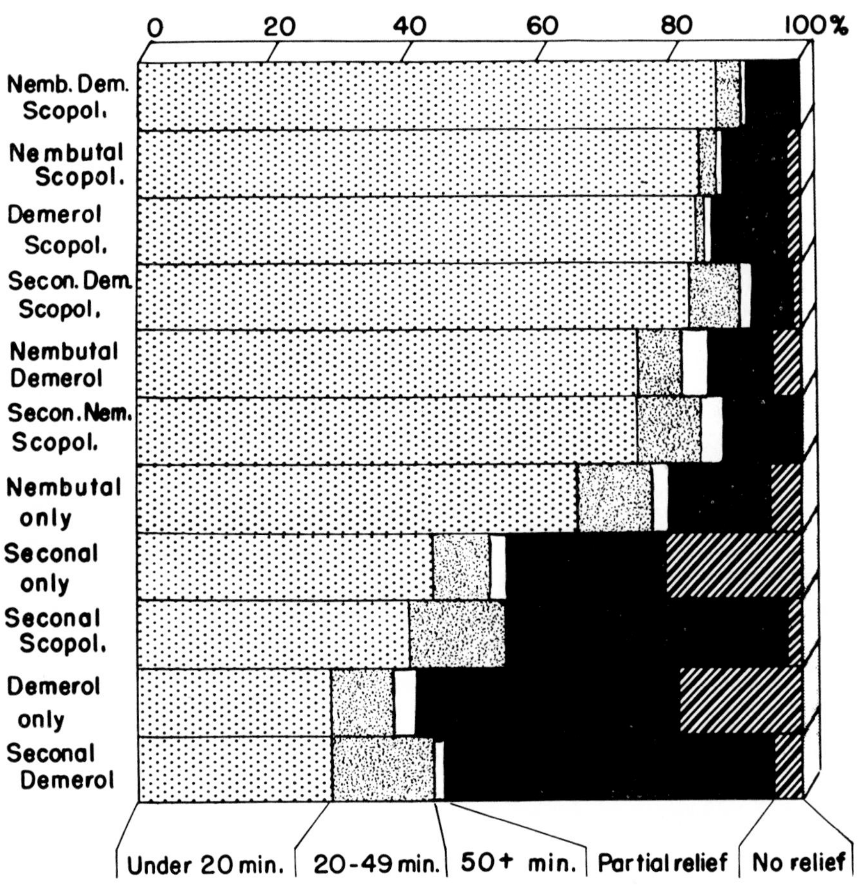

Fig. 8. This graph summarizes the low incidence of pain relief with single drugs reported by 9,347 mothers in the Baltimore obstetric anesthesia study, compared with the greatly improved incidence of relief when any of these drugs are used in synergistic combinations.

TABLE 4. PAIN RELIEF DURING ANALGESIA FOR SPECIFIED DRUGS EXPRESSED IN PERCENTAGES*

Drugs	Total Known as to Relief	No Relief	Partial Relief	Full Relief in:		
				Under 20 Min.	*20–49 Min.*	*50 + Min.*
Nembutal only	100	4.8	15.7	66.4	11.1	2.0
Nembutal and Demerol	100	4.0	10.0	76.0	6.0	4.0
Nembutal and scopolamine	100	1.7	10.0	84.9	3.1	0.3
Nembutal, Demerol and scopolamine	100	—	8.1	87.8	3.3	0.8
Seconal only	100	20.3	24.0	44.3	8.8	2.6
Seconal and Nembutal	100	—	10.5	79.0	10.5	—
Seconal and Demerol	100	4.2	48.8	29.7	15.5	1.8
Seconal and scopolamine	100	1.9	42.2	41.6	14.0	0.3
Seconal, Demerol and scopolamine	100	0.3	7.1	83.5	7.8	1.3
Seconal, Nembutal and scopolamine	100	—	11.8	75.3	9.7	3.2
All barbiturates, Demerol and scopolamine	100	0.2	7.1	84.7	6.9	1.1

* Baltimore Obstetric Anesthesia Study, *quoted by* Bryce-Smith, Roger, and Hingson, R. A.: Anesthesiology **15**:351-352, 1954.

of its longer and less intense action, is safer than the ultra short-acting barbiturates.

It may be administered safely in properly controlled doses to patients with cardiac, renal or liver disease. However, although barbiturates rarely produce marked changes in the blood pressure, the pulse or the respiratory rates, the tidal exchange commonly is reduced, and precipitous falls in blood pressure have been seen on occasions.

We concluded from the obstetric study that oral or parenteral administration of Seconal alone in the dosage described was inadequate in 38 to 65 per cent of women in labor, but when combined with Demerol, scopolamine or Nembutal, it provided a safe and satisfactory result in more than 80 per cent of cases (see Fig. 8). Its leading disadvantages were insufficient relief when used alone, delayed onset and occasional disorientation with some excitement during labor. A very rare condition of total apnea, which required active ventilation for 35 minutes, was observed in 2 of the 2,577 patients.

As with all depressant and narcotic drugs, measures and safeguards for controlling vasomotor and respiratory depression must be available at all times (Table 4).

COMBINATION OF AMNESIA, ANALGESIA AND SOPORIFICS

Table 2 (p. 18) illustrates the increasing efficiency of the combination over the high degree of failure as measured by patient dissatisfaction from the effect of one drug only. Thus the experience obtained in working with 8,000 mothers in the Johns Hopkins and the Sinai Hospitals in Baltimore was overwhelmingly in favor of 3 or more drugs used synergistically. This result indicates the inadequacies of all drugs used alone in obstetric labor through the encephalic approach. This is understandable when we consider the 2 billion brain cells grouped into subdivisions of specialized function.

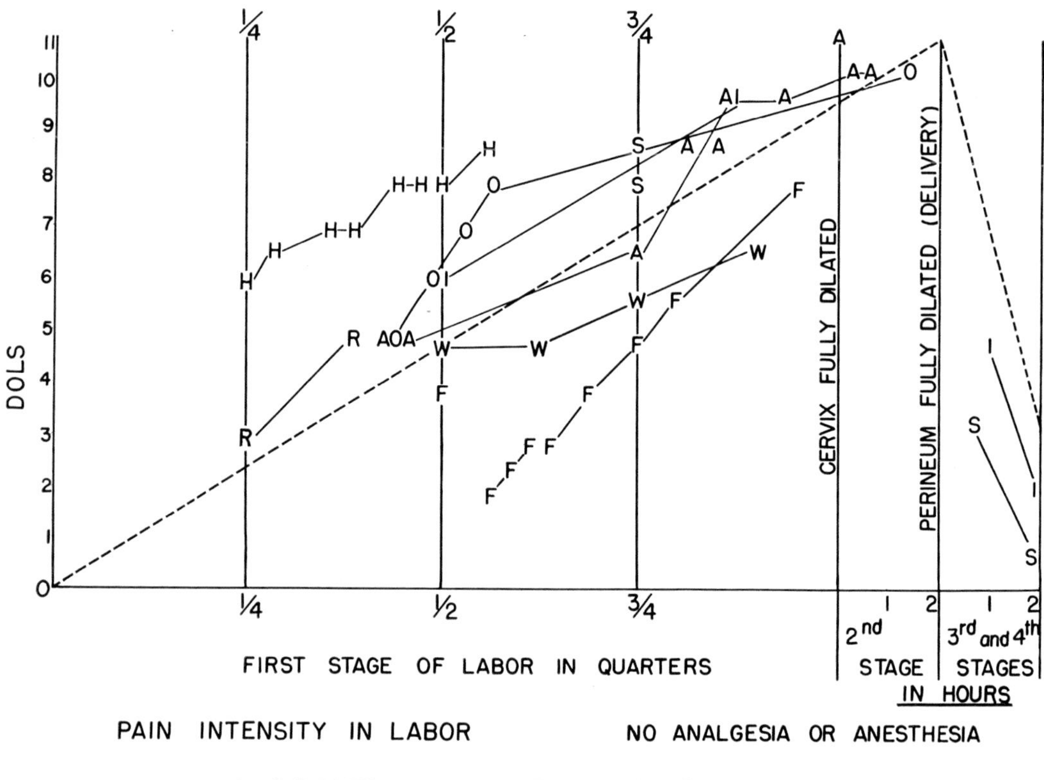

Fig. 9. Pain intensity in labor. (After Javert & Hardy: Anesthesiology **12**:189)

With the exception of scopolamine, which raises the basal metabolism, produces a peripheral vascular flush and possibly a visceral vasoconstriction and also a specific cortical state of confusion and amnesia; all other soporifics, analgesics and mixed amnesic drugs produce a depression first of the higher brain centers—and if given inexcessive dosage—of the lower brain and medullary centers as well, with resultant hypoxia and hypotension progressing toward anoxia and vasomotor collapse.

At this point we should give careful attention to the normal pattern of increasing intensity of obstetric pain as recorded by Hardy and Javert with the dolorimeter (Fig. 9). The subdivision of the first stage of labor by cervical dilatation significantly points out that dols of pain rise gradually from a relatively comfortable first quarter of the first stage to a veritable crescendo of maximum pain appreciation in the fourth quarter of the first stage.

While there is individual variation, 100 mg. of Demerol can reduce interpreted pain by an average of 3 dols for 1 to 2 hours. Obviously, this drug is not needed to relieve the 2 dols of pain of the first quarter of the first stage, but it alone without excessive dosage is insufficient to relieve the 11 dols of pain in the final quarter of the first stage. Yet scopolamine alone in extreme dosages has been used by Kirschbaum to obliterate the memory of not only the pain of labor but also of delivery as well without supplementary anesthesia. Undoubtedly, in these larger doses, there must be some analgesia or even anesthesialike states. A comparable state is achieved with large doses of magnesium sulfate alone, which has been used for surgical appendectomy. However, 2 recorded deaths stopped the use of this drug as an anesthetic and should give proper warning to obstetricians who rely on excessive intravenous doses of this drug in severe toxemia. This technic is not presented with the recommendations of the authors but rather as an illustrative pharmacologic pattern from extreme doses of a single agent.

Scopolamine and Apomorphine

Apomorphine was selected recently as the drug of choice at Boston Lying-in Hospital to counteract excitement resulting from scopolamine. Bert B. Hershenson and Elwood R. Brubaker (Harvard University) reviewed the records of 500 patients in whom this drug combination had been used.

The optimum routine of medication as finally established is as follows: Patients in labor are given 200 mg. (3 gr.) Seconal by mouth or rectum, after an enema on admission. When labor is progressing and the patient complains of pain, scopolamine and apomorphine are administered in doses of 0.6 mg. (1/100 gr.) each. In three quarters of an hour 0.4 mg. (1/150 gr.) scopolamine and 1.2 mg. (1/50 gr.) apomorphine are given again and then repeated at 2-hour intervals. Apomorphine is kept in sterile 20 cc. vials.

In 90 per cent of 300 patients in whom this regimen was used, effective amnesia resulted; the other 10 per cent received the drugs in insufficient quantity. Ninety-six per cent of patients receiving 3 or more doses had satisfactory amnesia. Vomiting occurred in 24.5 per cent of patients, but vomiting is common in labor when other premedication or no premedication is used. Excitement occurred in 21.5 per cent of patients as contrasted with 40 per cent when scopolamine alone was used. The average primiparous labor in this series was 11.3 hours as contrasted with 16 hours in primiparas who did not receive medication. Average multiparous labor was 6.5 hours in this series, contrasted with 12 hours in multiparas not receiving medication. No increase of blood loss was noticed. These drugs exerted no demonstrable depressant effect on full-term or late premature infants, even when administered shortly before delivery.

Scopolamine Only

H. M. Kirschbaum, of Woman's Hospital, in Detroit, has used scopolamine alone for the duration of labor and often for delivery with successful results. The initial dose is 0.6 mg. (1/100 gr.) of scopolamine, repeated at 30-minute intervals for a total of 3 doses. Then doses of 0.3 mg. (1/200 gr.) are repeated at intervals of 1 to 2 hours as long as is necessary.

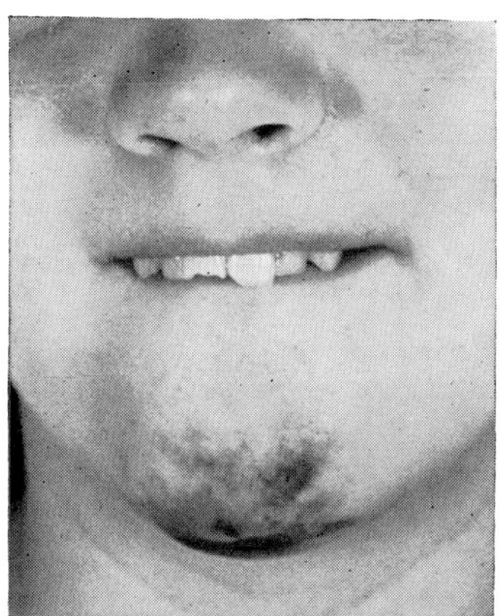

Fig. 10. This patient threw herself against a radiator near her bed when under analgesia with amnesic drugs. As a result, her right front tooth was chipped off and her chin bruised. Such patients never must be left for a second. (Zabriskie & Eastman: Nurses Handbook of Obstetrics, ed. 9, Philadelphia, Lippincott)

The disadvantages of this technic are: (1) faulty visual accommodation several days after delivery, (2) confused memory from one to several days, (3) edema of uvula, sore throat from excessively dry mouth and uncontrolled phonation and (4) profound excitement. The authors have investigated instances of self-injury produced by scopolamine in patients under inadequate surveillance during labor.

Chlorpromazine

Recently, chlorpromazine was introduced as a surgical premedicant, usually with some form of hibernation anesthesia. Early reports concerning its obstetric use indicate slight depression of the baby with maternal complications of hypotension and mental apathy extending over several hours. The authors wish to point out that at this writing this drug has not proved that it merits a place beside scopolamine, Demerol and the barbiturates, but it shows definite promise. Yet at least 9 cases of toxic hepatitis and 1 death associated with its use have been reported to the authors from 4 clinics. More recently we have observed 2 cases of tachycardia with electrocardiographic changes directly attributable to this drug.

Its schedule of dosage is as follows: 50 mg. each 4 to 6 hours, with or without scopolamine supplement. A few investigators are using 25 to 50 mg. Demerol each 2 hours after the chlorpromazine as an adjuvant analgesia.

THE PAIN FACTOR IN LABOR

The first step toward the alleviation of suffering during labor and delivery is the recognition of pain as a psychological interpretation of a physiologic entity. While it is true that frequently the intensity of pain in protracted labor is intensified by such factors as disproportion, cervical and birth canal rigidity, fatigue and emotional fear, even in physiologic labor the pain is real. James D. Hardy and Carl T. Javert have made a fundamental contribution in their standardization of the nature of pain in 13 unmedicated women throughout the various stages of labor. These patients, who knew well the principles of relaxation, volunteered to go through the major part of labor without medication in order that they might compare the discomfort from true labor pain with the pain of standard intensity produced by a 3-second exposure to thermal radiation on the dorsal surface of the right hand. The pain on the hand had been standardized previously into 10.5 units of painfulness (10.5 dols) between threshold and ceiling pain.

The mean intensity of the pain during the first quarter of the first stage of labor was no more than 2 dols. This was considered by all of the patients to be mild. However, the pain increased progressively in intensity, ranging from 3 to 5 dols in the second quarter of the first stage of labor, from 5 to 7 dols in the third quarter and from 7 to 10 dols during the final quarter and through the second stage of labor. This was considered by the patients to be the most intense pain in their experience. In the third stage the pain intensity ranged from 3 dols to threshold. The intensity of pain was roughly proportional to the extent of cervical dilatation and inversely proportional to the interval between contractions. Duration of pain was 15 per cent of contraction time of weak contractions and 95 per cent of contraction time for strong contractions.

On the basis of these data, summarized in Figures 9 and 11, it is evident that the use of major narcosis or major conduction anesthesia during the first half of the first stage of labor is seldom necessary. Except for the use of small doses of barbiturates and psychosuggestion therapy during the midnight hours when apprehensive patients are better off asleep, active analgesia at this time frequently can do more harm than good. Figure 12, from the Javert and Hardy report represents, in large measure, a resumé of their practices concerning the timing of the use of analgesia and anesthesia in the control of labor pain. This also represents our policy in the average case.

Finally, the following practical points should be observed for the best results:

1. All patients coming into the hospital at night in early labor can be given 100 mg. of barbiturate by mouth or by rectum unless contraindicated by prematurity, uremia, serious respiratory or heart lesion. This soporific eases emotional tension and permits naps between pains without obtunding labor.

2. During the day we have found that 50 mg. of Demerol by mouth is a safe sheet anchor for all normal cases and in this dose frequently produces a relaxing euphoric state. Never once in thousands of cases has this exploring initial dose caused any alarming complications. However, when used intravenously we give this warning. *Demerol in 100-mg. intravenous doses has produced sudden maternal death at least twice.* We strongly urge that initial intravenous dosage be limited to 25 mg. with at least an assessment period of 15 minutes reserved for evaluation of blood pressure and ventilation before a second 25 mg. is given for extreme pain. We condemn the practice of ever exceeding within a 2-hour period the 50 mg. total dose of intravenous Demerol.

As stated previously, both intravenous barbiturates and Demerol occasionally produce profound depression of the vital centers. Efficient oxygen ventilating apparatus must be at hand with a proper assortment of airways wherever these technics are used. Likewise, vasopressor and analeptic drugs for proper discriminatory use and intravenous fluids should be available.

These drugs, either alone or in com-

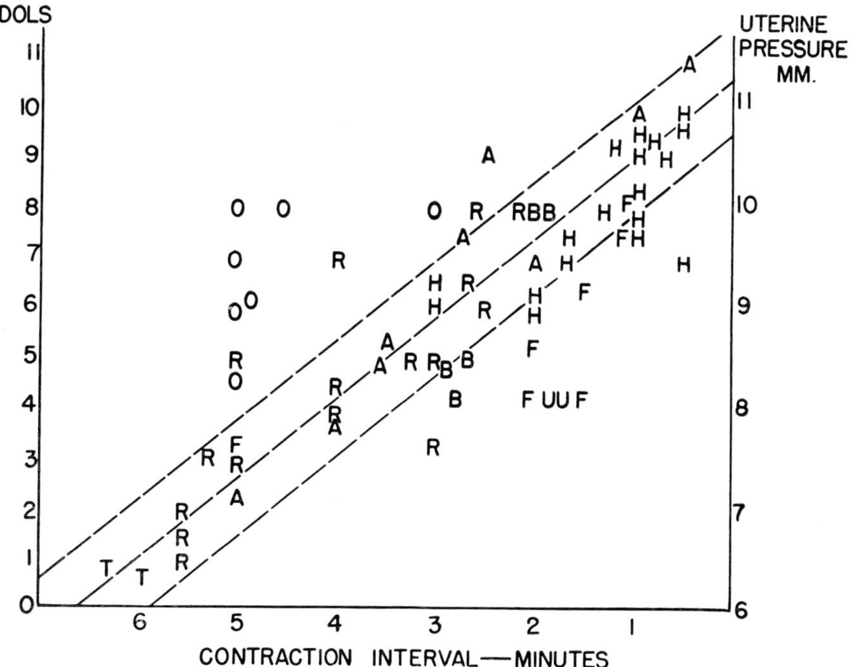

FIG. 11. Intensity of pain increases as interval between contractions decreases. (Javert & Hardy: Anesthesiology 12:189)

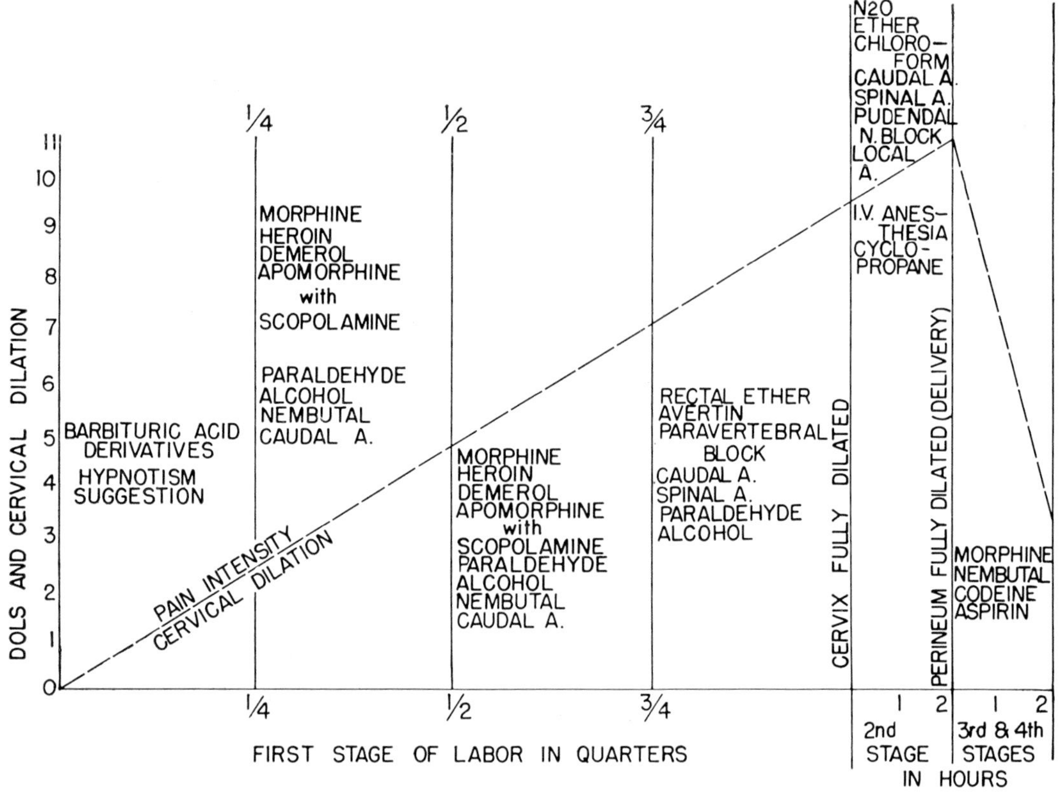

Fig. 12. Analgesia and anesthesia in labor. (Javert & Hardy: Anesthesiology **12**:189)

bination, are capable of producing excitement through obtunding the reasoning processes of the frontal lobe. In such cases nitrous oxide supplement with at least 30 per cent oxygen is better than carrying this systemic drug therapy to dangerous extremes.

Whenever possible in these cases the use of the anatomic approach of continuous caudal or peridural anesthesia is better for both mother and baby than general anesthesia and will permit immediate relaxation and also quiet sleep as soon as pain has been relieved.

Caution!

1. Do not leave sedated obstetric patients unattended.
2. Use side rails or restraining binders when indicated, since patients have broken arms, clavicles and ribs by climbing out of bed and falling to the floor.
3. Check frequently for hypoventilation and treat with oxygen inhalation and assist respirations in extreme cases.
4. Check for hypotension, particularly in hot weather, in patients with anemia and heart disease.
5. Should progress in labor be retarded, reduce dosage.
6. Always give 50 mg. of Demerol as first appraisal dose, and then add increments each 1 to 2 hours with 200 mg. top limit in any 8-hour period.
7. Give 100 mg. of barbiturate at night and to apprehensive patients by day early

in labor and limit total dose to 200 mg. in any 8-hour period.

8. Do not give barbiturates to patients with kidney disease, since confused states may persist for many hours thereafter.

9. Limit total dose of scopolamine to 1.2 mg. for entire labor and use the anatomic technics entirely for delivery after this amount is given rather than general anesthesia.

10. Try to avoid giving either systemic analgesics or soporifics within 2 hours of anticipated birth.

11. Use nitrous oxide, ethylene, cyclopropane or Trilene analgesia with contractions if additional systemic analgesia is indicated.

12. For premature births and for mothers with severe complicating disease, use reduced dosages of these drugs, if at all, and substitute caudal, spinal or peridural for both labor and delivery.

TECHNICS FOR ANALGESIA DURING LABOR AND FOR ANESTHESIA DURING DELIVERY

The technics currently advocated are presented in detail in Chapter 4, *Technics in Obstetric Amnesia, Analgesia and Anesthesia.* In some instances there will be a combination of one or more technics to produce the desired effect. No single measure is adequate for all cases. The technics are those used by the authors in the United States, as well as those gathered in personal tours of Europe, South and Central America and through consultations with anesthetists from Asia, Australia, New Zealand and Africa. Indications, cautions, contraindications and safety prerequisites are listed for each technic. Regardless of the technic selected there are basic principles common to all methods. Nevertheless, geography, topography, local economy and racial characteristics exert influences upon the choice of method and drug used; one must consider such things as environmental temperature, barometric pressure, oxygen concentration, humidity and availability of equipment, analgesic and amnesic drugs and anesthetics, and facilities for sterilization. Of like importance are physician and lay information and experience with the methods in final determination of procedure.

Examples illustrating these factors are represented by the following: Anemia with a red cell count of 2 million per cubic millimeter is an entirely different problem in Mobile, Ala., at sea level, from that upon the savanna between the northern Andes in Bogotá, Colombia, with an altitude of 8,000 feet above sea level. In the former city, oxygen in atmosphere is 21 per cent, and in the latter it is 15 per cent (almost a 30 per cent differential). Should toxemia with vasoconstriction or even eclampsia or hyperthyroidism or hyperpyrexia be superimposed upon this anemia, it is obvious that technics permitting the highest oxygen concentrations are of life-saving significance in both geographic areas—but particularly in Bogotá.

In like manner, the usual polycythemia of 6 million to 7 million red blood cells per cubic millimeter of blood in Mexico City and Denver at 5,000 to 6,000 feet altitude, present a different problem from the standpoint of fluid balance and need for hematocrit dilution in a cool external environment and those with low barometric pressure from what would be seen in the same circumstances in tropical Havana or subtropical New Orleans and Rome.

It is a well-known fact that open-drop ether technics are far more difficult, more expensive, if not impossible in the frequent 38°C. (100°F.) at Tucson, Ariz., and Caracas, Venezuela.

The dangers of electrostatic explosions with ether, cyclopropane, and ethylene are more real in arid Phoenix, Ariz.,

Needles, Calif., and Lima, Peru, than in the island cities of Britain, or in Panama City or Rio de Janeiro during the rainy season.

The standard dose of a conduction nerve block anesthetic for the Nordic women with an average height taller than 66 in. is far greater than that required by the Polynesian races, frequently 1 ft. shorter. The need for vasopressor prophylactic and therapeutic drugs is greater in maintaining a maternal systolic blood pressure of more than 80 in Philippine women who carry traditional hypotension than in Canadian woman who average from 10 to 30 mm. of mercury more.

The $6 per hour cost of a cyclopropane anesthetic is of prohibitive significance for the masses of Indian and Chinese women when a local or spinal or trichlorethylene anesthetic can be given for a few cents from a minute package or ampul.

The wasteful semiclosed nitrous oxide with oxygen at high minute volume flow rates might be accepted therapy in the United States, but vastly impractical in El Salvador, Greece and Poland, which must import these heavy cylinders from afar.

The curare, cyclopropane and Pentothal Sodium technics for cesarean section used in Cleveland and New York, where a Foregger or a Heidbrink anesthesia machine and equipment for airway management are found in every operating room, are not suited for the average clinic in Yugoslavia or in Albert Schweitzer's African hospital.

Some of the world's peoples fear needles as poison, and others fear the anesthesia machine as the gas chamber. Some prefer general anesthesia because their physicians and their mothers prefer general anesthesia; some prefer conduction block anesthesia for the same reason; some prefer uncomplicated childbirth without drugs—up to a point—because of fear of general and conduction anesthesia through lack of experience or because of prejudice or because they desire to pioneer a fad or a cult or pay an ecclesiastical penalty with pain during childbirth. A few either experience no pain through the gaping and adequate birth canal of the grand multipara, or their pain is so slight that they appear to be in no hurry to reach the birth room.

Happily, for all these people living in a world that will double its population in the present half century, medicine has developed many drugs, technics and agents as a result of the contributions of many countries, providing for mothers more safety and comfort than ever before toward the control of the *poena magna.*

BASIC PRINCIPLES FOR ALL TECHNICS

1. The most important single principle in the relief of obstetric pain is the experience of the anesthetist and the skill with which he applies the selected technic.

2. Today, because of the efficiency of many technics, it is never necessary nor should it be permitted to reduce the percentage of inhaled oxygen below 20 per cent.

3. All drugs given to relieve pain by inhalation, intravenous or intramuscular or in major nerve block injection, with the exception of spinal anesthesia, cross the placental barrier and may affect the baby adversely. Indeed, many of them stored in the fatty maternal depots not only cross the placenta but also traverse the lactating glands in the breasts and further depress the newborn for an additional 24 hours or more. For example, the barbiturate concentration in mother's milk may be several times that of her circulating blood.

4. All drugs that act through the en-

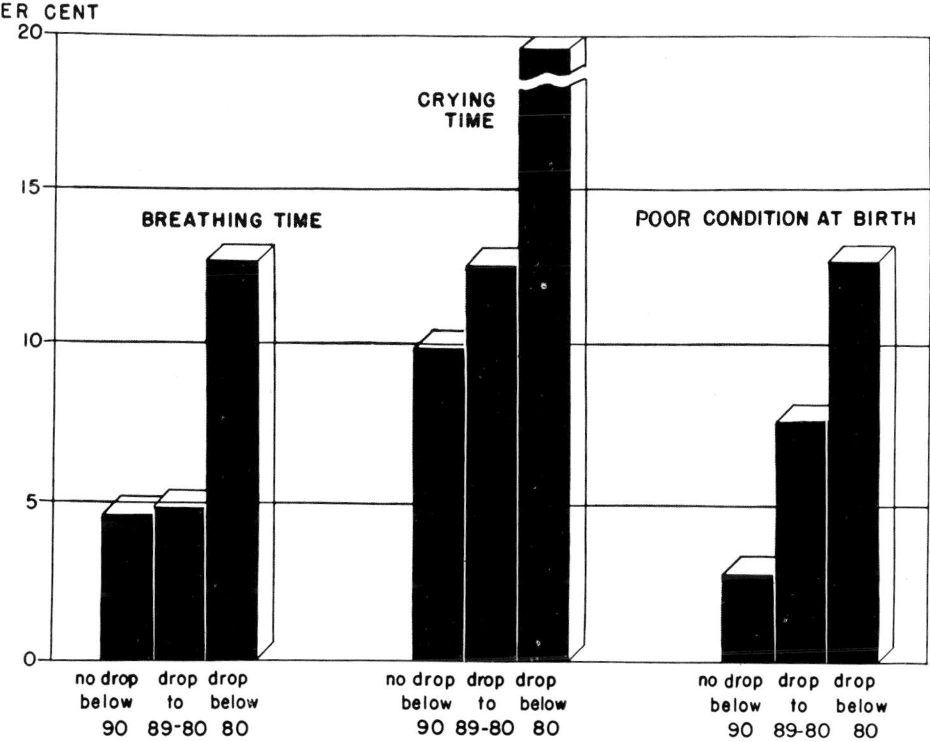

FIG. 13. The Negro infant at Johns Hopkins Hospital showed more significant depression of breathing time, crying time and physical well-being at birth as maternal blood pressure fell during delivery. Compare with white infants in Figure 14. (Baltimore Obstetric Anesthesia Study)

cephalic approach on the mother's brain depress the vital infant mechanisms and delay the breathing and crying time at least 12 to 15 per cent in full-term infants and at least 20 to 40 per cent in premature infants.

5. All drugs that depress the maternal blood pressure through sympathetic blockade are capable of producing fetal anoxia by reducing placental blood flow and transplacental filtration pressure during maternal hypotension. Figures 13 and 14 indicate that the Negro infants are in greater jeopardy from this factor. The drugs include not only the major vertebral block conduction anesthetics and general anesthetics but also magnesium sulfate, Demerol, morphine, sedative barbiturates, etc., as well as largactil and the methonium compounds. Likewise, the fetus suffers anoxia in maternal shock, anemia, premature separation of placenta and in hypoxic atmospheres. Nicholson Eastman's classic indictment of such factors as producing an analogous environment for the fetus as "delivery 2,000 feet above Mount Everest" should be given worldwide consideration.

6. Albeit, the placental barrier does offer some temporal and quantitative protection from fetal anesthetic poisoning. This seems to vary with the complexity of the chemical structure of the drug. For example, Hellman has demonstrated with spectroscopic methods that several of the barbiturates do not establish equilibrium between maternal and infant blood streams until 5 to 8 minutes after injection. We have demon-

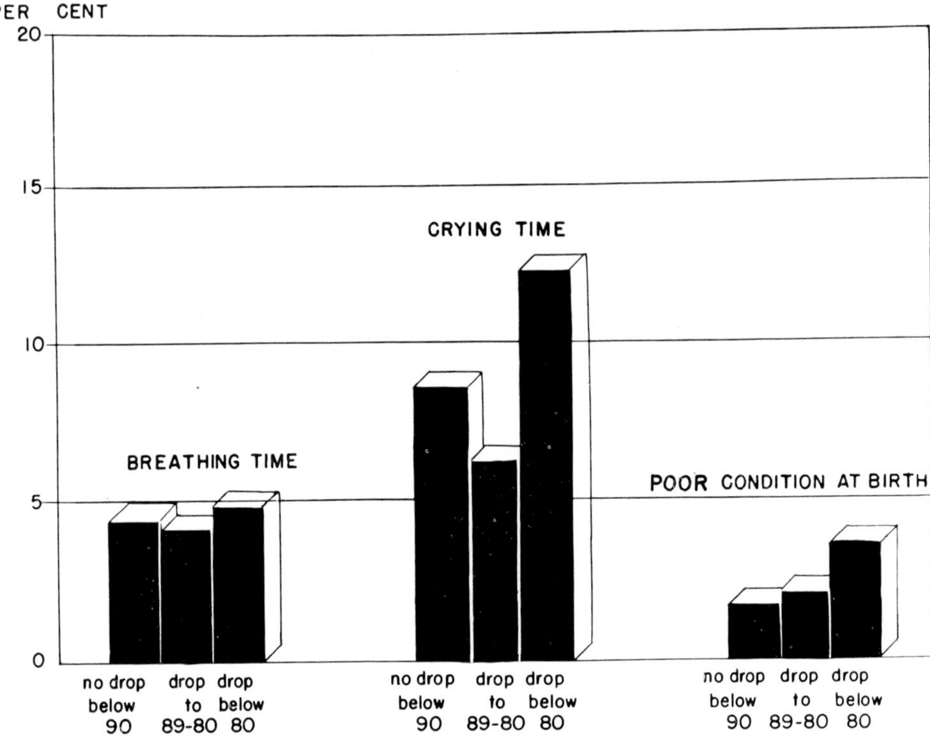

FIG. 14. As maternal blood pressure fell below 80 mm. Hg systolic, breathing time, crying time and incidence of poor condition at birth increased significantly for all white infants born from 1948 to 1951 at Johns Hopkins Hospital. (Baltimore Obstetric Anesthesia Study)

strated many times the birth of an active, awake, screaming baby to a mother deeply asleep with cyclopropane and, less frequently, ether.

7. Since most general anesthetics depress maternal respiration in both rate and depth, rich oxygen atmospheres are not enough. Assisted respiration and, in some cases, controlled respiration are essential to maintain adequate oxygenation with many technics. The obstetric patient with diminished respiratory volumes and increased metabolic activity, and a 12-pound gravid uterus riding on her diaphragm, is even more vulnerable to anoxia than the surgical patient. The infant is even more at the mercy of its mother's atmosphere and her anesthetist's skill.

8. It is unsafe to administer any anesthetic without proper equipment at hand to provide oxygenation and resuscitation.

9. In the absence of such equipment, mouth-to-mouth insufflation of both infants and mothers has been lifesaving.

10. The total number of milligrams of all agents, whether volatile or gaseous, solid barbiturates or local anesthetics, and their pharmacologic metabolism and method of elimination play a potentially deadly role in anesthesia for both mother and baby. An understanding of this role and of the safety mechanisms and antidotes concerning their use must be understood by both obstetricians and anesthetists if we are to reach the irreducible minimum death rate.

11. As all drugs depress the sensorium or nerve conduction so are they capable of depressing the power of uterine contraction and progress of labor in a varying degree related both to the power of the drug pharmacology and the individual patient susceptibility. At the same time the use of amnesic, analgesic and anesthetic drugs can correct or ameliorate unfavorable uterine dysfunction, tetany or cervical dystocia. Sometimes powerful relaxing anesthesia is essential to prevent fetal anoxia from uterine muscular arterial blockade. Therefore, pain relief must be of secondary significance to safety of mother and baby and to physiologic progress in labor. Also, its therapeutic applications must be understood.

INCOMPATIBILITIES OF VASOPRESSORS IN ANESTHESIA

Many incompatibilities exist in the use of the vasopressors. Chloroform, Trilene (trichloroethylene), and cyclopropane, because of the high frequency of cardiac irregularity with their use, through some direct pharmacologic cardiac muscle action, should not be used with the vasopressors.

Dripps, Kistler and Ruben (1949) determined that intramuscular injection of Vasoxyl produces a prompt and prolonged rise in blood pressure without central stimulation and without causing cardiac irregularities even during cyclopropane anesthesia. This fact is of utmost importance in providing a safeguard not hitherto available in event of circulatory collapse under cyclopropane anesthesia. The fact that ephedrine and particularly desoxyephedrine so stimulate the sensorium that postanesthesia sleep may not be forthcoming without heavy sedation for from 4 to 8 hours after administration presents another advantage of Vasoxyl. Moreover, hypotension after general narcosis responds more completely to the central nervous system stimulation of ephedrine and desoxyephedrine. Nevertheless, we emphasize a guarded caution in the use of Vasoxyl and an absolute warning against using the other vasopressors preceding, during or after cyclopropane anesthesia. Many publications in the past and many more anesthesia mortality commission studies have substantiated the incompatibility of most vasopressors. This includes the case of Pituitrin, because of its Pitressin fraction, with cyclopropane, and, now more recently, with Trilene. It is of utmost importance for the anesthetist to bear in mind the likelihood of development of auricular and even ventricular fibrillation when cyclopropane anesthesia is superimposed on or used concurrently with local or spinal anesthesia in which a vasopressor or a vasoconstrictor has been used. To test the validity of this adverse pharmacologic action in human beings, Adriani studied continuous electrocardiograms in dogs under spinal anesthesia in which epinephrine was incorporated with the spinal anesthetic. After 1 hour of control tracing he obtained a second hour of electrocardiograph when cyclopropane was superimposed in the same animal to anesthetic levels. As a final step in the experiment, he withdrew 1 cc. of cerebrospinal fluid and injected it intravenously in the same dog still anesthetized with cyclopropane. Immediately the animal exhibited profound arrhythmias, ventricular fibrillation and death. Therefore, it is encouraging to know that a vasopressor as efficient as Vasoxyl is being developed and is not producing this cardiac irritability when used with cyclopropane.

Ergot preparations should be used sparingly when indicated or not at all in patients who have received vasopressor drugs. This is particularly true in the

TABLE 5. PHARMACOLOGY OF THE VOLATILE AGENTS AND GASES USED IN ANESTHESIA

AGENT	ALIMENTARY SYSTEM				SKELETAL SYSTEM
	Mouth	*Tract*	*Liver*	*Elimination*	
Nitrous Oxide N_2O (80%)	Nil	Contractions increased ∝ Anoxemia N. or V.—23% Distention—3%	Nil (O_2)	Lungs (rapid) Skin	No relaxation unless O_2 ↓
Ethylene C_2H_4	Nil	Tone sl. ↑ Secretions ↓ N. or V.—35% Distention—7%	Nil	Lungs (rapid) Skin	Very slow relaxation
Cyclopropane C_3H_6	↑ ↓	Tone—Nil (deep ↓) N. or V.—39% Distention—13.5%	Nil	Lungs (rapid) Skin	Fair relaxation
Ethyl Ether $(C_2H_5)_2O$	Light sal. ↑ Deep sal. ↓	Tone ↓ Secretions ↓ N. or V.—41% Distention—16.5%	↓	Lungs (slow) Urine Milk Sweat	Good relaxation
Vinyl Ether $(C_2H_3)_2O$	Sal.	Peristalsis fairly active N. or V.—2%	Sl. ↓	Lungs (rapid) Urine Milk Sweat	Fair relaxation
Ethyl Chloride C_2H_5Cl	↑ ↓	Peristalsis ↓ N. or V. +		Lungs (rapid)	Poor relaxation
Chloroform $CHCl_3$	Sl. sal. ↓	Peristalsis ↓ N. or V. > E Dil. of stomach	Prol. ↓ ↓ ↓	Lungs (slow) Urine Milk Sweat	Good relaxation
Trichloroethylene $CHCl_3CCl_2$	Nil	N. or V.—rare	Sl. ↓ < E	Sl. ↓ < E	Poor relaxation

Code: ↑ Stimulation ↓ Depression ∝ Increased

TABLE 5. PHARMACOLOGY OF THE VOLATILE AGENTS AND GASES USED IN ANESTHESIA (*Continued*)

AGENT	METABOLISM			RENAL SYSTEM		PREGNANT UTERUS AND FETAL CIRCULATION	COMMENTS
	BMR	*Temp.*	*Adrenals*	*Kidney*	*Bladder*		
Nitrous Oxide N_2O (80%)	Sl. ↓	Sl. ↓	Nil	Nil	Nil	Effect on uterus nil Fetal cond. ∝ O_2	O_2 want N_2 content
Ethylene C_2H_4	Sl. ↓	Sl. ↓	Nil	Nil	Nil	No inhib. of contractions ↖x Placenta Fetal resp. not down Sl. incr. in bleeding	Nil $\bar{c}$ O_2 Pl Explosion risk
Cyclopropane C_3H_6	↓	↓	Nil	Nil	Ret.	Uterus light—Nil deep ↓ ↖x Placenta > 4–5 min. → Fetal resp. ↓	Exhaled dangerous 6-8 min. Resp. depress. Effect on heart D > L Resp. fail > heart Explosive
Ethyl Ether $(C_2H_5)_2O$	↓	↓	↓	↓	Ret.	Passes ↖x Placenta Contractions ↓ Fetal resp. ↓	Still safest agent Resp. fail > heart
Vinyl Ether $(C_2H_3)_2O$	↓	↓	Nil	Nil	Nil	Light—contr. not effect. ↖x Placenta	Not suitable for long proc. Good for induc. May → conv.
Ethyl Chloride C_2H_5Cl	↓	↓		Nil	Nil	? ↖x Placenta	Suitable for induction ? heart risk ? spasm
Chloroform $CHCl_3$	↓	↓	↓	↓ ↓	Ret.	Contracts ↓ ↖x Placenta Fetal resp. very slow ↓	
Trichloroethylene $CHCl_3CCl_2$	↓	↓		Nil	Nil	Contracts sl. effected ↖x Placenta Fetus ↓	Soda lime contraindic. Used in analg. conc.

Code: ↓ Depression ↖x Crosses Placenta ∝ Increased

TABLE 5. PHARMACOLOGY OF THE VOLATILE AGENTS AND GASES USED IN ANESTHESIA (*Continued*)

AGENT	CARDIOVASCULAR SYSTEM					
	Cardiac Output	*B.P.*	*Pulse Rate*	*Cardiac Muscle*	*Coronary Vessels*	*Peripheral Vessels*
Nitrous Oxide N_2O (80%)	Nil	Nil	Nil	Nil	Nil	Sl. V.D.
Ethylene C_2H_4	Sl. ↑	Sl. ↑	Nil	Nil	Nil	V.D.
Cyclopropane C_3H_6	↑	↑ (CO_2)	↓	Irrit. D > L Sens. by Adren.		V.D.
Ethyl Ether $(C_2H_5)_2O$	↑	Sl. ↑ Then ↓ P.P. ↑	Nil	Nil	V.D.	V.D. (1) Direct (2) via VMC
Vinyl Ether $(C_2H_3)_2O$	Nil	↑ ↓	Nil	Nil		V.D.
Ethyl Chloride C_2H_5Cl	↓	↓	↓ ↑ (Vagus)	↓ Arr. Adr.		V.D.
Chloroform $CHCl_3$	↓	↓ V.D. (Direct) P.P. ↓	Depressed	↓ Arr. L > D Adr.	V.D.	V.D.
Trichloroethylene $CHCl_3CCl_2$	Nil	Nil	Sl. ↑ Arr. Deep	Nil Arr. Deep Adr.		V.D.

TABLE 5. PHARMACOLOGY OF THE VOLATILE AGENTS AND GASES USED IN ANESTHESIA (*Continued*)

AGENT	RESPIRATORY SYSTEM						
	Minute Volume	*Respiratory Rate*	*Mucous Membrane*	*Bronchial Muscle*	*Alveoli*	*Stretch Receptors*	*Deflation Endings*
Nitrous Oxide N_2O (80%)	Nil ∝ O_2 ∝ CO_2	Nil	Nil	Nil	Nil	↑ Then Out	Nil
Ethylene C_2H_4	Sl. ↑	Sl. ↑	Nil	Nil	Nil	↑ Then Out	Nil
Cyclopropane C_3H_6	↓	↓	Nil	May give spasm	Nil	↑ Then Out	↑ ↓
Ethyl Ether $(C_2H_5)_2O$	↑	↑	↑ Secret Irrit.	Irrit. may cause spasm	↑ Secretion	↑ Then Out	↑ ↓
Vinyl Ether $(C_2H_3)_2O$	↑	↑	Slow Irrit.		Nil	↑ Then Out	↑ ↓
Ethyl Chloride C_2H_5Cl	↓	↑ ↓	Nil	May give spasm	Nil	↑ Then Out	↑ ↓
Chloroform $CHCl_3$	↓	↑ ↓	Slow Irrit.	Relaxed	Atel.	↑ Then Out	↑ ↓
Trichloroethylene $CHCl_3CCl_2$	Nil	Slow ↑ Deep Tach.	Nil	Relaxed	Nil	↑ Then Out	Prolonged ↑

TABLE 5. PHARMACOLOGY OF THE VOLATILE AGENTS AND GASES USED IN ANESTHESIA (*Continued*)

AGENT	CENTRAL NERVOUS SYSTEM							
	Cortex	*Medulla and Pons*	*Carotid Sinus*	*Carotid Body*	*Cerebral Vessels*	*Intracranial Pressure*	*Remarks*	*Reflexes*
Nitrous Oxide N_2O (80%)	↓	∝ O_2 T.R.C. ↓ R.C. C.C. V.C. V.M.C. Vagus	↑	∝ O_2	∝ O_2 ∝ CO_2 Nil	∝ O_2 ∝ CO_2 Nil		Pharynx ↓ Larynx +
Ethylene C_2H_4	↓	T.R.C. ↓ R.C. C.C. V.C. V.M.C. Vagus	↑	∝ O_2	∝ O_2 ∝ CO_2 Nil	∝ O ∝ CO_2 Nil		Pupils vary Pharynx ↓ Larynx +
Cyclopropane C_3H_6	↓ ↓ ↓	T.R.C. ↓ R.C. ↓ ↓ C.C. ↓ V.C. ↓ V.M.C. ↓	↑ ↓	↓	V.D.	Nil	Chol-inerg.	Pupils small till Plane IV Pharynx ↓ Larynx ↓
Ethyl Ether $(C_2H_5)_2O$	↓ ↓ ↓	T.R.C. ↓ R.C. ↑ ↓ V.C. ↓ C.C. ↓ V.M.C. ↓ ↓ ↓	↑ ↓	↑ ↓	V.D.	↑ ↓		Pupils classical Abolishes reflexes as depth increases
Vinyl Ether $(C_2H_3)_2O$	↓ ↓	T.R.C. ↓ R.C. ↑ ↓ V.C. ↓ C.C. ↓ V.M.C. ↓	↑ ↓	↑ ↓				Pupils usually roving
Ethyl Chloride C_2H_5Cl	↓ ↓	T.R. ↑ R.C. ↑ V.C. ↓ C.C. ↓ V.M.C. ↓ Vagus ↓	↑ ↓	↑ ↓		↑		Pupils vary Pharynx ↓ Larynx ↓ (spasm)
Chloroform $CHCl_3$	↓ ↓ ↓ ↓	T.R.C. ↓ R.C. ↓ C.C. ↓ V.C. ↓ V.M.C. ↓ Vagus ↓	↓	↑ ↓	V.D.	↑		Pupils classical
Trichloroethylene $CHCl_3CCl_2$	↓	R.C. ↑	↓	↓	Nil	Nil		

↑ Stimulation ↓ Depression ↖̸ Crosses placenta ∝ Increased > Before

TABLE 6. INTRAVENOUS DRUGS AND DOSAGES USED IN ANESTHESIA

DRUG, TRADE OR COMMON NAME	OFFICIAL OR CHEMICAL NAME	STRENGTH OF SOLUTION MG./CC.	AV. ADULT DOSE IN MG. (I.V., UNLESS STATED)	PRINCIPAL USE
Adrenalin	Epinephrine	1	0.1–0.5	Sympathetic stimulant
Aminophylline	Aminophylline	250	250–500	Bronchodilator, heart stimulant
Anectine	Succinylcholine	50	30–60	Skeletal muscle relaxant
Atropine	Atropine	0.4	0.4–1	Parasympathetic depressant
Benzedrine	Amphetamine	10	5–10	C.N.S. stimulant, vasopressor
Bistrium (C-6)	Hexamethonium	25	25	Vasodilator
Caffeine	Caffeine	250	200–500	C.N.S. stimulant
Cedilanid	Lanatoside C	0.2	0.4–0.8	Myocardial stimulant
Coramine	Nikethamide	250	500–1,000	C.N.S. stimulant
Demerol	Meperidine	50	25–100	Analgesic
Desoxyephedrine	(see Methedrine)			
d-Tubocurarine	Tubocurarine	3	3–15	Skeletal muscle relaxant
Ephedrine	Ephedrine	50	15–50	Vasopressor
Flaxedil	Gallamine triethiodide	20	20–100	Skeletal muscle relaxant
Heparin sodium	Heparin	10		Anticoagulant
Levophed	Norepinephrine	1	4 mg. in 1,000 cc.	Vasopressor
Methedrine	Metamphetamine HCl	20	5–15	C.N.S. stimulant, vasopressor
Metrazol	Pentylenetetrazol	100	100	C.N.S. stimulant
Morphine	Morphine		10–16 s.c.	Analgesic
Nalline	N-allylnormorphine	5	5–10	Morphine antagonist
Nembutal	(see Pentobarbital)			
Neosynephrine	Phenylephrine HCl	10	0.3–0.5	Vasopressor
Pentobarbital	Pentobarbital		100–200 p.o.	C.N.S. depressant
Pronestyl	Procaine amide	100	100–500	Myocardial depressant
Prostigmin	Neostigmine	1	1	Parasympathetic stimulant
Scopolamine	Scopolamine		0.4–0.6 s.c.	Parasympathetic depressant
Seconal (I.V.)	Secobarbital	50	100–150	C.N.S. depressant
Strophosid	K-strophanthoside	0.5	0.5	Myocardial stimulant
Syncurine	Decamethonium	1	1–3	Skeletal muscle relaxant
Thorazine	Chlorpromazine		25–50 I.M.	C.N.S. depressant
Viadril	2/OH Pregnandione Sodium Succinate	2	400	Amnesic soporific
Wyamine	Mephentermine	15	15–30	Vasopressor

presence of potential or labile hypertension and in obstetric toxemias. A major incompatibility or adverse summation of action of vasopressors is evident when ergot and some form of vasopressor are used concurrently. Therefore, it is particularly dangerous to use standard ergonovine for intravenous administration or ergotrate in the obstetric patient who has had a spinal anesthetic with ephedrine or some similar drug as a prophylactic or therapeutic vasopressor. Tyramine is a vasopressor with an organic structure similar to that of epinephrine. This compound, Tyramine, is an alkaloid of ergot and is a vasopressor twice as potent as ephedrine. Thus, when ephedrine and ergonovine are administered together or within a short space of time of each other to an unanesthetized patient or to a patient under spinal anesthesia, critical hypertension may develop. In one such patient receiving this combination in a Baltimore hospital, critical hypertension and total permanent hemiplegia developed immediately after administration. Six other near-fatalities have been reported to us in which this incompatibility was permitted to exist. Therefore, it is of particular importance for the anesthetist and the obstetrician to substitute Pitocin for standard ergonovine or ergotrate as an oxytocic in those patients delivered by cesarean section or vaginally with any form of vertebral conduction anesthesia. This is of even greater importance when the patient has hypertensive vascular disease or hypertension associated with toxemia of pregnancy.

In the diagrammatic illustrations depicting pharmacologic action of individual analgesic, amnesic and anesthetic agents on each maternal and fetal organ on the following pages, we have presented an epitome of present-day authoritative concepts from recognized authors.

Occasionally, opinions of various investigators concerning the specific effects of anesthetic and amnesic agents on body organs are controversial. It has been our policy to present the most authoritative and generally accepted opinion wherever possible. We have combined our own clinical observations with the opinions of pharmacologists, anesthesiologists and obstetricians in the final summary of this information.

In Plates 1 to 17 *blue* indicates depressing effects, and *red* indicates stimulating effects of the agents used, on both mother and baby.

BIBLIOGRAPHY

General

Bush, O. F., Penecost, P. S., and Adriani, John: Seconal Sodium as basal hypnotic and adjunct to anesthesia—evaluation of improved preparation for intravenous administration, Anesthesiology **12:**447-454, 1951.

Collins, R. M., and Rumbolz, W. L.: Unpublished report.

Stoelting, V. K., and Graf, J. P.: Intravenous sodium 5-allyl-5 (1-methylbutyl) barbiturate for hypnosis during nitrous oxide anesthesia, A.M.A. Arch. Surg. **64:**214-219, 1952.

Stoelting, V. K., Graf, J. P., and Rach, G. W.: Intravenous propyl-methyl-carbinyl allyl barbituric acid for hypnosis during nitrous oxide anesthesia, Anesth. & Analg. **29:**61-67, 1950.

Virtue, R. W., and Gootee, J. E.: Experimental and clinical evaluation of sodium allyl 1-methylbutyl barbiturate (Seconal) administered intravenously, Anesthesiology **12:**642-647, 1951.

Weitzman, C. C., and Davis, J. G.: Intravenous Seconal Sodium in obstetric labor, Am. Pract. & Digest Treat. **3:**712-716, 1952.

Weyl, R., Liu, W., and Lipp, E.: Evaluation of usefulness of intravenous Seconal Sodium in anesthesia, J. Internat. Coll. Surgeons **18:**365-371, 1952.

Anesthetic Drugs and Administration

Adriani, John: The Chemistry of Anesthesia, Springfield, Ill., Thomas, 1952.

———: The Pharmacology of Anesthetic Drugs, ed. 3, Springfield, Ill., Thomas, 1952.

Beecher, H. K.: The Physiology of Anesthesia, New York, Oxford, 1938.

Best, C. H., and Taylor, N. B.: Living Body: Text in Human Physiology, ed. 3, New York, Holt, 1952.

———: Physiological Basis of Medical Practice, ed. 5, Baltimore, Williams & Wilkins, 1950.

Dogliotti, A. M.: Anesthesia, Chicago, Debour, 1939.

Evans, F. T.: Modern Practice in Anesthesia, ed. 2, New York, Hoeber, 1954.

Flagg, P. S.: The Art of Anesthesia, ed. 7, Philadelphia, Lippincott, 1944.

Fulton, J. F.: Textbook of Physiology, ed. 17, Philadelphia, Saunders, 1955.

Goodman, Louis, and Gilman, Alfred: Pharmacological Basis of Therapeutics, ed. 2, New York, Macmillan, 1955.

Krantz, J. C., and Carr, C. J.: Pharmacological Principles of Medical Practice, ed. 3, Baltimore, Williams & Wilkins, 1954.

Lundy, J. S., and McQuillen, Florence, Editors: Anesthesia Abstracts, vol. 40, Minneapolis, Burgess, 1954.

Macintosh, R. R., and Bannister, F. B.: Essentials of General Anesthesia, ed. 5, Springfield, Ill., Thomas, 1952.

Minnitt, R. J., and Gillies, M. C.: Textbook of Anesthetics, ed. 7, Baltimore, Williams & Wilkins, 1948.

Sollman, Torald: A Manual of Pharmacology, ed. 7, Philadelphia, Saunders, 1948.

CHLOROFORM

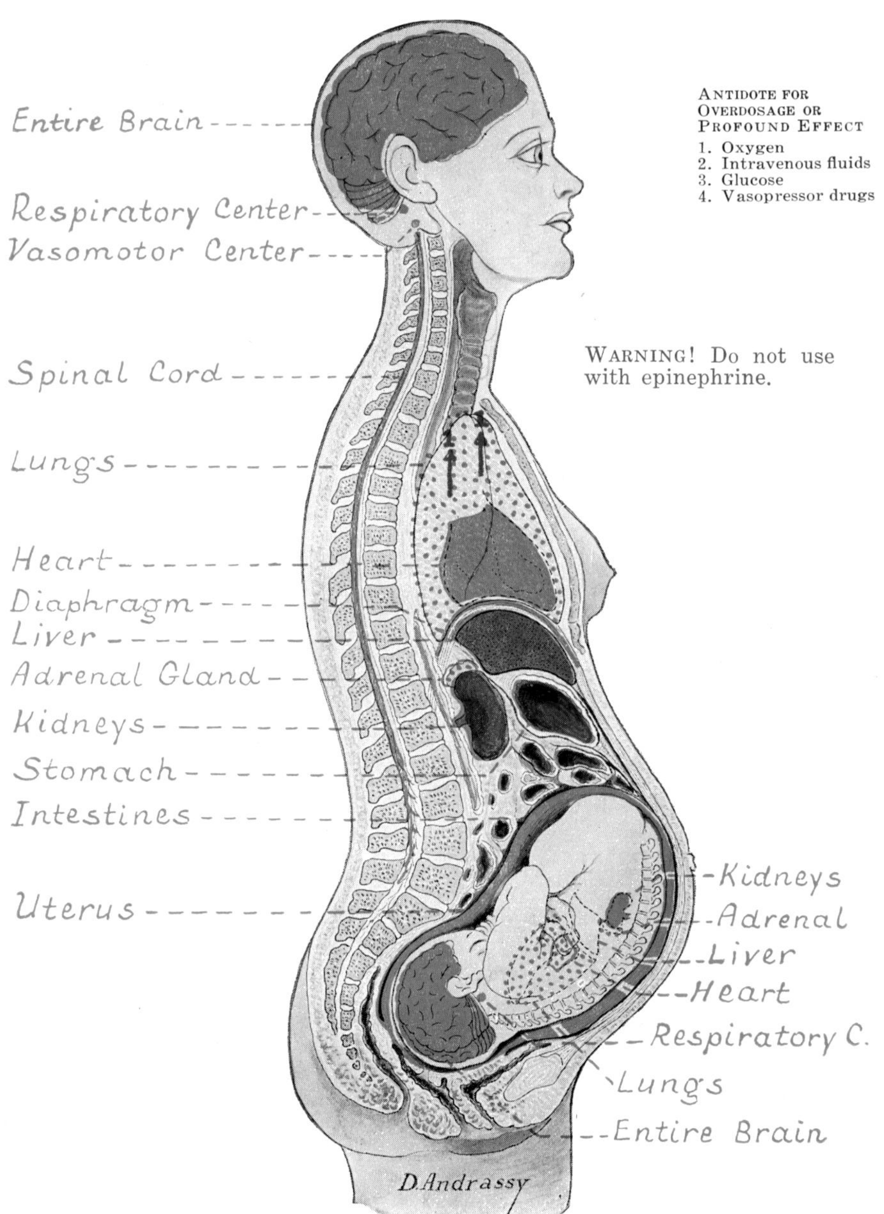

ANTIDOTE FOR OVERDOSAGE OR PROFOUND EFFECT

1. Oxygen
2. Intravenous fluids
3. Glucose
4. Vasopressor drugs

WARNING! Do not use with epinephrine.

PLATE 1. The action of chloroform. The *blue* indicates *depression* of maternal and fetal organs. Solid color indicates intensified action. Dotted color indicates moderate action. The numbers on the ascending *red* arrows indicate sequence of *stimulation*.

ETHYL ETHER

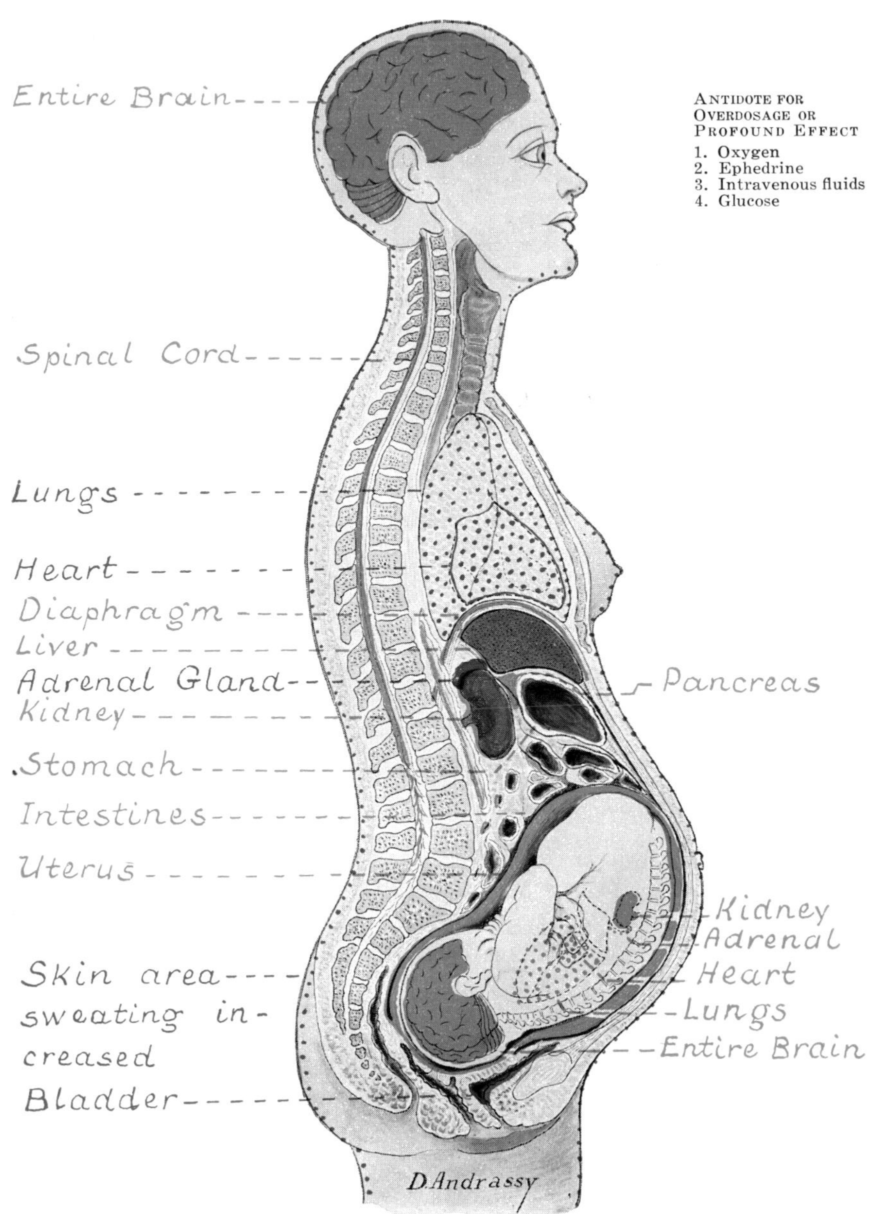

ANTIDOTE FOR OVERDOSAGE OR PROFOUND EFFECT

1. Oxygen
2. Ephedrine
3. Intravenous fluids
4. Glucose

PLATE 2. The action of ethyl ether. The *red* indicates *stimulation* and *blue* indicates *depression* of maternal and fetal organs. Solid color indicates intensified action; dotted color indicates moderate action; outline dots indicate minimal action.

DIVINYL ETHER
(Vinethene)

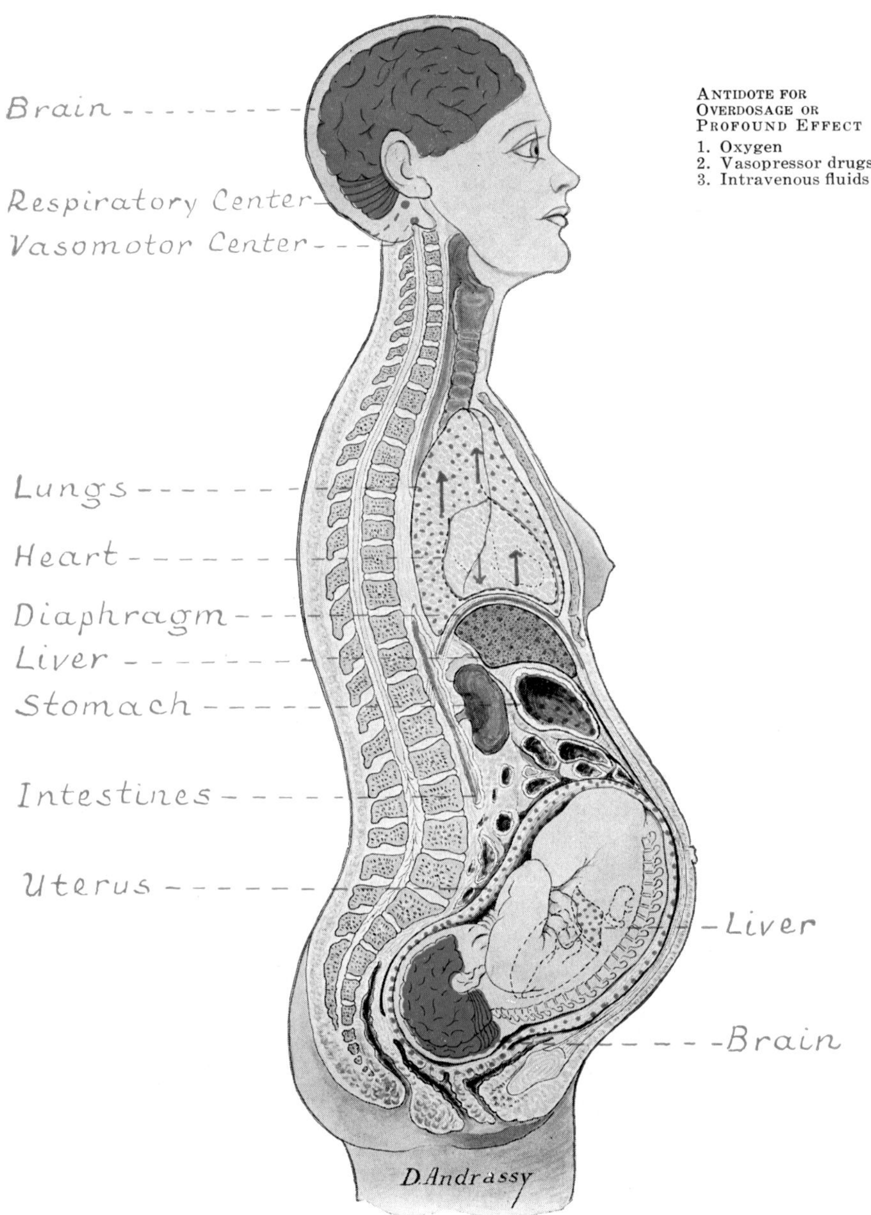

PLATE 3. The action of divinyl ether. *Blue* indicates *depression* of maternal and fetal organs. Solid color indicates intensified action; dotted color indicates moderate action; outline dots indicate minimal action. The *red* ascending *arrows* indicate the sequence of *stimulation* and the *blue* the *depression*.

NITROUS OXIDE

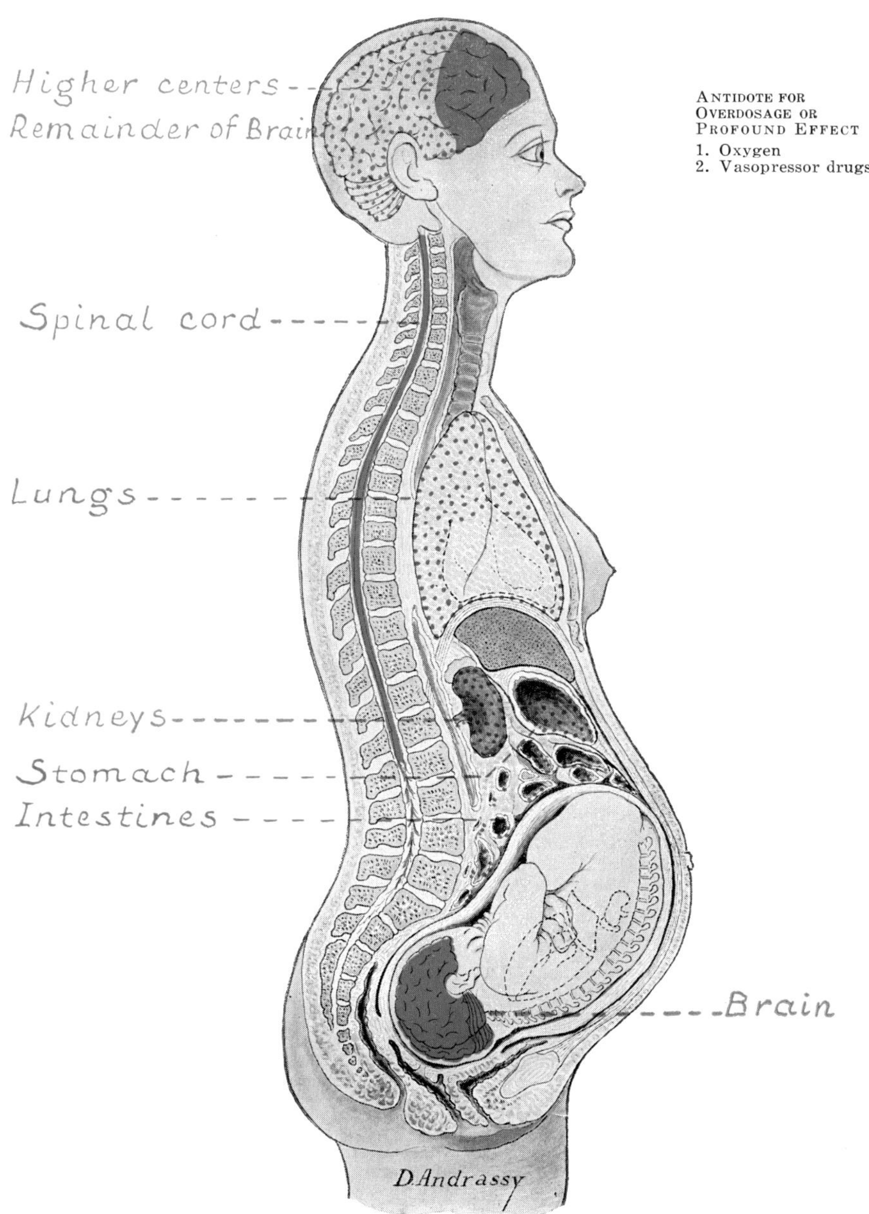

ANTIDOTE FOR OVERDOSAGE OR PROFOUND EFFECT

1. Oxygen
2. Vasopressor drugs

PLATE 4. The action of nitrous oxide. The *red* indicates *stimulation*, and the *blue* indicates *depression* of maternal and fetal organs. Solid color indicates intensified action; dotted color indicates moderate action.

ETHYLENE

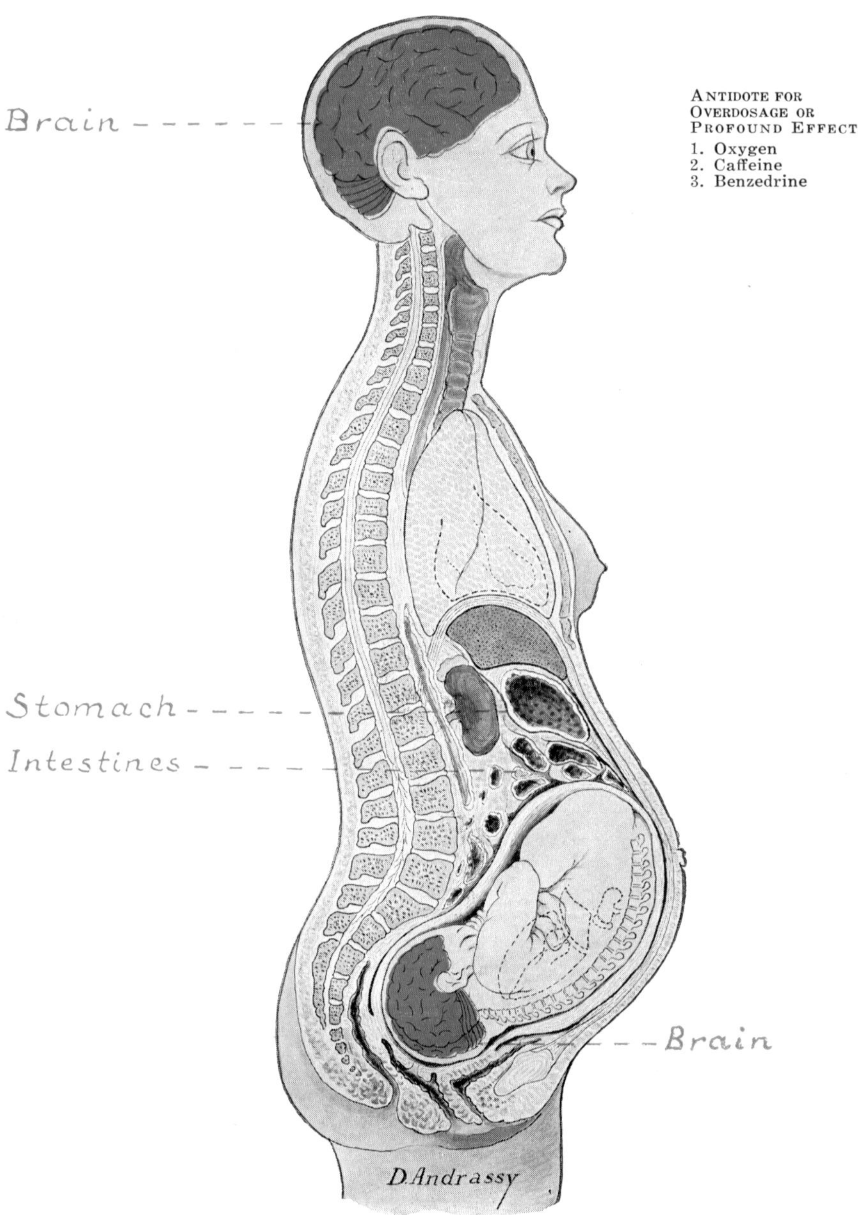

PLATE 5. The action of ethylene. The *blue* indicates *depression* of maternal and fetal organs. Solid color indicates intensified action; dotted color indicates moderate action.

CYCLOPROPANE

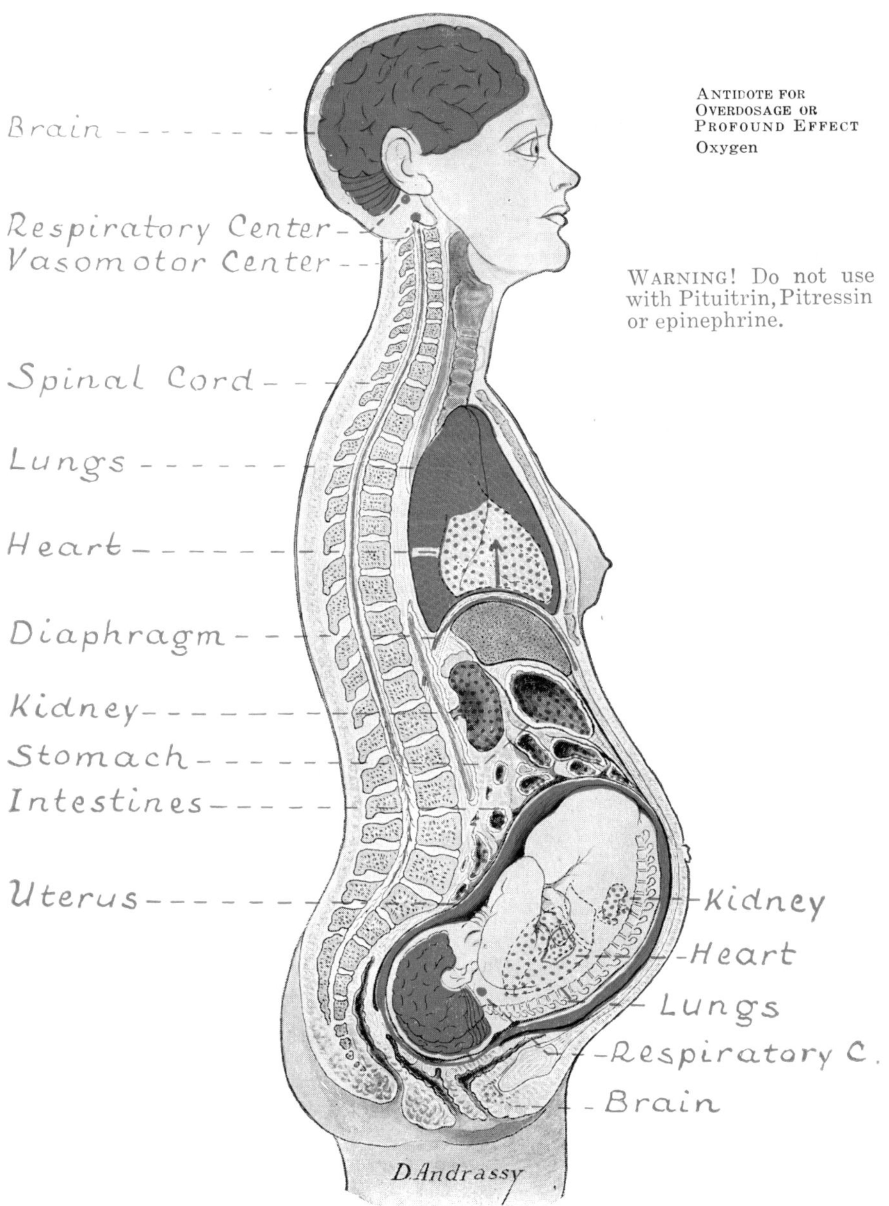

ANTIDOTE FOR OVERDOSAGE OR PROFOUND EFFECT
Oxygen

WARNING! Do not use with Pituitrin, Pitressin or epinephrine.

PLATE 6. The action of cyclopropane. The *blue* indicates *depression* of the maternal and the fetal organs. Solid color indicates intensified action; dotted color indicates moderate action. The ascending *red arrow* indicates *stimulation*.

TRICHLOROETHYLENE
(Trilene)

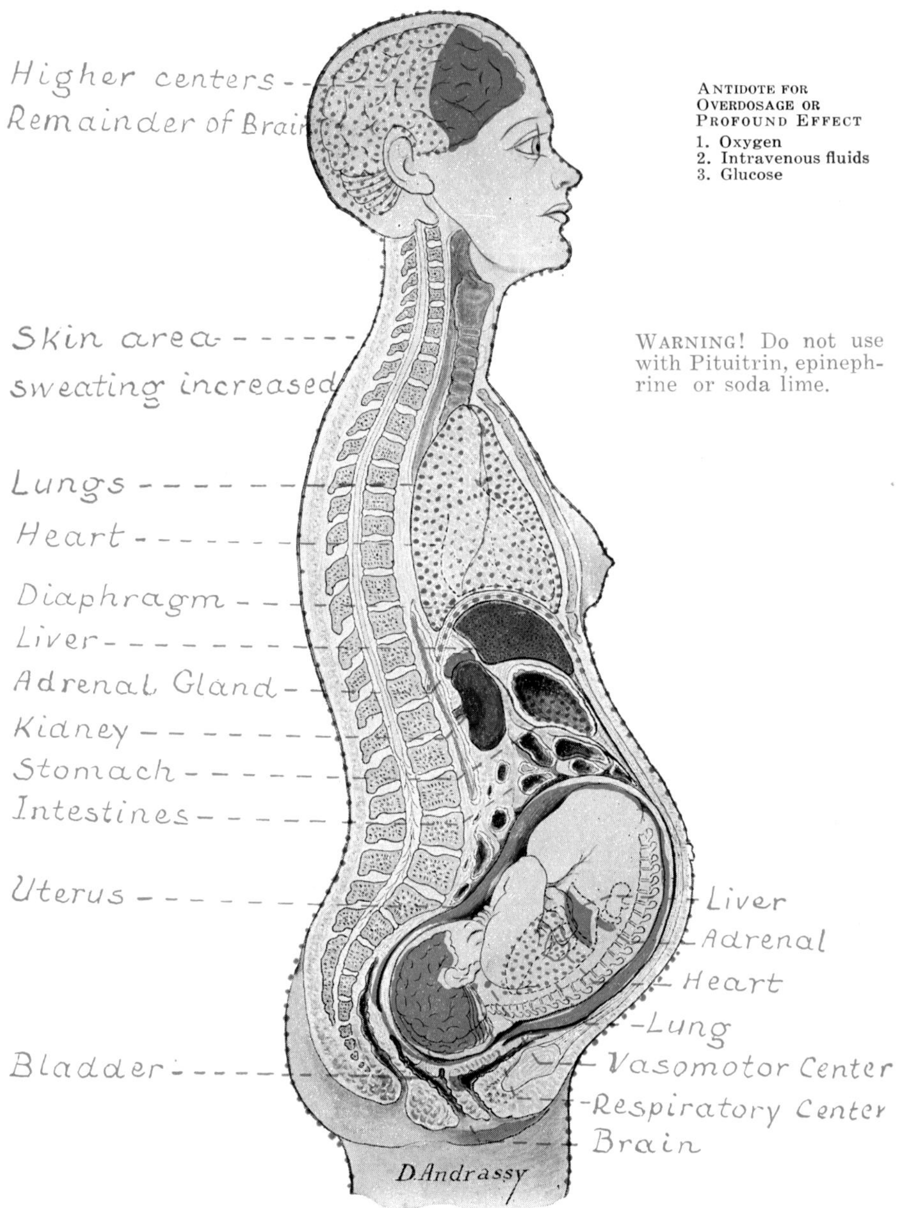

Plate 7. The action of trichloroethylene. The *red* indicates *stimulation* and the *blue* indicates *depression* of the maternal and the fetal organs. Solid color indicates intensified action; dotted color indicates moderate action; outline dots indicate minimal action. The number 2 on the descending arrow indicates the sequence of depression.

BELLADONNA
(Atropine or Scopolamine)

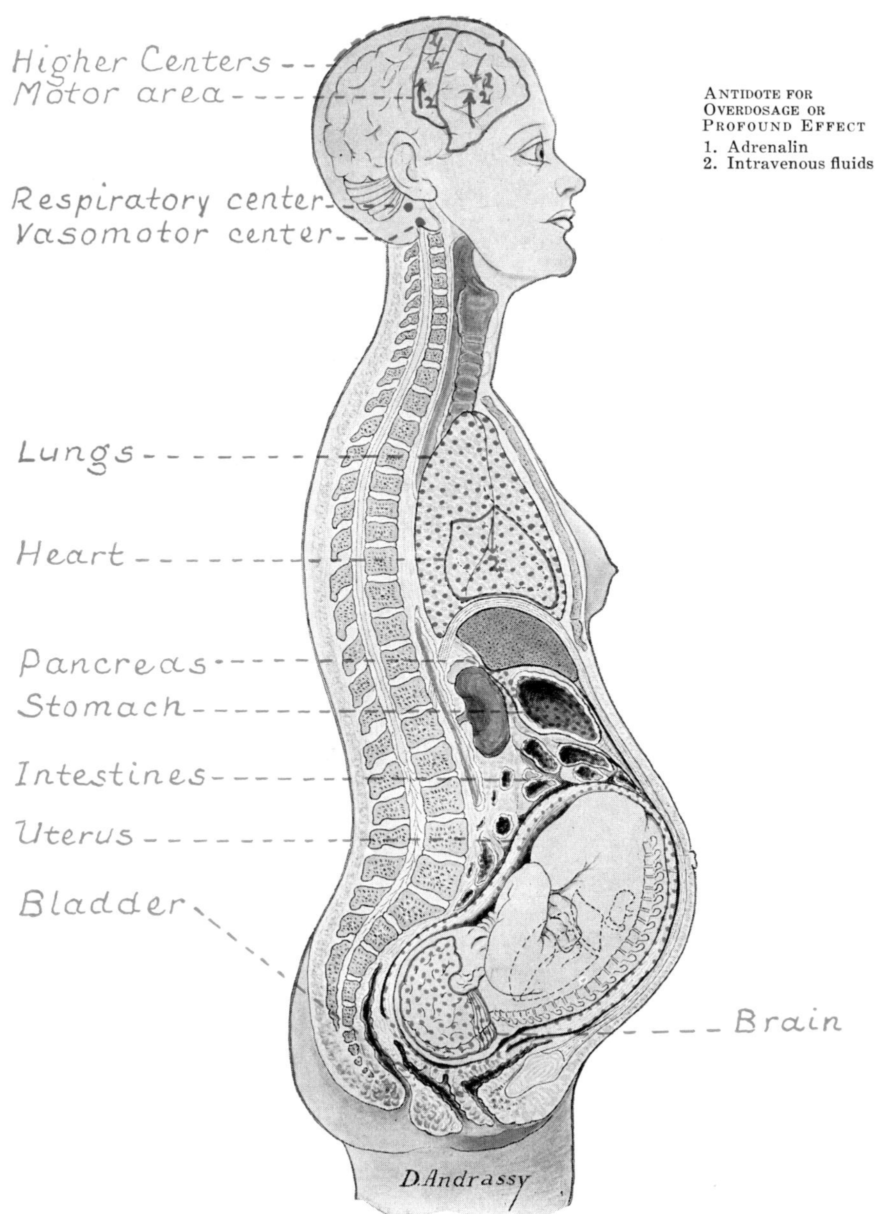

ANTIDOTE FOR OVERDOSAGE OR PROFOUND EFFECT
1. Adrenalin
2. Intravenous fluids

PLATE 8. The action of belladonna. The *red* indicates *stimulation,* and the *blue* indicates *depression* of the maternal and the fetal organs. Dotted color indicates moderate action; outline dots indicate minimal action. The numbers on the ascending and the descending arrows indicate the sequence of stimulation and depression.

TRIBROMOETHANOL
(Avertin)

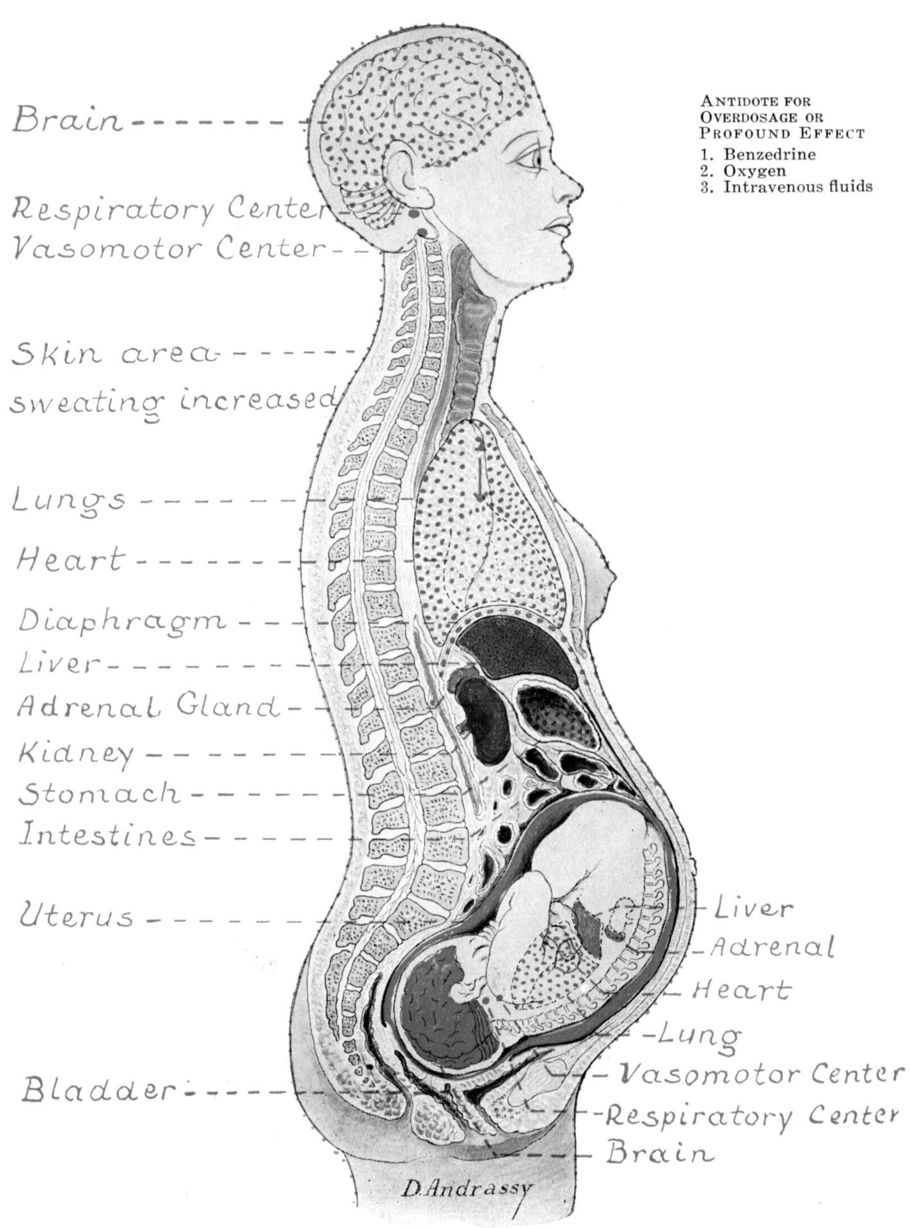

Antidote for Overdosage or Profound Effect

1. Benzedrine
2. Oxygen
3. Intravenous fluids

Plate 9. The action of tribromoethanol (Avertin). The *red* indicates *stimulation,* and the *blue* indicates *depression* of the maternal and the fetal organs. Solid color indicates intensified action; dotted color indicates moderate action; outline dots indicate minimal action. The number 2 on the descending arrow indicates the sequence of depression.

PARALDEHYDE

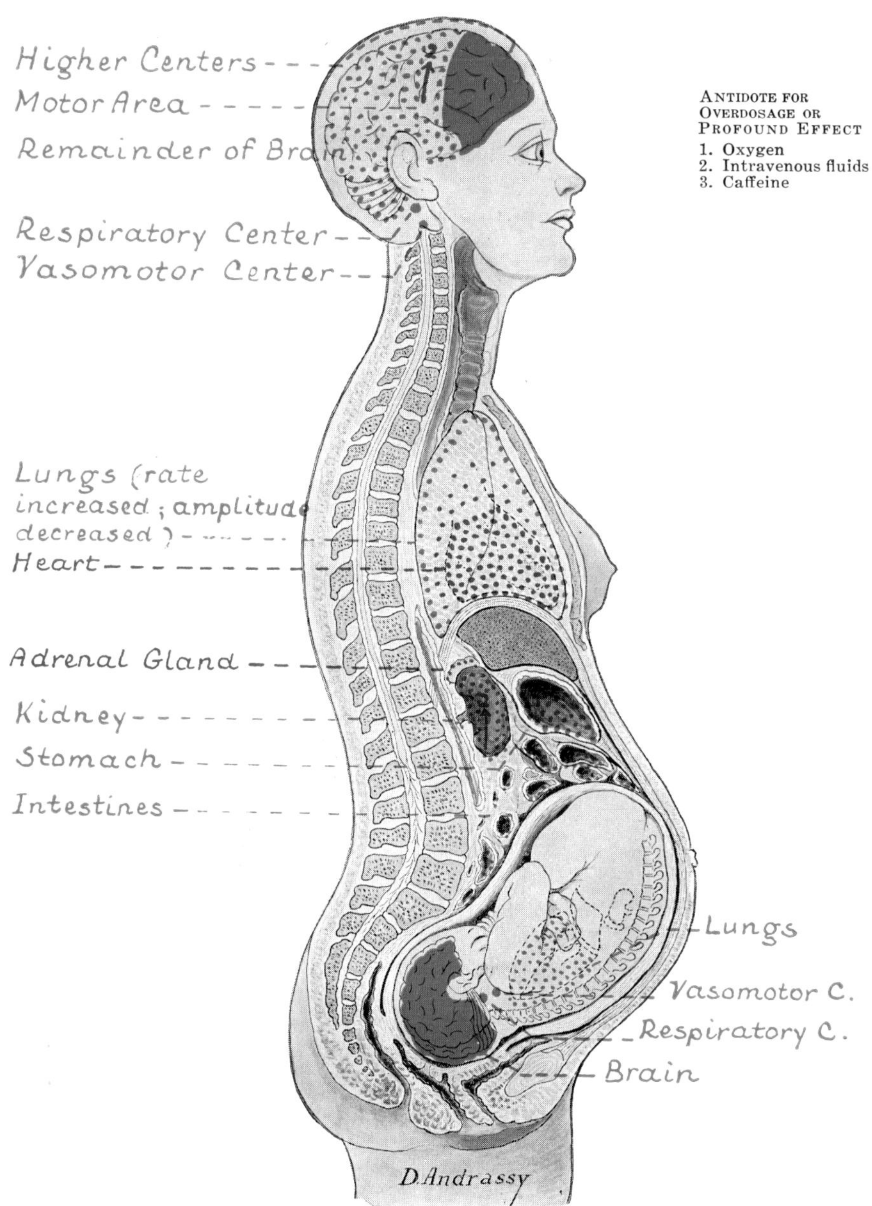

ANTIDOTE FOR OVERDOSAGE OR PROFOUND EFFECT

1. Oxygen
2. Intravenous fluids
3. Caffeine

PLATE 10. The action of paraldehyde. The *red* indicates *stimulation* and the *blue* indicates *depression* of maternal and fetal organs. Solid color indicates intensified action; dotted color indicates moderate action; outline dots indicate minimal action. The number 2 on the ascending red arrows indicates the sequence of stimulation.

BARBITURATES

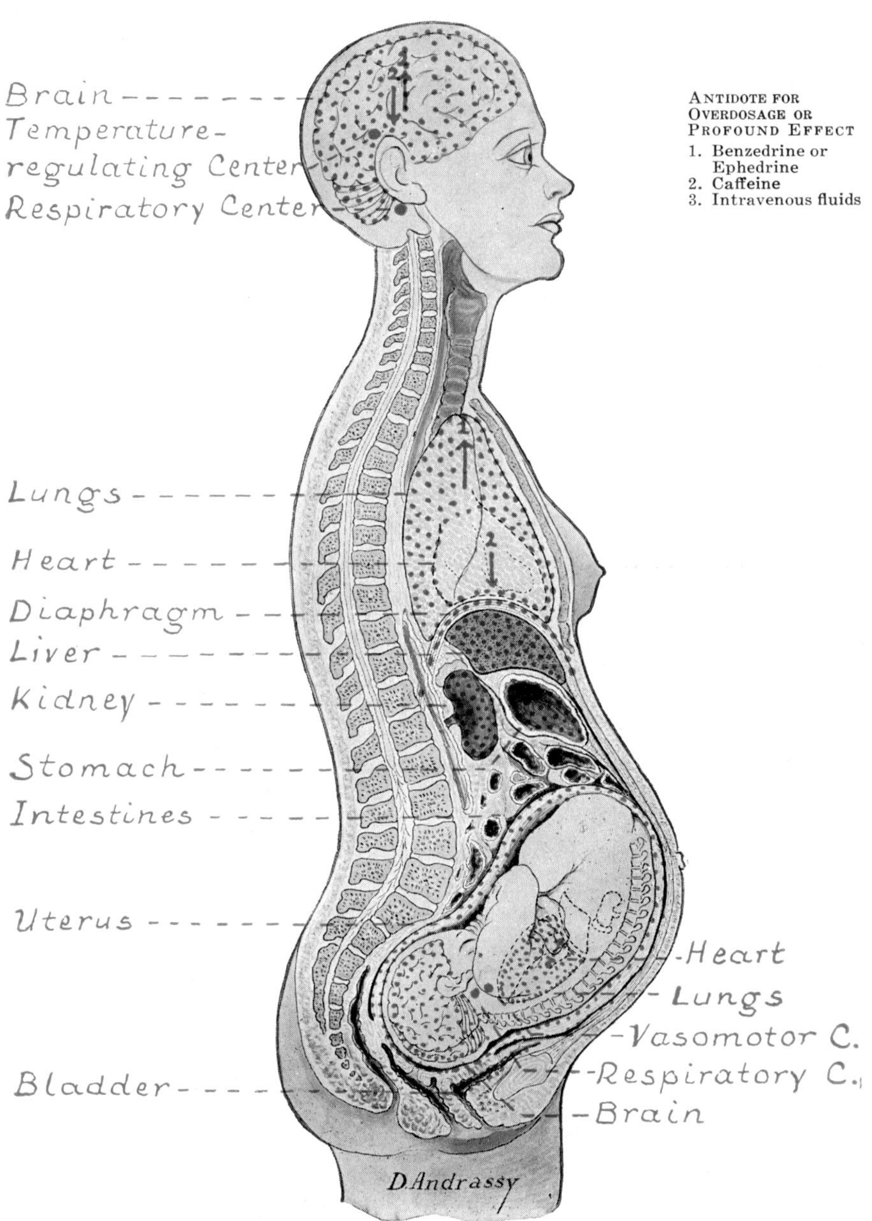

ANTIDOTE FOR OVERDOSAGE OR PROFOUND EFFECT

1. Benzedrine or Ephedrine
2. Caffeine
3. Intravenous fluids

PLATE 11. The action of the barbiturates (Delvinal, Seconal, Amytal, phenobarbital). The *red* indicates *stimulation* and the *blue* indicates *depression* of maternal and fetal organs. Dotted color indicates moderate action; outline dots indicate minimal action. The numbers 1 and 2 on the ascending and the descending red and blue arrows indicate the sequence of stimulation and depression.

INTRAVENOUS BARBITURATES

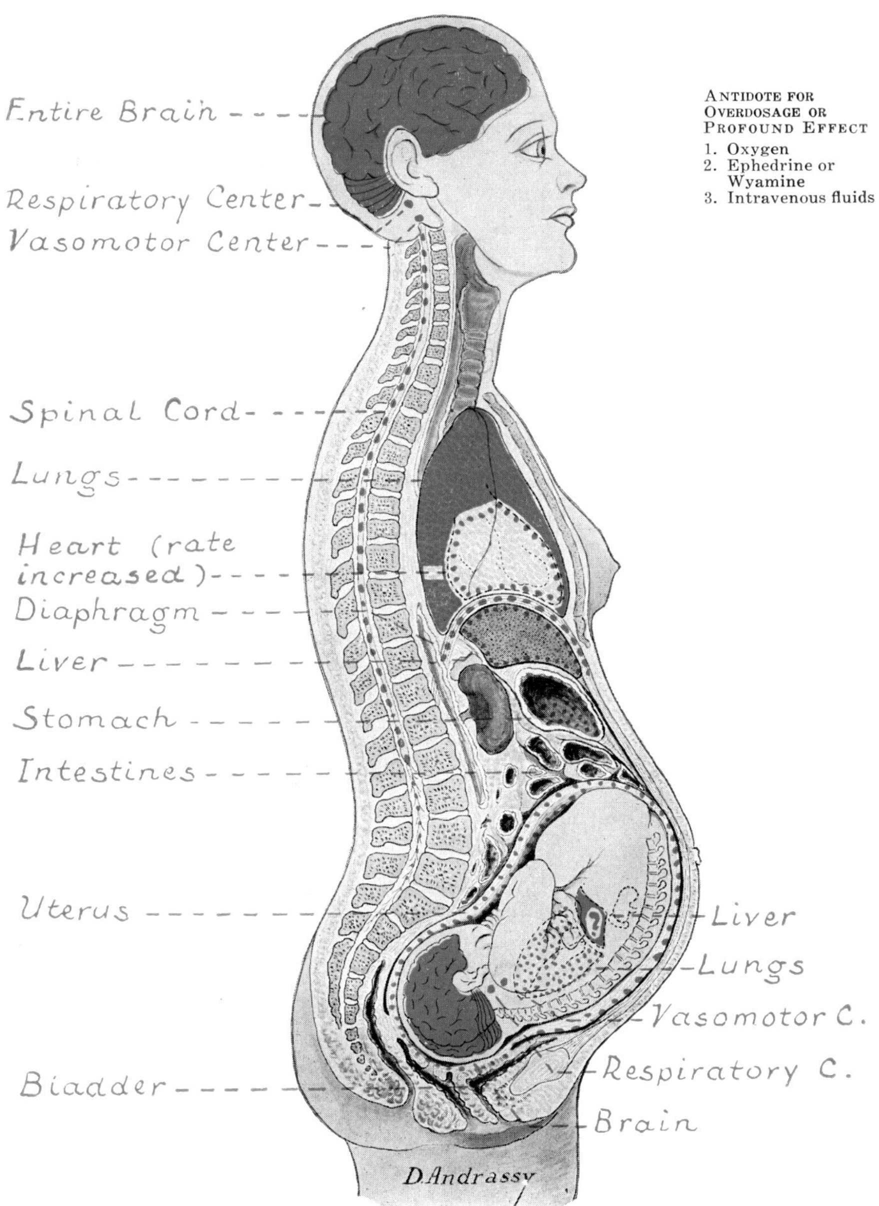

ANTIDOTE FOR OVERDOSAGE OR PROFOUND EFFECT

1. Oxygen
2. Ephedrine or Wyamine
3. Intravenous fluids

PLATE 12. The action of intravenous barbiturates (Pentothal Sodium, Surital Sodium, Kemithal and Evipal Sodium). The *red* indicates *stimulation* and the *blue* indicates *depression* of maternal and fetal organs. Solid color indicates intensified action; dotted color indicates modified action; outline dots indicate minimal action.

OPIATES

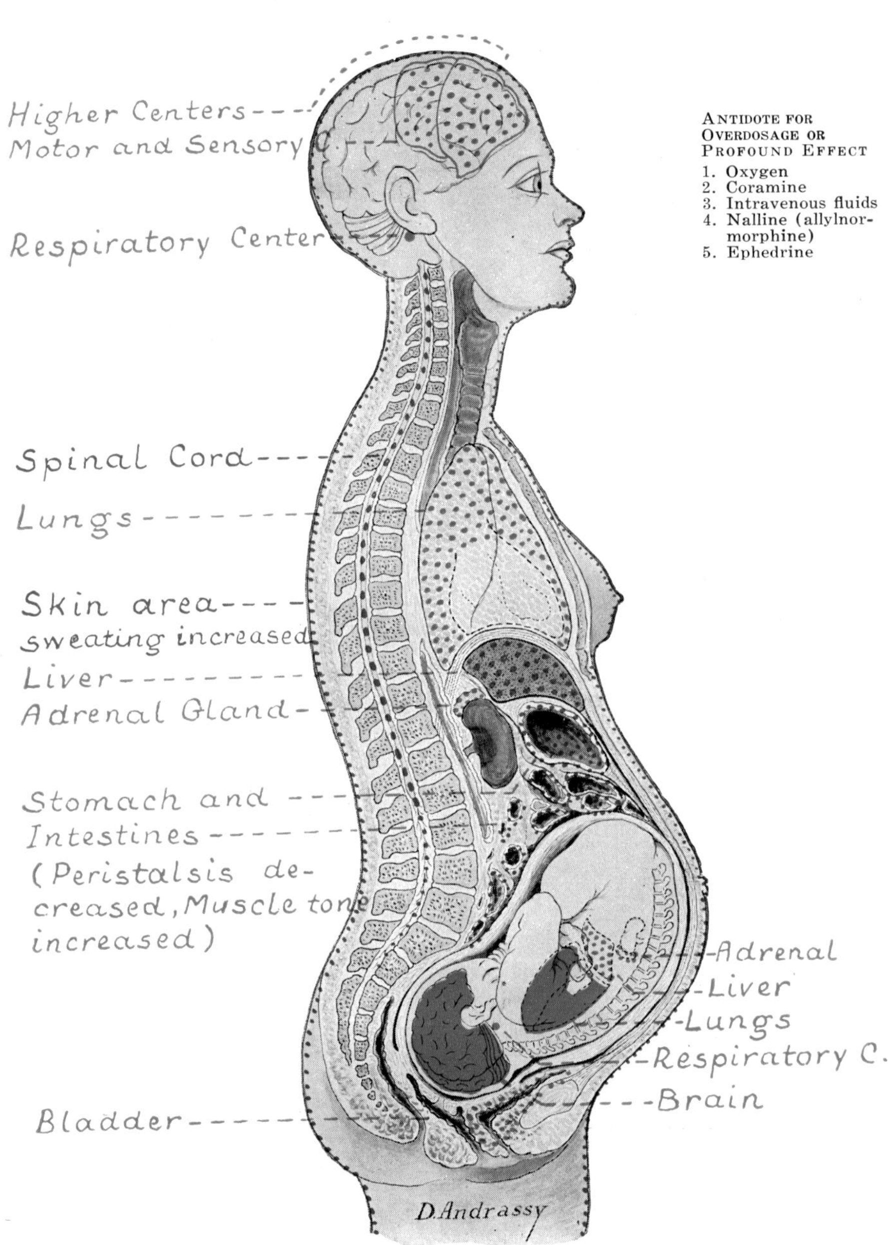

PLATE 13. The action of the opiates (morphine, heroin, codeine, Dilaudid, Pantopon). The *red* indicates *stimulation* and the *blue* indicates *depression* of maternal and fetal organs. Solid color indicates intensified action; dotted color indicates moderate action; outline dots indicate minimal action.

DEMEROL
(Pethidine)

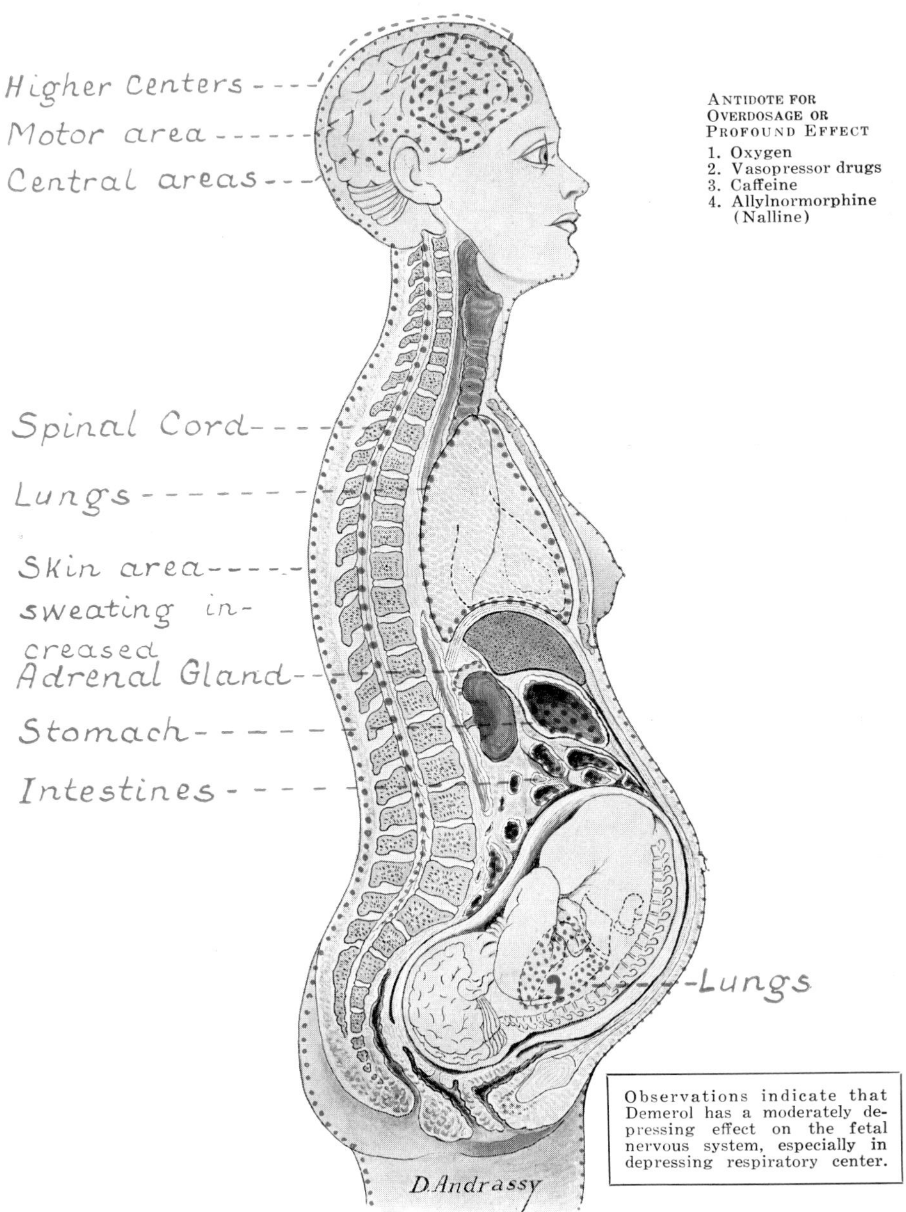

ANTIDOTE FOR OVERDOSAGE OR PROFOUND EFFECT

1. Oxygen
2. Vasopressor drugs
3. Caffeine
4. Allylnormorphine (Nalline)

Observations indicate that Demerol has a moderately depressing effect on the fetal nervous system, especially in depressing respiratory center.

PLATE 14. The action of Demerol. The *red* indicates *stimulation* and the *blue* indicates *depression* of the maternal and the fetal organs. Dotted color indicates moderate action; outline dots indicate minimal action.

LOCAL AND REGIONAL ANESTHESIA

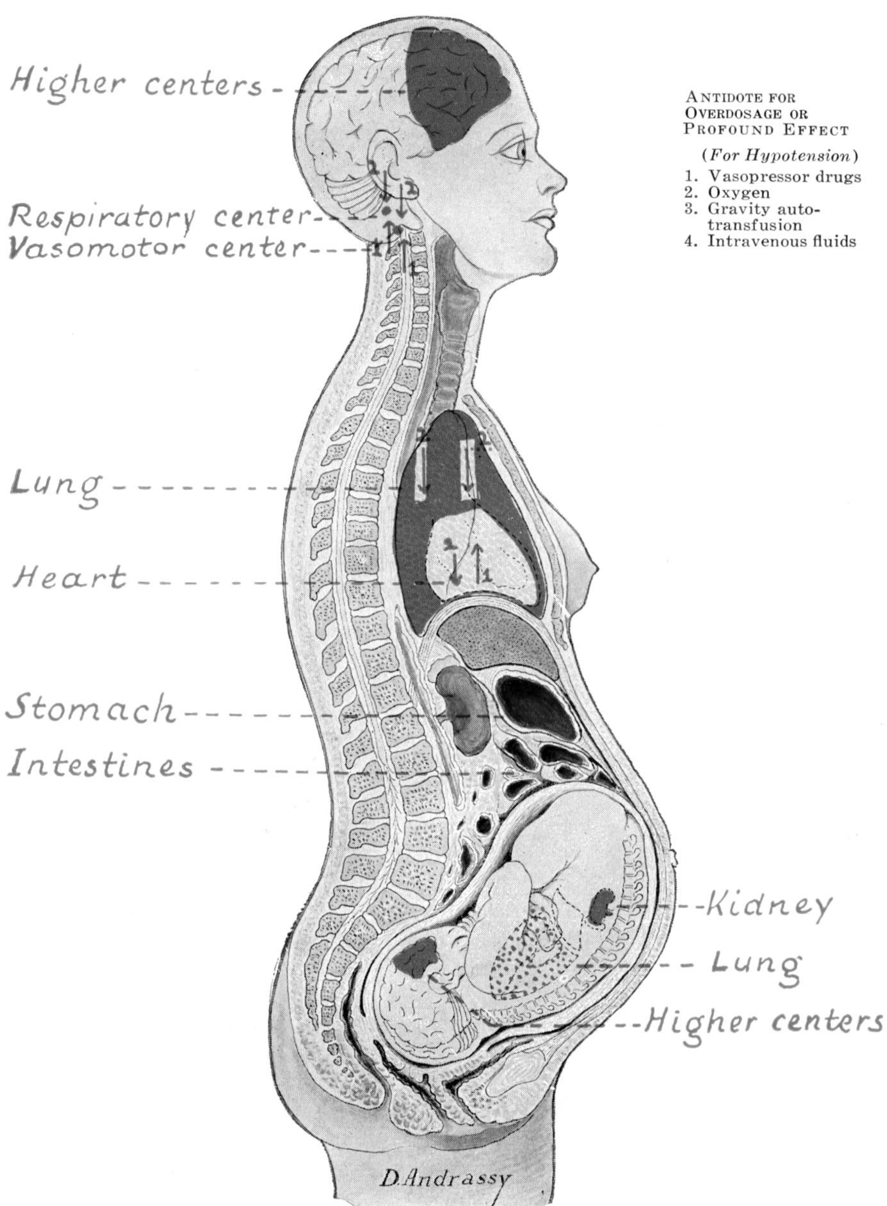

ANTIDOTE FOR OVERDOSAGE OR PROFOUND EFFECT

(*For Hypotension*)

1. Vasopressor drugs
2. Oxygen
3. Gravity auto-transfusion
4. Intravenous fluids

PLATE 15. The action of local and regional anesthesia (Metycaine, procaine and Xylocaine). The *red* indicates *stimulation* of maternal and fetal organs. Solid color indicates intensified action; dotted color indicates moderate action. The number 1 on the ascending red arrows indicates the sequence of stimulation and the number 2 on the descending blue arrows indicates the sequence of depression.

SPINAL AND CONTINUOUS SPINAL ANESTHESIA

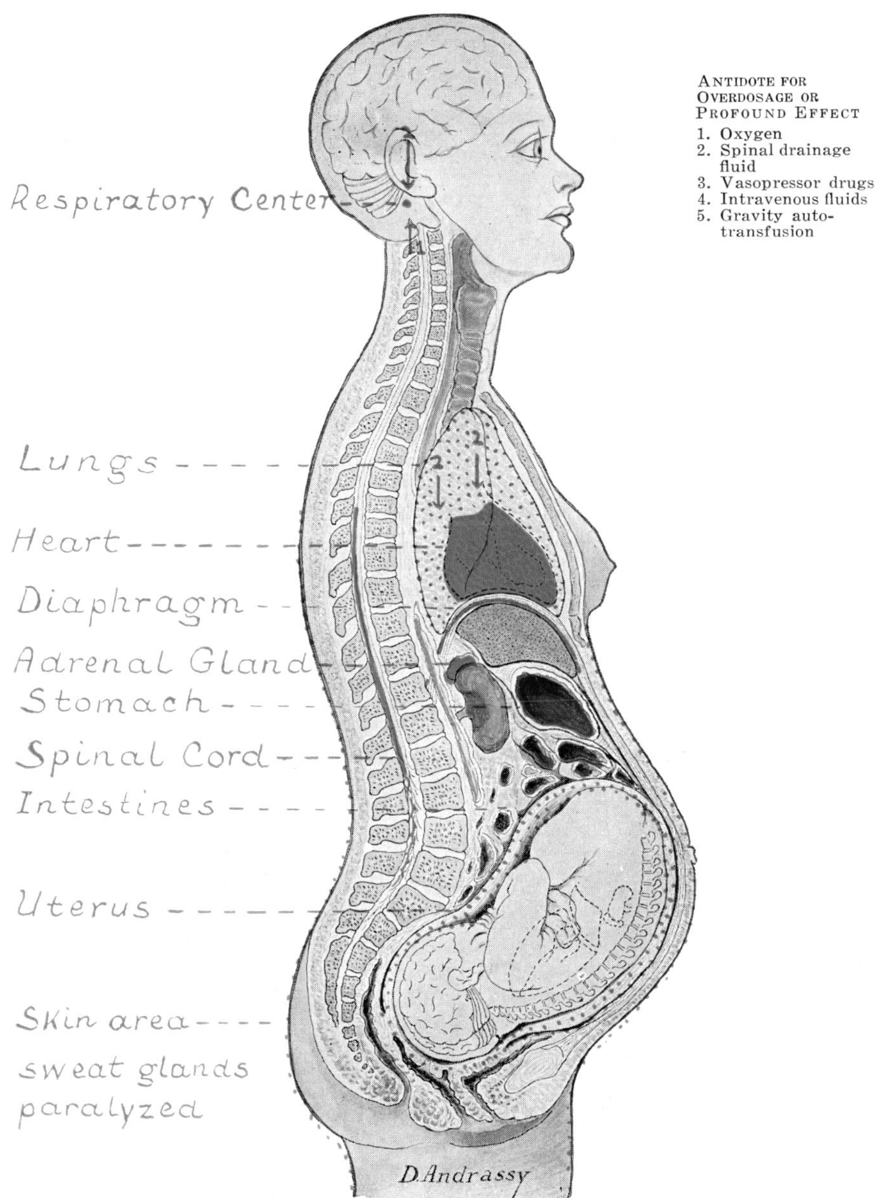

ANTIDOTE FOR OVERDOSAGE OR PROFOUND EFFECT

1. Oxygen
2. Spinal drainage fluid
3. Vasopressor drugs
4. Intravenous fluids
5. Gravity autotransfusion

PLATE 16. The action of spinal and continuous spinal anesthesia (Metycaine, procaine, Pontocaine, Nupercaine, Xylocaine). The *red* indicates *stimulation* and the *blue* indicates *depression* of maternal and fetal organs. Solid color indicates intensified action; dotted color indicates moderate action; outline dots indicate minimal action. The number 1 on the ascending and the number 2 on the descending arrows indicate the sequence of stimulation and depression.

CAUDAL AND CONTINUOUS CAUDAL ANALGESIA

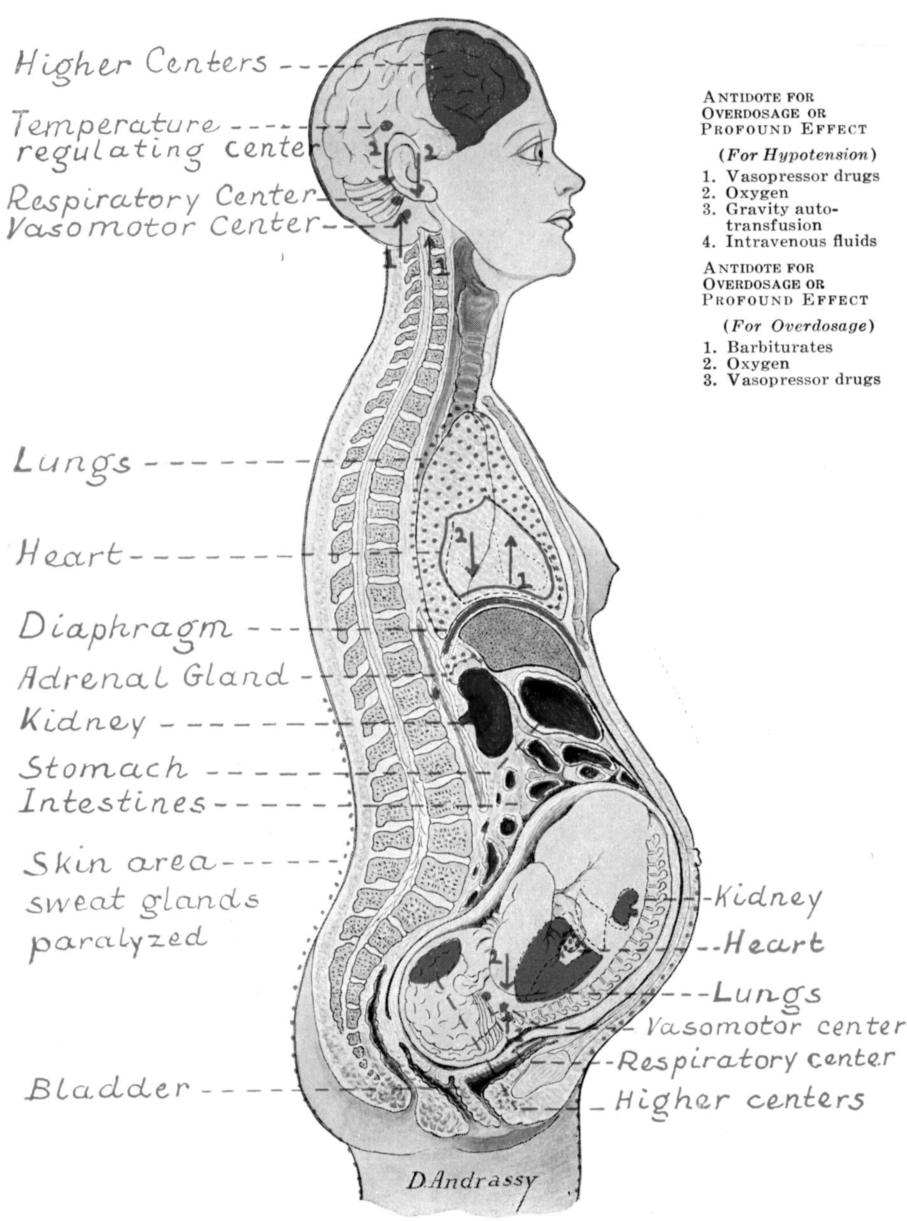

PLATE 17. The action of caudal peridural and continuous caudal analgesia (Metycaine, procaine, Pontocaine, Xylocaine). The *red* indicates *stimulation* and the *blue* indicates *depression* of maternal and fetal organs. Solid color indicates intensified action; dotted color indicates moderate action; outline dots indicate minimal action. The number 1 on the ascending and the number 2 on the descending blue arrows indicate the sequence of stimulation and depression.

»» 2 «« Obstetric Amnesia, Analgesia and Anesthesia in Historical Perspective

For the understanding of new technics or a proper utilization and standardization of old ones in obstetric anesthesia and their impact upon cultural mores, it is necessary for the student to have a sense of continuity with the past.

CHILDBIRTH BEFORE ANESTHESIA

The use of anesthetics to alleviate the pain of surgical operations and of childbirth was unknown before the middle of the nineteenth century. Nevertheless, historical manuscripts from all the early civilizations describe the pains concomitant with childbirth.

Early Chinese history records the use of opiates and soporific potions for relief of pain in childbirth.

From the Egyptian Polydamna, wife of Thor, Helen of Troy is said to have learned how to prepare herbal remedies that banished sorrow from the memory. When the hero Rustam, son of Zal and Rudabah, was being born, an eagle soared round the bed of the lying-in woman and dropped a remedy that made it possible for the babe to come out of his mother's body painlessly.

The fulfillment of the Biblical prophetic curse—"In sorrow shalt thou bring forth"—was described in many of the books of the Old Testament during the 4,000 years of recorded Hebrew history before Christ.

King David, who had several wives and numerous concubines, probably spoke with authority when he wrote in Psalm 48: 6, "Fear took hold upon them there, *and* pain, as of a woman in travail." The prophet Isaiah, in the thirteenth chapter of his writings, said, ". . . they shall be in pain as a woman that travaileth. . . ." Again, in Chapter 21 he graphically stated, "Therefore are my loins filled with pain: pangs have taken hold upon me, as the pangs of a woman that travaileth: I was bowed down at the hearing *of it;* I was dismayed at the seeing *of it.*"

The prophet Jeremiah has written more on the subject of the pains of childbirth than any other early writer. A few of his descriptions follow:

> For I have heard a voice as of a woman in travail, *and* the anguish as of her that bringeth forth her first child, the voice of the daughter of Zion, *that* bewaileth herself, *that* spreadeth her hands, *saying,* Woe *is* me now. . . . (4:31)
>
> . . . our hands wax feeble: anguish hath take hold of us, *and* pain, as of a woman in travail. (6:24)
>
> . . . shall not sorrows take thee, as a woman in travail? (13:21)
>
> . . . wherefore do I see every man with his hands on his loins, as a woman in travail, and all faces are turned into paleness? (30:6)
>
> . . . the mighty men's hearts in Moab at that day shall be as the heart of a woman in her pangs. (48:41)
>
> . . . anguish and sorrows have taken her, as a woman in travail. (49:24)
>
> The king of Babylon hath heard the report of them, and his hands waxed feeble: anguish took hold of him, *and* pangs as of a woman in travail. (50:43)

The Greek goddess Actemia, terrified by her mother's suffering at her own birth, besought from Zeus the favor of eternal virginity. Subsequently, she seduced Endymion and was punished for

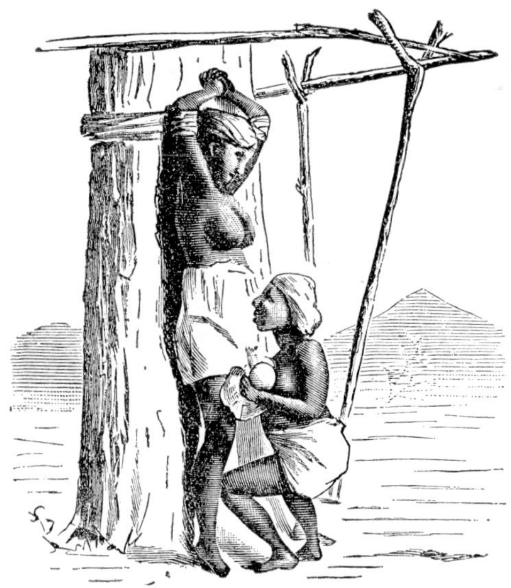

Fig. 15. A woman of the Serang Islands delivering while standing erect. (Ploss & Bartels: Das Weib in der Natur- und Völkerkunde, Leipzig, Th. Grieben's Verlag)

her early prudery by a truly godlike superfecundation; she became the mother of 50 daughters all at one time.

According to Sir James Simpson:

> The ancients appear also to have attempted to relieve the pain attendant upon parturition by anesthetizing agents, as we may learn from the various Greek writers. Such a practice is mentioned by Platus in his *Ophelion* and I may also quote the following passage. Theocritus says, "For then the daughter of Antigone, weighed down with throes, called out for Lucina, the friend of women in travail, and she with kind favour stood by her, and in sooth poured down her whole limbs an insensibility to pain, and so a lively boy, like to his father, was born.

The early civilizations devised various mechanical torture devices to be used as aids in bring on childbirth. Women in the Serang Islands were delivered while standing erect, bound to a tree, with their arms together above their heads. The Apache Indian squaws sometimes were delivered suspended from a tree by a rope under the armpits. The strong braves of the tribe would grasp the parturient above the fundus of the uterus and would swing all their weight against it.

Women in some Asiatic tribes had a practice of kneeling in labor with one or more assistants standing on their shoulders. From this position they would try to pull themselves into a standing one by grasping a pole.

In the Pago Pago Island, of the Samoa group in the Pacific, where the tribal civilization is older than the European, for generations women in labor have been treated with pressure anesthesia. These women kneel in labor, and during each uterine contraction the strong man of the tribe sits behind them and presses his heels into their short ribs. These natives are convinced that such pressure lessens their pain.

(It is interesting to note that the area selected for pressure anesthesia is the identical one which Cleland, in 1926, found to be the pathway of uterine pain as it entered the cord in the eleventh and the twelfth thoracic segments.)

Black were the moments in the civilization of mankind when, in many parts of the world, men of great weight would jump up and down upon the abdomen of a woman in labor to hasten the childbirth.

Figure 16 illustrates two of the barbaric practices imposed upon women in labor.

The apostle Paul used a striking metaphor with reference to the better world for which the people were striving when he said in Romans 8:22, "For we know that the whole creation groaneth and travaileth in pain together until now."

The Romans of Paul's day, as with the rest of the world, did nothing to relieve the sufferings of childbirth from which Paul drew his comparison.

The Dark Ages, which followed the fall of Rome, not only provided no relief for the travail of childbirth but also established a tradition of "hands off" for the medical profession that precluded attempts at giving relief. The care of woman in labor was left to ignorant midwives.

The Renaissance of Western Civilization brought no relief from the sufferings of the superstitious Middle Ages for women in labor. As late as 1591, Enfame Macalyane was burned at the stake by the ecclesiastics in Edinburgh for attempting to assuage the pangs of labor.

In the records of the trials of the sixteenth century, we find many cases in which witches were prosecuted for attempting to abolish the pains of labor by charms and other means. One method that was practiced was to hold a sword before the patient, who was directed to look at it steadily, in the same way that Latina is said to have held a palm branch and brought forth Apollo without suffering. In reality, this was a form of mesmerism. Another way employed was to hang the husband by his feet in the next room until the labor was accomplished.

America produced one of the first physicians to challenge the reign of the midwives, by offering a prescription for relieving painful childbirth. It is set forth in a manuscript of Zerubbabel Endecott, of Salem, Mass. Zerubbabel was a son of Governor Endecott by his second wife, but the records provide little information as to his life other than that he was a physician, that he served on an occasional jury and that he was fined, in

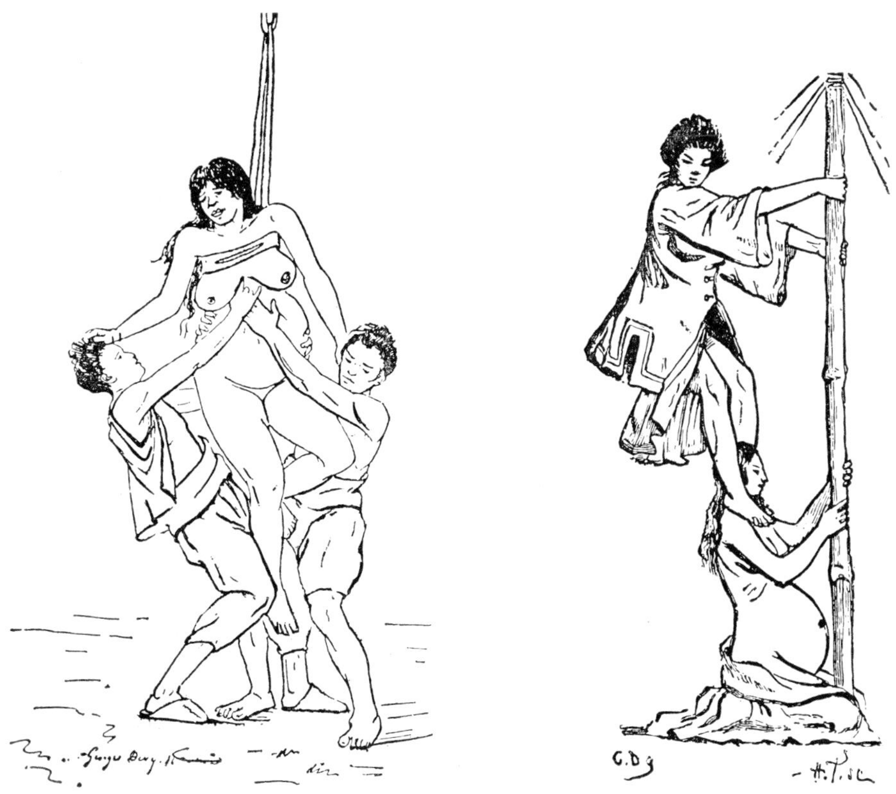

FIG. 16. (*Left*) Delivery of a Siamese woman. (*Right*) The Kalmuks hasten labor. (After Witlowski)

1659, by the Quarterly Court, for excessive drinking. Endecott's prescription is given here in full:

> For Sharpe and Difficult Travel in Women with child Take a Lock of Vergins haire on any Part of ye head, of half the Age of ye Woman in travill. Cut it very smale to fine Powder then take 12 Ants Eggs dried in an oven after ye bread is drawne or other wise make them dry and make them to powder with the haire, give this with a quarter of a pint of Red Cows milk or for want of it give it in strong ale wort.

In France, there are recorded instances of painless childbirth during profound intoxication that was not induced for this purpose. One such case occurred in a woman brought into the Hôtel Dieu of Paris, in 1818. Also, there is the celebrated case of the Comtesse de St. Geran, who was rendered insensible by a draught given to her by the midwife; she was delivered, and her child was abducted before she regained consciousness.

These are those rare exceptions when a woman has delivered without "feeling" what always has been her heritage—pain. The Black Hole of Calcutta was no more horrible in the history of mankind than have been some of the abuses of womanhood in her hour of travail. The forgotten woman in the history of civilization has been the woman enduring the most intense of all human sufferings—the pain of childbirth.

It was not until the eighteenth century that midwives began to be replaced by physicians, a process that was accelerated by the establishment of chairs of midwifery in the European universities, led by Edinburgh in 1726.

The primary objective of all of this effort was the humanitarian desire to relieve pain. Such an aim becomes evident in the thinking of a society only when human life becomes of value and in obstetrics when the status of women begins to improve. Today, when anesthesia is accepted as a matter of course, how many of us give thought to obstetrics of a hundred years ago? Can we picture the scenes of operative deliveries in those days?

It would be easy to recount the hideous suffering endured in those seemingly far-off days, for there is vast material to choose from. Kerr and Moir present two extracts from accounts of actual episodes that took place in preanesthesia days.

The first is from a letter addressed to Simpson; it was written by a doctor who himself had submitted to a major operation.

> Suffering so great as I underwent cannot be expressed in words, and thus fortunately cannot be recalled. The particular pangs are now forgotten; but the black whirlwind of emotion, the horror of great darkness and the sense of desertion by God and man, bordering close upon despair, which swept through my mind and overwhelmed my heart, I can never forget, however gladly I would do so. . . . I watched all that the surgeons did with a fascinated intensity. I still recall with unwelcome vividness the spreading out of the instruments; the twisting of the tourniquet; the first incision; the fingering of the sawed bone; the sponge pressed on the flap; the tying of the blood vessels; the stitching of the skin; and the bloody dismembered limb lying on the floor.
>
> Before the days of anesthetics, a patient preparing for an operation was like a condemned criminal preparing for execution. He counted the days till the appointed day came. He listened for the echo on the street of the surgeon's carriage. He watched for his pull at the doorbell; for his foot on the stair; for his step in the room; for the production of his dreaded instruments; for his few grave words, and his last preparations before beginning. And then he surrendered his liberty, and revolting at the necessity, submitted to be held or bound, and helplessly gave himself up to the cruel knife.

The other is from that gem of medical reminiscence, *Rab and His Friends,* by Dr. John Brown.* It refers to an operation by James Syme, in the Minto House

* Brown, John: Rab and His Friends, Boston, Page.

Hospital, on Ailie, the wife of James, a carter, who had a breast removed for a malignant tumor.

Next day, my master, the surgeon, examined Ailie. There was no doubt it must kill her, and soon. It could be removed—it might never return—it would give her speedy relief—she should have it done. She curtsied, looking at James, and said, "When?" "Tomorrow," said the kind surgeon, a man of few words. She and James and Rab and I retired. I noticed that he and she spoke little, but seemed to anticipate everything in each other. The following day, at noon, the students came in, hurrying up the great stair. At the first landing-place, on a small well-known blackboard, was a bit of paper fastened by wafers, and many remains of old wafers beside it. On the paper were the words, "An operation today. J. B., Clerk."

Up ran the youths, eager to secure good places: in they crowded, full of interest and talk. "What's the case?" "Which side is it?"

Don't think them heartless; they are neither better nor worse than you or I: they get over their professional horrors, and into their proper work; and in them pity—as an emotion, ending in itself or at best in tears and a long-drawn breath lessens, while pity as a motive, is quickened, and gains power and purpose. It is well for poor human nature that it is so.

The operating theatre is crowded; much talk and fun, and all the cordiality and stir of youth. The surgeon with his staff of assistants is there. In comes Ailie: one look at her quiets and abates the eager students. That beautiful old woman is too much for them; they sit down, and are dumb, and gaze at her. These rough boys feel the power of her presence. She walks in quickly, but without haste; dressed in her mutch, her neckerchief, her white dimity shortgown, her black bombazeen petticoat, showing her white worsted stockings and her carpet-shoes . . .

Ailie stepped up on a seat, and laid herself on the table, as her friend the surgeon told her; arranged herself, gave a rapid look at James, shut her eyes, rested herself on me, and took my hand. The operation was at once begun; it was necessarily slow; and chloroform—one of God's best gifts to his suffering children—was then unknown. The surgeon did his work. The pale face showed its pain, but was still and silent . . .

It is over: she is dressed, steps gently and decently down from the table, looks for James; then, turning to the surgeon and the students, she curtsies—and in a low, clear voice, begs their pardon if she has behaved ill. The students—all of us—wept like children; the surgeon helped her up carefully—and, resting on James and me, Ailie went to her room, Rab following.

In Philadelphia, in 1804, 7 years before Sir James Simpson, of Edinburgh, was born, Peter Miller wrote a thesis as a requirement toward his doctorate to an examining board of University clergy entitled *The Means of Lessening the Pains of Parturition.* After quoting the authorities of his day who described the necessity of obstetric pain, Dr. Miller proposed that women be relieved by one of the three following methods:

1. The use of nauseating emetics to distract a woman in labor. Thus, the spasmodic contractions of the diaphragm were used to propel and hasten delivery as described by the ancient medical axiom: "a sick labor is a rapid one."
2. Vigorous exercise and semistarvation to simulate the living conditions of certain tribes of primitive people, such as the Congo native or the early American Indian, who had been reported as having rapid and almost painless labors.
3. Phlebotomy of 400 to 800 cc. of blood during labor as a means of relieving pelvic congestion and of producing relaxation of the perineum. An added advantage, said Dr. Miller, is that bloodletting in labor reduces blood loss after delivery of the placenta.

No greater boon has ever come to mankind than the power to induce a temporary but complete insensibility to pain. So far as surgery is concerned, the means of inducing anesthesia are highly developed and extremely effective. Our goal in obstetrics should be to provide safely for the parturient during labor and delivery and without harm to the child, the comparable freedom from pain that is now enjoyed by the patient undergoing surgery. In appraising the following account of some of the at-

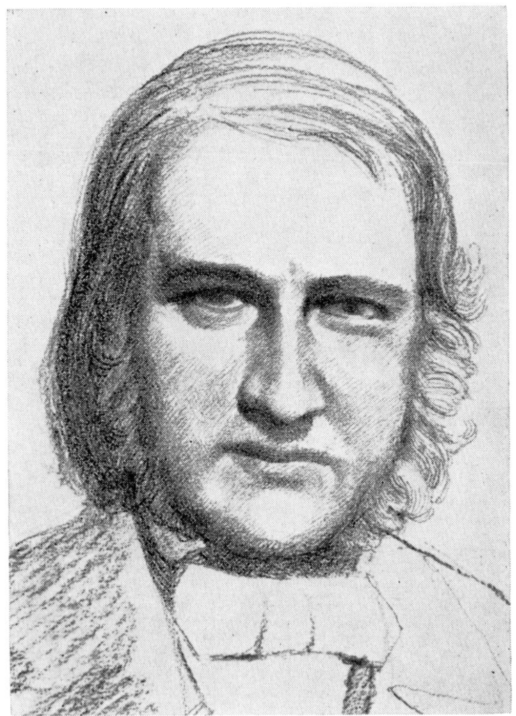

Fig. 17. Sir James Y. Simpson (1811-1870), Scottish contemporary of Snow and Channing, who did much toward the acceptance of anesthesia in obstetrics. (Sharp & Dohme: Seminar, Vol. 17, No. 1, p. 4)

tempts made to achieve this goal one must bear in mind:

1. The difficulty of finding a brain-drugging agent powerful enough to narcotize the mother while not endangering the more delicate baby;

2. The relatively short space of time that has elapsed since the nerve supply of the uterus was understood, thus permitting the scientific use of regional anesthesia.

CHILDBIRTH AFTER ANESTHESIA

The Encephalic Approach

General Anesthesia

It was not by chance but by years of effort that Dr. James Y. Simpson was able to overcome the worst pains of labor and delivery by general anesthesia. Graduated from Edinburgh, in 1832, with the avowed purpose of finding a means of relieving the sufferings of women in labor, he had risen to occupy the chair of midwifery and had tested various agents, including ether, before he eagerly followed up Bell and Florens' reports of success in animal experimentation using chloroform with an immediate trial of this fluid on human beings. Dr. Simpson first tried the new drug with his assistants, Duncan and Keith, Mrs. Simpson, her niece and a friend of the family. The effect of chloroform inhalations upon these voluntary participants of that famous experiment on Nov. 4, 1847, convinced Dr. Simpson that "this is far stronger and better than ether." Six days later he reported to the Edinburgh Medical-Chirurgical Society the use of chloroform in 30 painless deliveries. Very soon the physician who had discovered the means of conquering the horrible pains of childbirth was defamed by the Scottish Calvinists as a blasphemer, heretic and agent of the devil. The clergy sent a circular to the physicians of the town containing these words: "To all seeming, Satan wishes to help suffering women but the upshot will be the collapse of society, for the Fear of the Lord, which depends upon the petitions of the afflicted, will be destroyed. For tens of thousands of years births have taken place without any means of allaying pain. Has not Nature disclosed the wisdom of God in her conduct of the process of birth?" The ministers read from the pulpit Genesis 3:16: ". . . in sorrow thou shalt bring forth children." Simpson, who was also a student of the Bible, quoted Genesis 2: 21: "And the Lord God caused a deep sleep to fall upon Adam, and he slept: and he took one of his ribs, and closed up the flesh instead thereof." "What

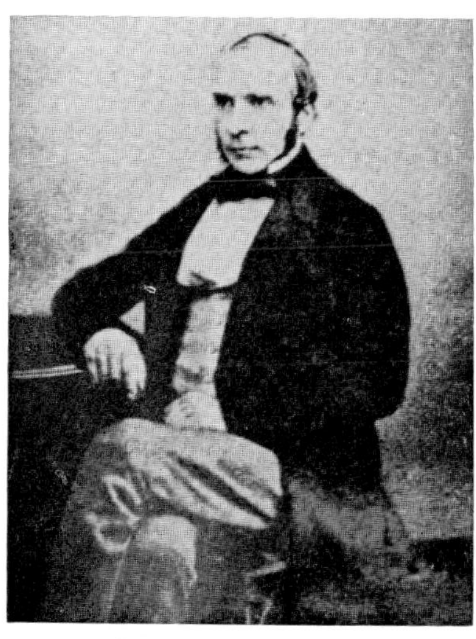

Fig. 18. Dr. John Snow, one of the earliest English anesthetists, who administered chloroform analgesia to Queen Victoria.

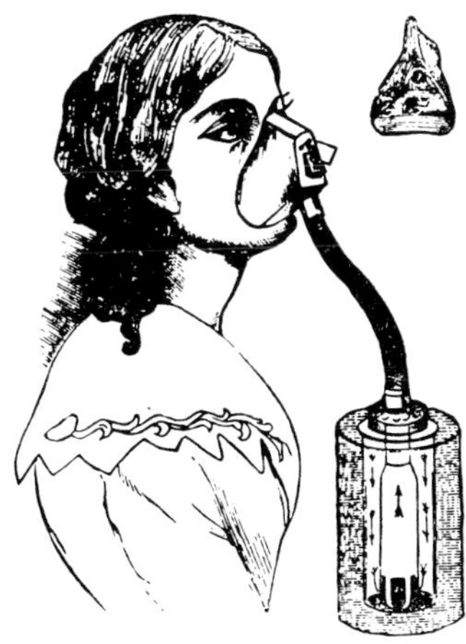

Fig. 19. Snow's inhaler.

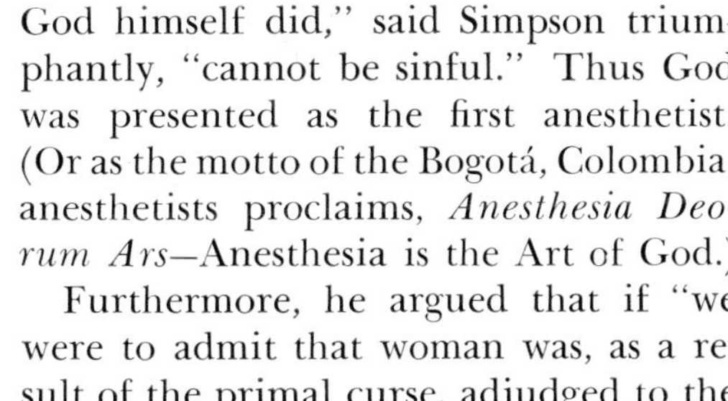

God himself did," said Simpson triumphantly, "cannot be sinful." Thus God was presented as the first anesthetist. (Or as the motto of the Bogotá, Colombia, anesthetists proclaims, *Anesthesia Deorum Ars*—Anesthesia is the Art of God.)

Furthermore, he argued that if "we were to admit that woman was, as a result of the primal curse, adjudged to the miseries of pure physical pain and agony in parturition, still, certainly under the Christian dispensation, the moral necessity of undergoing such anguish has ceased and terminated."

On April 19, 1853, Simpson received a letter from Queen Victoria's obstetrician, Sir James Clark, which read in part:

> I am almost forgetting to notice the chief object of my writing to you, which was to tell you that the Queen had chloroform exhibited to her during her late confinement. . . . It acted admirably. It was not at any time given so strongly as to render the Queen insensible, and an ounce of chloroform was scarcely consumed during the whole time. Her Majesty was greatly pleased with the effect and she certainly never has had a better recovery. . . . I know this information will please you, and I have little doubt it will lead to a more general use of chloroform in midwifery practice in this quarter than has hitherto prevailed.

This use of chloroform was during the

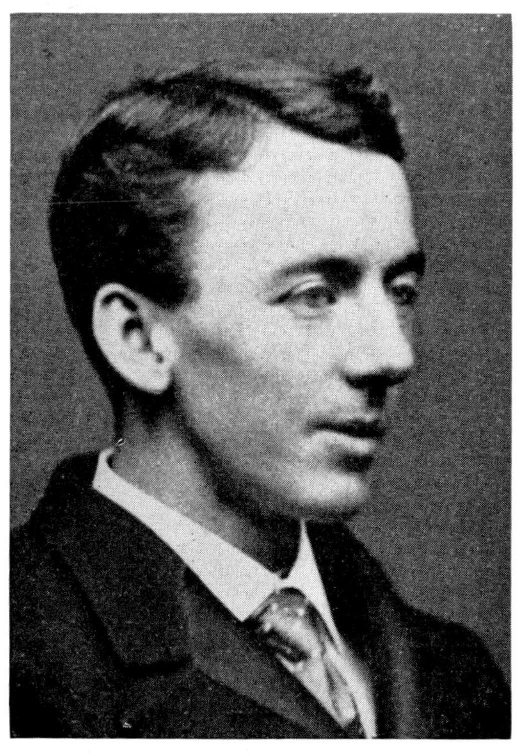

Fig. 20. Walter Channing (1786-1876), Boston physician, who pioneered in the use of anesthesia in obstetrics in America. (Sharp & Dohme: Seminar, Vol. 17, No. 1, p. 4)

birth of the Queen's eighth child, Prince Leopold. John Snow, the first physician to devote his full time to anesthesia, administered the drug.

Since the time of Simpson, every new remedy that has been introduced to relieve the pains of childbirth has been criticized by both the profession and the laity and, more especially, by the ecclesiastics.

In the 3 decades following, the use of chloroform analgesia became one of the most important possessions of medicine throughout the world, but this is now considered to be too powerful a drug for common use.

Nitrous Oxide

In 1880, Klikowitsch, of St. Petersburg, Russia, applied nitrous oxide and oxygen inhalation analgesia to 25 obstetric cases. He observed that 3 or 4 inhalations rendered the uterine contractions "painless" without clouding the consciousness. Dr. J. Clarence Webster, of Chicago, was one of the first in America to use nitrous oxide and oxygen in obstetric practice, in 1909. Since then it has achieved widespread popularity, although studies by Eastman have shown the danger of asphyxia neonatorum if the anesthetic is not given correctly. Courville has proved that such asphyxia may cause irreparable damage to the higher centers of the baby's brain. However, this method has proved its worth, and nitrous oxide is used in some combination in almost one half of present-day deliveries.

Trichloroethylene

Trichloroethylene, first described in 1864 by Emil Fischer, was developed as an anesthetic by Lehmann in the laboratory. Jackson, of Cincinnati, in 1933, studied it as an anesthetic in dogs. His colleague, Striker, introduced it in clinical anesthesia in the same year. But it was not until 1941 that Langston Hewer, of England, because of its nonflammability, low cost and high analgesic efficiency, was able to reintroduce it on the battlefield in World War II. From these beginnings, it was first accepted in surgery and later more widely in obstetrics, first in Britain and Canada and recently in some parts of the United States.

Twilight Sleep

Twilight sleep, from the German word *Dämmerschlaf,* was a term used by Carl Gauss, of Freiburg, in his report, *Geburten in künstliche Dämmerschlaf,* published in 1906, to describe that "state of clouded consciousness" induced by the use of scopolamine-morphine.

The combination of scopolamine and morphine had been in use in surgery for some time, and, in 1903, the obstetrician von Steinbüchel, of Graz, used it in obstetric cases. Subsequent experiments with it were carried on in a number of clinics without notable success, until, in 1905, Bernhard Krönig and Carl Gauss began large-scale experiments with the drug combination at the Frauenklinik of the State University of Freiberg with the hope of working out a fixed dosage, so that all the delicate adjustments could be dispensed with. However, it was soon clear that no routine method could be developed. "If you could trust to having an average woman," Gauss said, "you could use an average dose; but the dose is easier to standardize than the woman."

Following publication of the 1906 report, experiments with scopolamine-morphine were widely undertaken. The Berlin Charité sent Hocheisen to Freiburg to study the method. Returning to his hospital, he made numerous experiments and at a meeting of the Society for Obstetric Practice and Gynecology, in Berlin, reported on 100 cases. He found that "the expulsion period averaged 6 hours and 15 minutes against the normal 1 hour and 45 minutes," and he concluded that "Scopolamine causes protraction of birth and protraction of birth causes asphyxia." As the Berlin Charité stood high in the medical world, this report received wide attention and had a profound effect on the profession.

In turn, Gauss pointed out several deviations in Hocheisen's method from his own. He said he could take no responsibility when his directions were not followed. And Preller, of the Mannheim Klinik, affirmed that "only by systematically following Gauss's directions can a correct *Dämmerschlaf* be obtained."

Even in the hands of skillful practitioners of the Freiburg method the treatment was by no means sure. An analysis of Gauss's report on 3,000 cases treated at the Frauenklinik up to 1911 shows an important relationship between the degree of care obtained and the effectiveness of twilight sleep. Eighty-two per cent of the patients in well-furnished rooms experienced perfect twilight sleep, as against 56 per cent of the patients in open wards. Thus, in the conditions obtaining at the Freiburg clinic, only 2 in 3 who received morphine-scopolamine were blessed with "painless" delivery.

In 1918, the use of the famous *Dämmerschlaf* was discovered by the lay press. Within a few months babies by "twilight" became a fad, and the relief of pain during labor became one of the chief problems of the average physician practicing obstetrics. William H. Knipe, in 1914, was the first to report on a relatively large number of cases so managed in this country.

Broadhead, of the Harlem and Postgraduate Hospitals in New York, Hellman, Beach, Rongy and Livingston were American obstetricians who first used this method and modifications of it.

Jaeger was the first to use Pantopon alone and in combination with scopolamine in obstetrics. The method has fallen into disrepute because of the high incidence of asphyxia (or apnea) in the newborn.

The Introduction of Demerol

In 1938, Benthin, of Germany, introduced into obstetrics the use of Demerol, a synthetic substitute for morphine. Immediately, it was determined from its use that a high grade of analgesia at the thalamic level was produced with a much smaller incidence of fetal and respiratory depression than that seen with morphine or the other opium derivatives. This work was confirmed by de Senarclens, of Switzerland, Gilbert and Dixon, of Baltimore, and Irving, of Boston. The impetus of Irving's thorough evaluation and enthusiastic reports from the Boston Lying-in Hospital rapidly developed this agent as an analgesic of the first magnitude in most of the obstetric clinics in the United States.

Development of the Barbiturates

In 1902 Emil Fischer, of Berlin, one of the greatest physiologic chemists of all time, synthesized barbital (Veronal), the first of the barbiturates. In 1921 Hamblen and Hamlin, of Virginia, first reported the use of barbiturates in 50 cases. In 1923 Cleisz, a Frenchman, used barbital and allylisopropyl barbituric acid or Numal in obstetrics. During the next 2 decades, reports came from both European and American clinics concerning the use of a great variety of barbiturates in labor. Drabkin, Ravdin, Hirst, Lapham, McCallum, Mendenhall and Zerfas made early contributions to the knowledge relating to the use of these drugs.

As usual, the early opinions on the use of these drugs in obstetrics were controversial. The descriptive phrase, "the battle of the barbiturates," helps to describe some of the bitter feelings on this subject.

In January, 1933, Irving and his associates reported on a year's clinical research with a number of the more popular analgesic methods. They observed groups of cases under Sodium Amytal and scopolamine; Pantopon, magnesium sulfate and rectal ether; Pernocton; pentobarbital and scopolamine; Sodium Amytal and rectal ether; pentobarbital and rectal ether; pentobarbital and paraldehyde. The Pantopon and scopolamine series followed the technic of twilight sleep; the Pantopon, magnesium sulfate and rectal ether series followed Gwathmey's synergistic analgesia. He found that apnea occurred in from 35 to 67 per cent of the babies, depending upon the drugs used, as compared with 2 per cent for a series with no analgesic drugs. He concluded that Nembutal with scopolamine was the most effective method.

Charles Hunt in a survey of opinions of 80 obstetricians in every state in the Union found that 87 per cent of them were using some form of barbiturates in various combinations. Later, Ralph Waters measured the volume of gases respired by the mother after barbiturates and found that as little as 4.5 gr. lowered the respiratory exchange by 23 per cent, indicating danger of anoxia to the baby in the absence of clinically observable effects on the mother.

Hellman, at Johns Hopkins University, in 1946, reported the use of Sodium Pentothal in 3,000 deliveries. Bryce-Smith and Hingson, in 1954, reported the use of intravenous and intramuscular Seconal Sodium in 2,500 obstetric deliveries. Milton Lewis, of Nashville, has reported the use of oral and intravenous Delvinal Sodium in a large successful series for labor and delivery. Rucker, in Virginia, Calvo, in Bogotá, Colombia, Dipple, of Texas, and Gustavson, of Indiana, also have championed the use of intravenous Sodium Pentothal for labor and delivery. Lundy and Hunt, at the Mayo Clinic, have combined local block with intravenous Sodium Pentothal anesthesia in cesarean section. Nearly all the investigators on the subject have concluded that the use of the barbiturates is favorably supplemented by the synergistic application of scopolamine or one of the opiates.

Combinations of Anesthesia and Narcosis

After Gwathmey's experience during World War I, when he found that if ether was administered into the alimentary tract, it exerted some analgesic and anesthetic effect, he devised the use of rectal ether in a vehicle of olive oil for pain relief during labor and delivery. His method was supplemented by the addition of quinine to the ether–olive oil mixture for rectal instillation and by intramuscular injection of morphine and magnesium sulfate early in labor. In 1931 he presented convincing statistics on the use of this method of pain relief in 20,000 cases. He proposed that this method had factors of safety for both home and hospital deliveries not obtained with the other general anesthetics. Since that time the method has been used widely in hospitals throughout the country and has been modified by various investigators. The most popular modification was that of McCormick, who substituted the use of barbiturates by mouth for the intramuscular injection of morphine and magnesium sulfate. McCormick also devised an instrument that has worked satisfactorily for the rectal instillation of the mixture. Irving, Berman and Nelson condemned combinations of rectal ether with hypnotic drugs because of the high incidence of apnea of the baby and the necessity for constant supervision of the mother, and Drane found the incidence of apnea to vary from 15 to 47 per cent.

In 1926 Willstätter and Duisberg introduced a type of basic anesthesia with the rectal instillation of minute quantities of tribromethyl alcohol (Avertin). Parsons, Straub, Raginsky and Bourne have contributed valuable pharmacologic data supplementing the work of the originators in the use of this method in obstetrics. Their method of pain relief in labor enjoyed a temporary wave of enthusiastic approval but now is almost entirely abandoned in obstetrics because of the mounting death rate from its use.

In America, one of the most popular methods of producing obstetric amnesia has been the oral and the rectal administration of paraldehyde. This drug was introduced by Cervello in 1882. Its use has been championed by Kane and others, who reported large series of cases so managed with relative safety for the mother and with a very good degree of amnesia produced. Nevertheless, the depressing effects of this drug on the vital mechanism of the fetus have been reviewed critically by the medical profession. Ralph Waters concluded that opiates, barbiturates and other nonvolatile drugs, as well as inhalation agents in sufficient dosage, all cause depression of the respiratory center of both mother and child; and with the increase in pain relief there is a decrease in safety.

ANATOMIC APPROACH TO THE CONTROL OF PAIN

The year 1901 will be remembered as the beginning of the use of conduction anesthesia in obstetrics. In this year Kreis, of Germany, first used spinal anesthesia for operative delivery. In this same year the French urologist, Cathelin, instituted into clinical practice the technic of caudal analgesia, which he had discovered independently with M. A. Sicard, of Paris.

Even though Cathelin was not an obstetrician, he envisioned the use of caudal analgesia in obstetrics. He included the following prophecy in his first scientific paper on the subject.

> En somme, l'injection épidurale et la pénétration par le canal sacré constituent une méthode nouvelle qui mérite d'être étudiée par les chirurgiens et par les médecins, comme procédé d'analgésie opératoire ou simplement comme procédé pour calmer les douleurs (accouchement douloureux, douleurs de cancers inopérables).

Caudal Anesthesia (Single Injection)

In 1909, von Stoeckel, of Marburg, Germany, was the first to apply Cathelin's technics in obstetrics by injecting cocaine solutions in the peridural space, through the approach of the sacral hiatus. He blocked the painful impulses from the pelvic organs during labor and delivery. Even though he secured considerable relief for most of his 134 patients, he was able to record that only 9 patients in this series were completely relieved of all pain in delivery. He concluded erroneously that no pain came from the uterus itself but from pull on ligaments of the lumbar region and from the anterior abdominal wall. Except for the small series of deliveries conducted by Kreis, of Germany, in 1901 with spinal anesthesia, this was the first attempt to relieve the pains of labor by the anatomic approach. Schlimpert, Läwen and von Gaza continued the application of caudal analgesia to obstetrics. Schlimpert made sure of reaching all pain-carrying nerves by a block to the costal margin. By 1920, Erwin Zwiefel had collected 4,000 cases of caudal block from the literature. In America the technic was used successfully for obstetrics by Meeker and Bonar in 1923. Oldham reported his series in 1925, Lundy in 1928, Henry and Jaur in 1929, Rucker in 1930, Campbell in 1935, Johnson in 1936. In 1939 Baptisti reported the successful use of caudal analgesia in 200 obstetric cases. Hopp reported the use of 2 caudal injections in 3 obstetric cases in 1941. Lahmann and Mietus, in January, 1942, reported 400 obstetric cases in which caudal analgesia was used for delivery. Robert M. Mitchell was the silent collaborator in this study.

In 1933, John G. P. Cleland reported his experiences with the use of paravertebral block and low caudal analgesia to control the pains of both labor and delivery. Cleland began his studies on the neurology of the uterus at McGill University in 1927. He was the first to identify the pathway of uterine pain. Thus, upon his work is based the logical, accurate application of conduction anesthesia to obstetrics.

In 1935, Graffagnino, of New Orleans, first reported the use of epidural anesthesia in obstetrics, through a modification of the original technic of Pagés, of Spain, and Dogliotti, of Italy.

Spinal Anesthesia

In 1928 George Pitkin introduced the use of hyperbaric spinal anesthesia for obstetric delivery. He called his method "controllable spinal anesthesia in obstetrics."

From 1927 until the present, S. A. Cosgrove, of the Margaret Hague Maternity Hospital in the Jersey City Medical Center, has been the leading proponent of spinal anesthesia in obstetrics. His series includes more than 10,000 cases, in which he has pointed out the accrued benefits of this method of management for the handicapped patient during terminal labor and also for delivery. Masson and Randall, of the Mayo Clinic, have found spinal anesthesia satisfactory for cesarean section.

Continuous Spinal Anesthesia

Lull and Ullery used the safety mechanism of Lemmon's continuous spinal anesthesia in over 1,000 consecutive cesarean sections without maternal mortality. Since 1940 the authors have used this technic in more than 2,000 cesarean sections without mortality at operation or within the first week postpartum. There can be no question but that spinal anesthesia, in safe adequate doses, produces total relief from pain in the terminal part of labor. In small doses the anesthetic may have no influence on uterine contractions, but doses sufficient to produce complete anesthesia of the abdomen usually diminish and, frequently for a time, suppress contractions. The total paralysis of the abdominal muscles is responsible for failure of the fetus to advance through the birth canal.

Saddle-Block Spinal Anesthesia

In 1946, Adriani and Parmley and Roman-Vega modified and improved Pitkin's method of saddle-block spinal anesthesia in obstetrics with hyperbaric Nupercaine. This method and modifications of it, because of its simplicity and relative safety, now are utilized in more than half the obstetric clinics in the United States as the indicated method in at least one fifth of the nation's deliveries.

Continuous Regional Anesthesia

In 1931, Eugene Aburel, of Rumania, reported to the Société d'Obstétrique et de Gynécologie de Paris his technic of continuous (protracted) local anesthesia in obstetrics. He inserted a 14-cm. needle to the left of the lumbar vertebral column just anterior to the lumbo-aortic nerve plexus. Through this needle he introduced a fine elastic silk catheter, which remained in place after the withdrawal of the needle. Through this catheter he made serial injections of

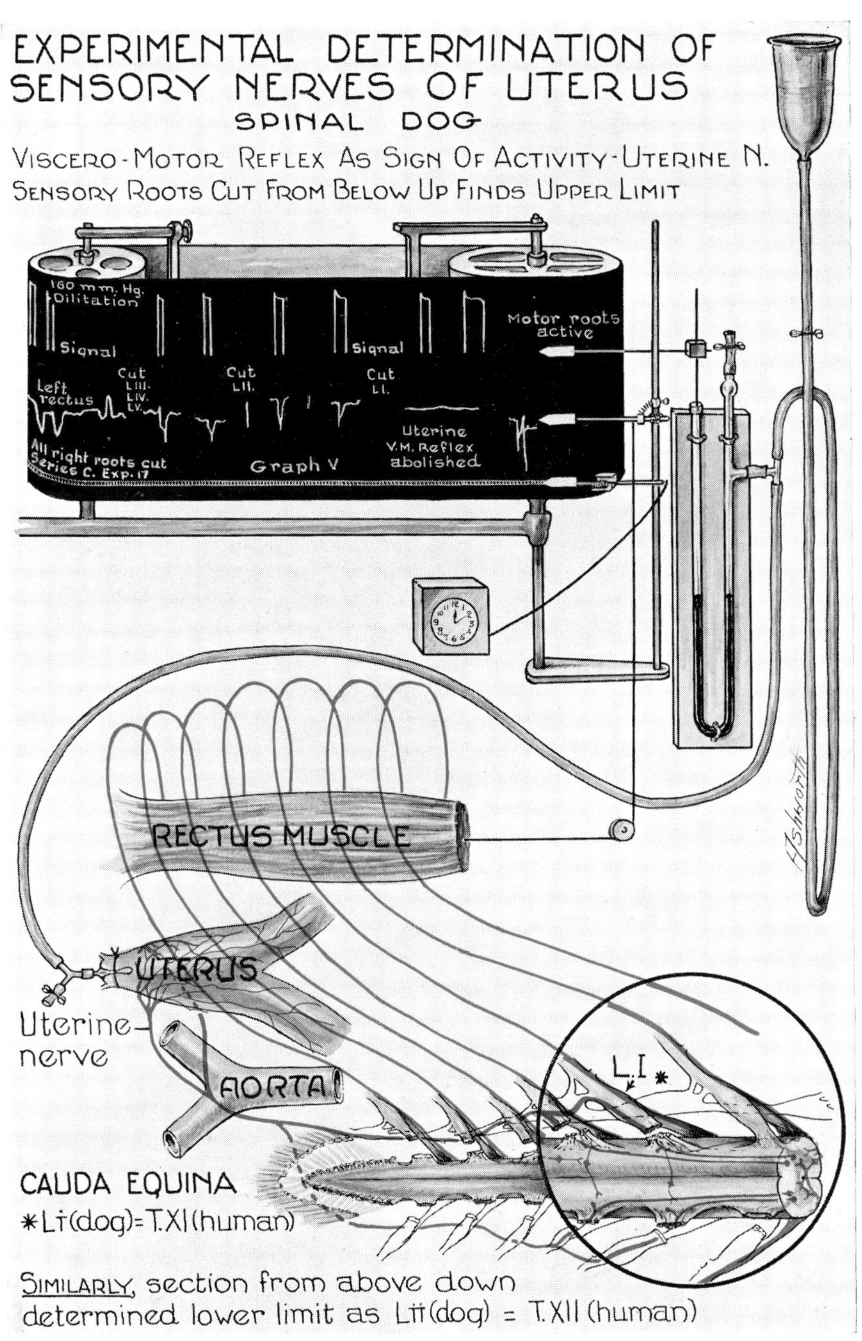

PLATE 18. Sensory nerves of uterus are shown in red. Motor nerves of rectus are shown in blue. (From John G. P. Cleland, M.D.)

0.005 per cent Percaine to control the pain of uterine contraction for the duration of travail. Thus, he antedated Lemmon and Hingson and Edwards in the use of a continuous device for prolonged anesthesia.

Continuous Caudal Analgesia

In 1940, Hingson and Edwards began the use of sacral caudal block for obstetric delivery in the Staten Island Marine Hospital. After first using epidural lumbar anesthesia, advocated on the European continent by Dogliotti and in America by Graffagnino, they abandoned this method temporarily because of its potential hazard of massive spinal anesthesia from injecting a solution in such close proximity to the subarachnoid space. Because of Hingson's familiarity with the continous spinal anesthesia of Lemmon and Paschal, with Southworth he applied continuous caudal analgesia in surgery in 1941, and with Edwards he first applied it in obstetrics on January 6, 1942. Since that time, more than 3 million babies have been delivered with this technic, effecting a startling reduction in infant mortality and stimulating the entire medical profession to re-evaluate all methods of pain relief in labor.

Low Dose Spinal Analgesia

During the period between 1940 and 1944, Hingson and the physicians of the Philadelphia Lying-in Hospital began the use of low dosage isobaric spinal anesthesia in obstetrics with Metycaine and procaine. This method, like the hyperbaric saddle-block technic, is now used widely in obstetric clinics.

In 1946, Curbello, of Cuba, and Hingson, Cleland, Flowers and Hellman independently introduced and adapted continuous peridural anesthesia for obstetric delivery and cesarean section by means of the polyethylene and divinyl plastic catheters. Cleland further refined this technic by using both continuous peridural and continuous caudal analgesia with the double catheter insertion.

Regional and Local Anesthesia

In developing perineal local, pudendal block and presacral anesthesia, the work of Greenhill, Benaron and Tucker during the period 1936 to 1950 is noteworthy.

Almost every drug that has been found to possess pain-relieving properties in any branch of the medical sciences has been used at one time or another in obstetrics. Many of the investigators with these drugs and methods, in discouraging the use of certain technics, have contributed as much to the safety of mother and baby as have the proponents of many of these measures in their efforts to relieve the suffering and distress of parturition. The fact that any patient undergoing obstetric management with amnesia, analgesia, and anesthesia should be surrounded by all the safeguards of a modern hospital with a trained personnel cannot be overlooked.

It would be a premature conclusion that the pains of labor and delivery can be controlled completely by the existing technics of present-day medicine. The day of the panacea is not yet in sight. However, tremendous strides have been made toward this end in the last 4 decades. The Old Testament curse of womankind may be repudiated some day in the New Testament prophecy from I Timothy 2:15: ". . . she shall be saved in childbearing, if they continue in faith and charity and holiness with sobriety."

"Divinum est opus sedare dolorem" (Divine is the work to subdue pain), said Hippocrates. This still is the challenge to the chemist, the pharmacologist, the obstetrician and the anesthetist, who are uniting their efforts toward the safe control of pain in childbirth.

3 Anatomic and Physiologic Considerations

NEUROPATHWAYS OF PARTURITION*

Control of pain during labor and delivery has become a major factor in obstetric practice. Thus it is necessary to have a full understanding of the topographic location and the specialized functions of the neuro-afferent pathways to all organs and structures involved in the birth act. Furthermore, the obstetrician is faced many times with a need to maintain the uterine activity or to plan a co-ordinated augmentation of the expulsive forces in which the striated abdominal and intercostal muscles are involved, including the diaphragm.

The periodic, rhythmically increasing and fading pain that occurs synchronously with the uterine contraction every 3 to 4 minutes in the average case lasts from 30 to 40 seconds, but in tumultuous labor it may occur every 1½ to 2 minutes, lasting from 40 to 80 seconds. In desultory labor the contractions occur every 6 to 10 minutes, with the pain lasting not more than 20 to 30 seconds. This pain has been found to be transmitted first over the sensory fibers from the corpus and the fundus of the uterus (blue solid lines in Plate 19) to the large circumcervical ganglionic network (Frankenhäuser), and thence over the hypogastric nerves and the lower aortic postganglionic sympathetic fibers to the paravertebral sympathetic chain at the level of the second and the third lumbar vertebrae. Continuing without synapse in a cephalic direction, these nerves transverse the gray rami of the eleventh and the twelfth thoracic and probably also the first lumbar nerve to enter the communicating system of these 3 dorsal root ganglia with the preganglionic afferent system in the lateral spinothalamic fasciculus of the spinal cord to the thalamic pain center and its cortical radiations. Whenever these pathways are interrupted by eleventh and twelfth paravertebral segmental block, by second and third lumbar sympathetic block, by low lumbar aortic plexus block, by peridural eleventh thoracic through first lumbar block, by ascending caudal block or by saddle spinal block anesthesia, the labor contraction pain is alleviated.

The second component of labor pain is the backache associated with cervical dilation. These stimuli are transmitted through the parasympathetic system of the second, the third and the fourth sacral nerves (blue dotted lines). The resulting sensation of sacral and sacroiliac pain has been interpreted as pain reflexes over the skin and fascia distribution of the somatic segmental branches of these nerves. Low saddle spinal, caudal or presacral block will relieve this pain.

The third component of childbirth pain is that transmitted from the stimulus of stretching the lower birth canal and the perineum. Pressure upon the bladder and the rectum through the pudendal nerve or its perineal and hemorrhoidal branches (see p. 76) may be involved also.

* This section, and the section on "Innervation of External Genitalia and Perineum," prepared by author (Hingson), which follows, are taken from pp. 104 and 105 of The Ciba Collection, Vol. 2, Ciba Pharmaceutical Products, Inc., Summit, N. J.

This pain can be relieved by pudendal and perineal nerve block, anesthetizing the nerves indicated in the picture by the broken lines. These blocks, of course, produce also a flaccid paralysis of the perineal musculature, which, however, greatly facilitates operative or obstetric maneuvers.

Correctly performed saddle spinal anesthesia produces a more or less complete analgesia from the perineum and the sacral plexus ascending to the tenth thoracic segment (see p. 55, *The Ciba Collection,* Vol. I). The more heavily myelinated nerves of the lower abdominal musculature and, depending on the position and its timing after injection of the anesthetic, the entire anterior roots continue to function and permit intentional co-operation of the individual by increasing the intra-abdominal pressure.

INNERVATION OF EXTERNAL GENITALIA AND PERINEUM

The musculature and the integument of the perineum are innervated mainly by the *pudendal nerve.* Derived from the anterior rami of the second, the third and the fourth sacral nerves, it leaves the pelvis through the greater sciatic foramen, between the piriformis and the coccygeus muscles, and crosses beneath the ischial spine on the mesial side of the internal pudendal artery. It then continues within Alcock's canal in the obturator fascia on the lateral wall of the ischiorectal fossa, toward the ischial tuberosity. The pudendal nerve divides into 3 branches: (1) The inferior hemorrhoidal nerve pierces the medial wall of Alcock's canal, traverses the ischiorectal fossa and supplies the external anal sphincter and perianal skin. (2) The *perineal nerve* runs for a short distance in Alcock's canal and divides into a deep and a superficial branch. The deep branch sends filaments to the external anal sphincter and the levator ani muscles and then pierces the base of the urogenital diaphragm to supply the superficial and the deep perineal muscles, the ischiocavernosus and the bulbocavernosus muscles and the membranous urethral sphincter. The superficial branch divides into medial and lateral posterior labial nerves, which innervate the labium majus. (3) The *dorsal nerve of the clitoris* passes through the urogenital diaphragm to the glans of the clitoris.

The following nerves contribute to the innervation of the perineal skin: The *anterior labial branches* of the *ilio-inguinal nerve* (L-1) emerge from the external inguinal ring to be distributed to the mons veneris and the upper portion of the labium majus. The *external spermatic branch* of the *genitofemoral nerve* (L-1, 2) accompanies the round ligament through the inguinal canal and sends twigs to the labium. The *perineal branches* of the *posterior femoral cutaneous nerve* (S-1, 2, 3) run forward and medialward in front of the ischial tuberosity to the lateral margin of the perineum and the labium majus. *Branches* of the *perineal nerve* (S-2, 3, 4) include the dorsal nerve of the clitoris and the medial and the lateral posterior labial branches to the labium majus. The *inferior hemorrhoidal branch* of the *pudendal nerve* (S-2, 3, 4) contributes to the supply of the perianal skin. The *perforating cutaneous* branches of the second and the third sacral *nerves* perforate the sacrotuberous ligament and turn around the inferior border of the gluteous maximum to supply the buttocks and the contiguous perineum. The *anococcygeal nerves* (S-4, 5 and coccygeal nerve) unite along the coccyx and then pierce the sacrotuberous ligaments to supply the anococcygeal area.

THE SENSORY INNERVATION OF THE UTERUS

A knowledge of the course of the sensory paths to the pelvic parts is a

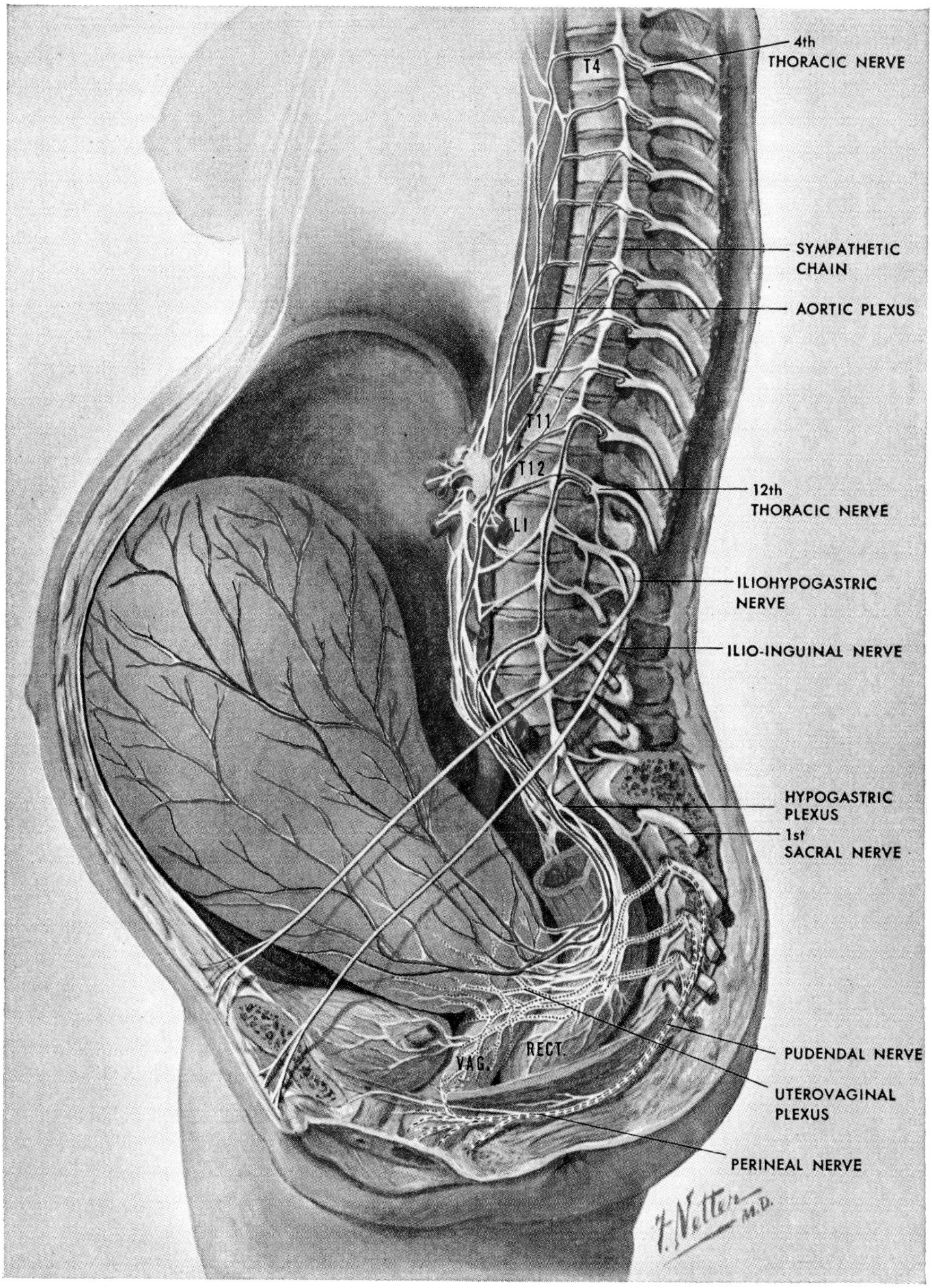

PLATE 19

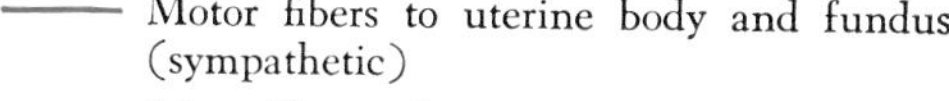

——— Motor fibers to uterine body and fundus (sympathetic)

········· Motor fibers to lower uterine segment, cervix and upper vagina (parasympathetic)

– – – – Motor fibers to lower vagina and perineum (somatic)

——— Sensory fibers from body and fundus of uterus (sympathetic)

········· Sensory fibers from cervix and upper vagina (parasympathetic)

– – – – Sensory fibers from lower vagina and perineum (somatic)

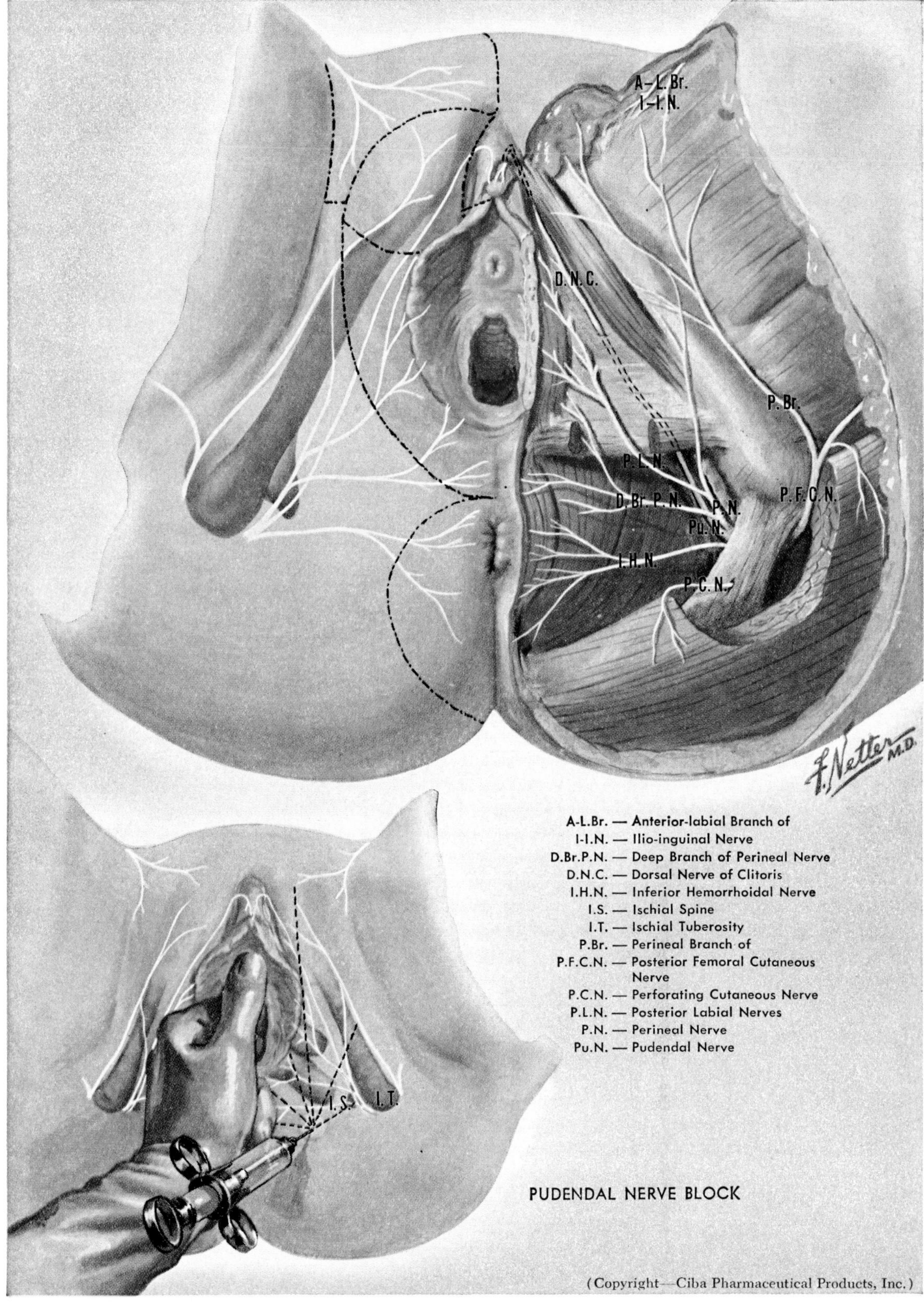

PUDENDAL NERVE BLOCK

prerequisite for understanding the principles that underlie the block of afferent impulses propagated from the contracting uterus during the first stage of labor and from those pelvic structures that are stretched as an incident to the expulsion of the child. *All* primary sensory nerve cells are located in the dorsal root ganglia (Plate 19). The latter are grayish swellings upon the dorsal roots of each of the successive spinal nerves. The nerve cell bodies of these ganglia are ovoid in shape. Each cell issues a single process that divides T-like to send one branch fiber distally through the spinal nerve to end in a sensory receptor, and another branch fiber centrally through the dorsal root into the spinal cord. The sensory ganglion cells vary in size and can be classified conveniently into categories of *large* and *small.* The diameter of the fiber of a dorsal root ganglion cell is roughly proportionate to the size of the cell body. Large dorsal root ganglion cells have wide diameter axons surrounded by thick myelin sheaths. Therefore, these cells provide the largest sensory fibers in the spinal nerves. The smallest ganglion cells have fine axons that are either thinly myelinated or nonmyelinated. Study of the rate of conduction of nerve impulses in nerves having a relatively pure content of sensory fibers indicates that the large myelinated fibers are the most rapidly conducting ones from (80 to 120 m. per second). The composite of sensory conducting units also contains a group of small, thinly myelinated fibers with a conduction rate of from 16 to 30 m. per second. The fibers of this group are from 2 to 6 microns in diameter, and their myelin sheaths are somewhat thinner than those of the smaller preganglionic, myelinated, efferent fibers described earlier. Finally, the sensory nerves contain a numerically large group of fibers that are of tiny size and do not have myelin sheaths. These conduct at the very slow rate of from 1/4 to 2 m. per second. These 3 groups, large, small and thinly myelinated and nonmyelinated, in addition to conducting at different rates, appear to serve the sense modalities differently. For example, pain, which is our chief concern at the moment, is carried both by the small, thinly myelinated fiber component and by the nonmyelinated component. Thus, one of the fiber components of the pain pathway in peripheral nerves is *relatively fast* and the other *slow*. Component fibers of both groups are distributed through the visceral as well as the somatic nerves.

The 3 groups of fibers also respond differently to conduction block caused by application of pressure and that caused by procaine. The inference from experimental work on procaine block is that the small fibers (associated with "pain" conduction) are blocked earlier than the larger ones concerned with conduction of "touch" and "pressure." In block by pressure, the large fibers associated with touch and pressure sensations are blocked more readily than the small ones associated with pain.

The aggregate of all sensory fibers proceeding centrally from the dorsal root ganglion form the dorsal root. Ranson has shown that as the dorsal root fibers break through the covering pia-glial membrane of the spinal cord at the cord's posterolateral sulcus, they aggregate into medial and lateral root divisions which may be identified histologically by the sizes of the nerve root fibers that they contain. The medial division is composed of large, myelinated fibers (therefore, fast-conducting); the lateral division has small thinly myelinated and nonmyelinated fibers. Ranson has shown also that section of the lateral division of a dorsal root experimentally abolishes reflexes that in man are associated with the experience of pain. The axons of the pain pathway through the lateral division of the dorsal root terminate almost immediately in the substantia gelatinosa which forms the cap of the gray matter of the dorsal column of the spinal cord. Here they form synaptic relations with the cells of origin of the spinothalamic neuron, the axons of which cross the mid-line of the spinal cord and ascend to the ventral nuclei of the thalamus. Thus, nervous activity initiated in the uterus as a result of its physiologic contractions during the first stage of labor, or that which is initiated by stretching of the perineum, and so on, would be propagated into the spinal cord, and thence after synaptic relay across the sagittal plane of the nervous system to the opposite thalamus. There, evidence would indicate, the activity is registered in consciousness as pain by activation of a thalamocortical circuit mechanism. To the best of present knowledge, this central course for nervous activity associated with pain applies to the superficial pain of pin prick, pain arising from stimulation of endings in muscle and periosteum and pain arising from sensory receptors in the viscera. It is obvious that all of these origins for pain must be contemplated in considering the effectiveness of a regional block that is to alleviate the pangs of labor.

Insofar as the visceral pain paths distributed through the sympathetic chain are concerned, it has been the general tendency to believe that nervous activity initiated in a viscus enters the cord by way of a large number of dorsal roots. To trace the specific afferent path of sensation arriving from the uterus, Cleland utilized a visceromotor reflex activated by stimulation of the uterus.* This stimulation results in a contraction of the rectus abdominus muscle. He used the experimental method to determine which dorsal roots, when sectioned, abolished this reflex. He deduced from his experiments that the afferent fibers from the human uterus enter the cord over the T-11 and the T-12 dorsal roots. If the afferent routes for reflexogenic activity and for pain parallel one another, these should be the segmental

* AUTHORS' NOTE. One of the authors remembers an occasion when he was called into consultation for the delivery of 2 patients with spinal-cord lesions.

The first patient was a primipara who had a malignant tumor of the spinal cord. A gradual paralysis of both motor and sensory components developed until a clinical syndrome similar to transection of the spinal cord distal to the tenth thoracic segment was produced. A sharp zone of skin anesthesia from the umbilicus downward resulted. Despite the pathology, the patient continued her pregnancy. She went into a painless, spontaneous labor and was delivered of a living child, with a minimum of blood loss.

In February, 1946, in the Methodist Hospital in Memphis, a patient who was permanently paralyzed from an automobile accident entered the hospital for delivery. She had a motor and sensory paralysis of both lower extremities, which had persisted for the period of 5 years since the accident. There was considerable muscular atrophy and wasting of the lower half of the body. The skin over the perineum was thin and of a poor texture, as is often seen in patients who survive crushing injuries of the spinal cord. It was determined that the level of sensory anesthesia extended on the left to the tenth thoracic segment and on the right to the eleventh thoracic segment. Obstetric and roentgen examination revealed that the patient was pregnant at term with twins. Because of the atrophic condition of the perineum and the birth canal, with the possibility of slow healing powers, a cesarean section was decided upon as the optimum method for delivery. Local infiltration of the abdominal wall with an anesthetic solution was carried out throughout the thoracic segments of the tenth and the eleventh on the right and throughout the tenth thoracic on the left. With only 2½ in. of such local block anesthesia it was possible to perform a classic cesarean section for the delivery of 2 healthy and vigorous babies without pain. The uterus contracted promptly with little blood loss.

These two cases, together with the patient who had a transection of the spinal cord at the tenth thoracic segment from an automobile accident, and the patient with a transection of the cord at the sixth thoracic segment, as reported by DeLee, confirm the hypothesis of Cleland, namely, that there is a dissociation between the sensory and the motor components of the uterus. He determined that the sensory afferent fibers entered the spinal cord through the eleventh and the twelfth thoracic somatic nerves.

The 4 clinical cases described and referred to, and the several thousand cases in whom we have blocked the impulses with regional analgesia of these segments, have confirmed the fact that the work of Cleland has become a monumental milestone in the understanding and the control of childbirth pain.

levels for transmitting to the central nervous system the pains of labor that are associated with uterine contractions. Other evidence indicates that section of the superior hypogastric plexus in the human female alleviated the pains of the first stage of labor in several of the patients who had this operation for dysmenorrhea and subsequently became pregnant (Rutherford). Histologic study has shown that the hypogastric plexus contains a significant number of small, thinly myelinated fibers of a type that in various experimental studies have been shown to be concerned with the "transmission of pain"; it may contain nonmyelinated pain fibers as well. The nervus erigens, arising from the S-2, 3 and 4 spinal nerves and containing the chief parasympathetic outflow to the pelvic viscera, shows a significant complement of small, thinly myelinated sensory fibers. However, it would not appear that the sensory fibers of the nervus erigens transmit pain from the body of the uterus in the human female, although they may do so from the cervix and the vagina. The pudendal nerve, and its branch, the *perineal,* also must be remembered as containing a significant complement of sensory fibers. Since this nerve, which has an S-2, 3 and 4 segmental origin, like the nervus erigens, has both deep and superficial branches, it may be presumed that its sensory fiber component plays an important role in transmitting to the central nervous system the painful effects of stretching of the perineum during the expulsion of the child. Henry Head, basing his observations on the referred pain concept, states that when the cervix begins to dilate, pain is felt over the sacrum and the coccyx and the S-2, 3 and 4 dermatome areas. When the cervix has dilated and the contractions are forcing the head through the pelvis, there are many causes of pain:

1. Traction upon adjacent and associated organs, such as the tubes or the ovaries;
2. Drag upon ligaments attaching the uterus to the pelvis;
3. Pressure upon the bladder, the urethra, the rectum and the pelvic sling of musculature;
4. In some cases, projection of a fetal part against the uterine wall and
5. Obstruction of one or both ureters occurring from pressure of the presenting part. Thus, hydro-ureter, with its consequent pain, may result.

In summary, it would appear that two widely separated series of dorsal roots are concerned with the transmission of pain from the organs of parturition during labor. The higher group, believed on the basis of clinical experience and deductions from experimental evidence to be chiefly those of the T-11 and 12 segments, is concerned with the labor pains that arise from the rhythmic contractions of the uterine musculature. The lower group, those of the S-2, 3 and 4 segments, is concerned with the pain pathway from the lower uterine segment and the structures of the anatomic perineum. Clinical study of the continuous caudal analgesia method (Lull and Hingson) has indicated that: (1) blocking the sacral nerve roots abolishes the pain of distention of the birth canal, paralyzes the skeletal musculature of the perineum and abolishes tone in the smooth muscle of the cervix and (2) extending the block to include the T-11 root level abolishes the pain of uterine contractions without impairing their force. Thus, in 5,000 carefully observed cases in labor it was reported that without exception patients who had skin analgesia over the cutaneous distribution of the T-11 and 12 roots on both sides experienced surcease from pain even in the presence of strong uterine contractions.

UTERUS MOTOR NERVE SUPPLY

Uterine contractility is initiated either through sympathetic stimulation of the thoracolumbar outflow conducted by white rami communicantes (probably T-6 through L-2) or by the humoral pitocinlike stimulation of the intrinsic nerve endings within the uterus itself. The rhythmicity of the Broxton Hicks contractions is considered to be an alternate balance between sympathetic contraction effect and parasympathetic relaxation effect.

INNERVATION OF THE BLADDER

Both the sympathetic and the parasympathetic subdivision contribute to the involuntary (visceral) efferent innervation of the bladder. The pudendal (S-2, 3 and 4 origin) nerve provides the voluntary innervation of the external sphincter.

The sympathetic outflow arises chiefly from the L-2 to 5 motor roots, passes through the sympathetic chain, the hypogastric plexuses and the subsidiary vessical plexus of the bladder. Learmonth has observed that following stimulation of the superior hypogastric plexus there is a contraction of the internal sphincter of the bladder, constriction of the urethral orifice and increased tone in the trigone. It is stated by others that the hypogastric plexus contains efferent inhibitory fibers to the bladder as well. The inferior mesenteric ganglion has been said to be the prepostganglionic relay point in the sympathetic outflow.

The parasympathetic outflow arises from S-2, 3 and 4 cord segments, and its preganglionic fibers are distributed through the nervus erigens to the pelvic plexus. After the prepostganglionic synapse in the pelvic plexus, the path reaches the bladder wall. Stimulation of the nervus erigens is said to produce contraction of the detrusor muscle and relaxation of the internal sphincter. This action usually results in expulsion of urine under experimental conditions. The parasympathetic outflow may also contain efferent inhibitory as well as motor fibers.

There are 3 routes for afferent impulses from the bladder and the urethra to the central nervous system. One of these, through the hypogastric plexus, the lumbar components of the sympathetic chain, the rami communicantes and the lumbar dorsal roots, would appear to be concerned chiefly with the mediation of pain. Learmonth, handling the superior hypogastric plexus with a forceps in a patient under spinal anesthesia, noted that the patient experienced crushing pain referred to the bladder. Rutherford noted no bladder difficulties following presacral neurectomy other than those that might be noted following any ordinary laparotomy, which suggests that the hypogastric route does not play an important role in the transmission of reflexogenic activity from the bladder. However, presacral neurectomy has been noted to relieve vesical pain.

The second afferent route from the bladder utilizes the nervus erigens and the dorsal roots of the S-2, 3 and 4 dorsal roots. This route appears also to convey some pain, for, when the sacral nerves are blocked, manipulation with a cystoscope is no longer painful, although distention of the bladder still causes suprapubic discomfort. It is believed that one third of the nerve fibers in the nervus erigens are afferent in nature. The afferent impulses conveyed by this route serve muscle stretch and some pain, touch and temperature sensations from the bladder and the posterior urethra.

The third route for afferent impulses is over the pudendal nerve. There are many small, myelinated fibers in this

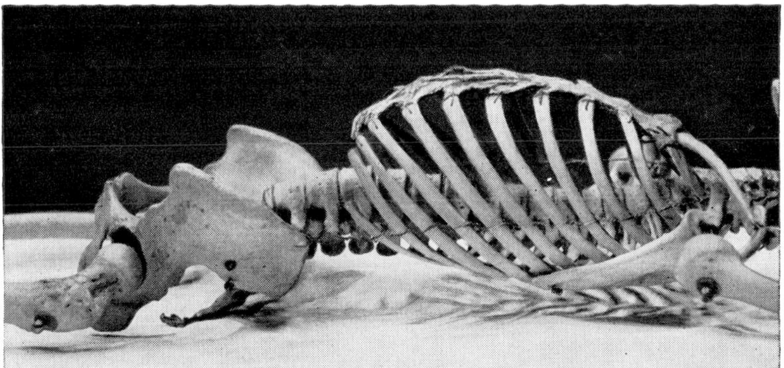

Fig. 21. Skeleton lying on back showing normal curves of spine. (Maxson, Louis H.: Spinal Anesthesia, Philadelphia, Lippincott)

nerve, and proof is given of the reflexogenic action of some of the afferents upon the bladder mechanism by the contraction of the bladder, which results from stimulation of the cut distal end of a pudendal nerve.

Under continuous caudal analgesia, the spontaneous emptying by the musculature of the bladder is severely crippled temporarily. This is readily understood when the levels of innervation for the bladder mechanism and for the organs of parturition are compared. In explaining this phenomenon, it should be understood that the peripheral nervous mechanism controlling the bladder operates through reflex arcs that may be interrupted, or blocked, on their motor side, their afferent side or through disturbance of the intrinsic cord mechanism. Brock summarizes clearly the effects of these interferences. Disturbance of sacral parasympathetic action at the cord level produces a flaccid paralysis of the bladder wall. Evacuation becomes difficult, and residual urine is apt to collect. With involvement of the sympathetic pathway as the spinal cord center, it is the storage capacity of the bladder that is interfered with. Finally, when the afferent bladder pathways are involved, voluntary urination may be normal, but absence of the feeling of distention permits of a large accumulation of urine. Depletion of afferent inflow from the bladder wall, which normally operates through reflex arcs to maintain bladder tone, may cause the internal sphincter to be relaxed and dribbling to occur. A combination of these factors may be expected to disturb temporarily normal bladder emptying during the effective period of continuous caudal analgesia.

COMPONENTS OF THE VERTEBRAL COLUMN*

Topographic Anatomy

The parts of the vertebral column are classed in 5 major divisions:

1. The cervical vertebrae: 7, sometimes 8 in number
2. The thoracic vertebrae: 12 in number, sometimes 11 or 13

* Maxson, L. H.: Spinal Anesthesia, Philadelphia. Lippincott, 1938.

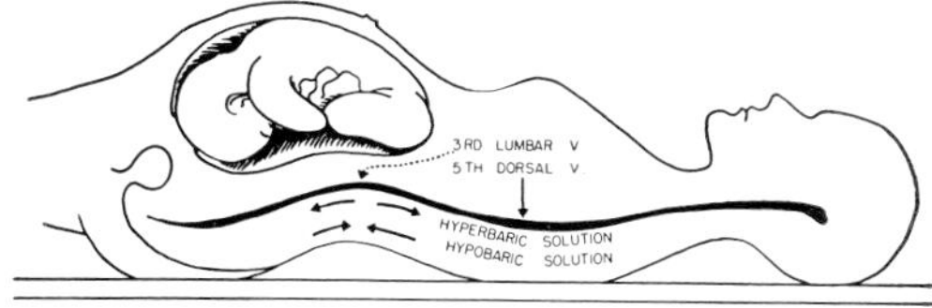

Fig. 22. High and low points of spinal curves with pregnant patient lying on back. (Maxson, Louis H.: Spinal Anesthesia, Philadelphia, Lippincott)

3. The lumbar vertebrae: 5, sometimes 6. Occasionally there is complete sacralization of the fifth lumbar vertebra

4. Sacrum: 5 separate vertebrae in childhood, fused in adult.

5. Coccyx: 4 or 5 rudimentary vertebrae, fused after middle life into 2 or 3 segments

These vertebrae differ greatly in size and form. There seems to be an increase in structural strength and size in a progressive manner inferior from the atlas of the cervical vertebrae to the large triangular fused sacrum. In understanding the structure of a typical lumbar vertebra, one knows the structure of the other vertebral segments in the spinal column. A typical lumbar vertebra has the following parts:

A. A body, or centrum, of cancellous bone, roughly cylindrical but broader from side to side

B. 2 pedicles, short and strong

C. 2 laminae, meeting posteriorly and forming the arch

D. A spinous process, projecting posteriorly, rising from the union of the laminae

E. 2 transverse processes, 1 on each side, rising from the junction of the pedicles and laminae

F. 4 articulating processes, 2 on each side, superior and inferior, for articulating with the vertebrae above and below

G. 2 mammillary processes. 1 on each side, on the upper surface

The vertebrae are separated by the

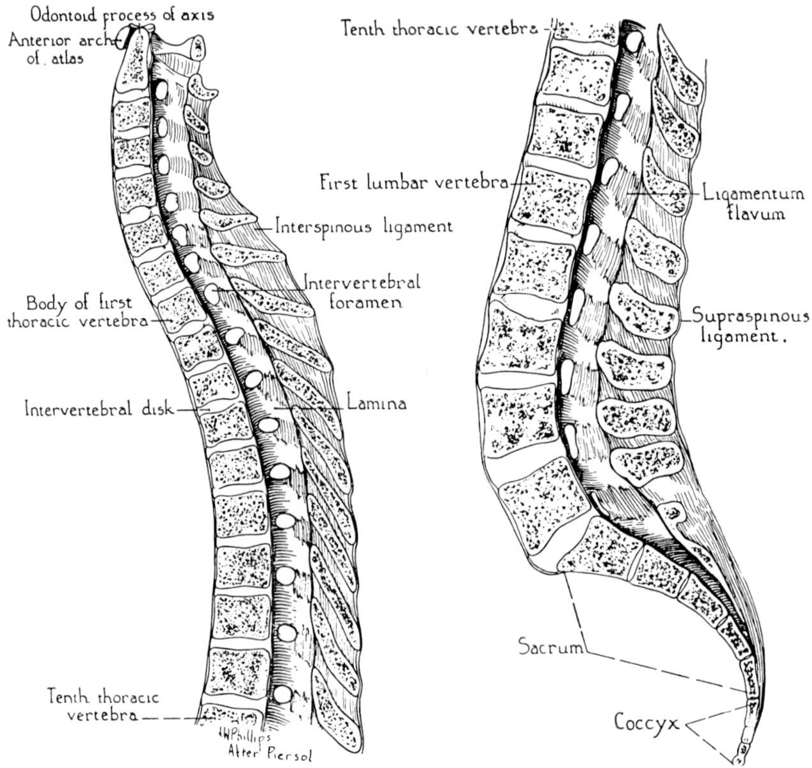

FIG. 23. Sagittal section of spinal column, showing the direction of the spinous processes, their relationship to the vertebral bodies, the intervertebral foramina and the posterior spinal ligaments. (Maxson, Louis H.: Spinal Anesthesia, Philadelphia, Lippincott)

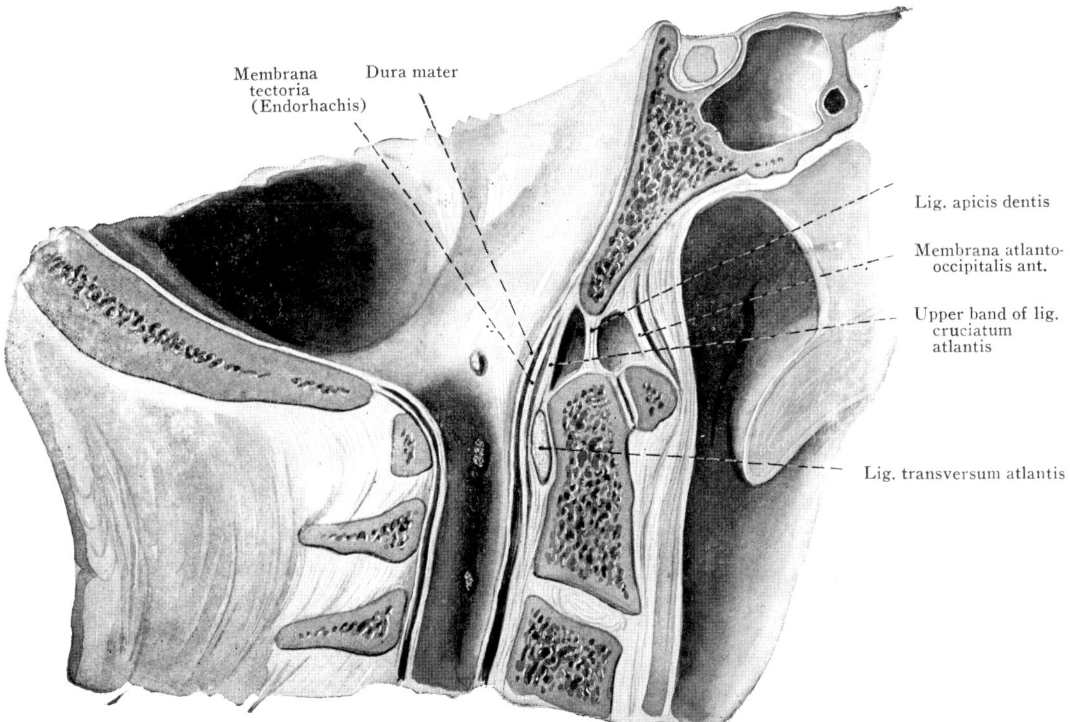

FIG. 24. Median-sagittal section through the base of the skull and the first 3 cervical vertebrae, showing the topography of the epidural cavity (cranial extremity). The epidural cavity is shown ending at the foramen magnum; it is bounded anteriorly by the spinal dura mater and the tectorial membrane (specialized part of posterior longitudinal ligament) and posteriorly by the spinal dura mater and the fusion of ligamenta flava and interspinous ligaments. The subdural cavity within the vertebral canal is continuous at the foramen magnum with the subdural cavity within the cranial cavity. (Peham & Amreich: Operative Gynecology, vol. 1, Philadelphia, Lippincott)

intervertebral disks, cylindrical pads of fibro-elastic cartilage. These disks are the somatic mesodermal derivative of the embryonic notocord. The elasticity of these disks gives the spine its flexibility.

CURVES

After infancy, the spine has 4 normal curves:

Cervical curve: convexity anterior
Dorsal curve: convexity posterior
Lumbar curve: convexity anterior
Sacrococcygeal curve: convexity posterior (generally, the sacral curve)

The degree of curvature varies in different individuals, and owing to the flexibility of the spine it may be modified greatly by posture. During the latter months of pregnancy, the adjustment of the weight-bearing lines produces the so-called "strut of pregnancy," which is a great anterior exaggeration of the lumbar curve and a posterior exaggeration of the dorsal curve. When the head is bent forward as far as possible and the knees meet the chin, the cervical and the lumbar curves are reversed so that the spine becomes one continuous curve with convexity posterior just as in fetal life.

These curves play a part in the pooling or laking of fluid injected into the peridural space.

The peridural space* is that portion of the vertebral canal not occupied by the dura and its contents. This space surrounds the dura like a sleeve below the foramen magnum and separates the dura from the ligaments and the periosteum which form the wall of the vertebral canal. Superiorly, it ends at the foramen magnum where the dura mater divides into 2 layers, one becoming the endosteum of the skull and the other the pachymenix over the brain. Within the canal, the dura lies in close apposition to the periosteum of the posterior aspects of the bodies of the vertebrae, and laterally it extends with each nerve root. Posteriorly, it has no connections. As the nerve trunks emerge from the intervertebral foramina, a curtain is formed over the opening by connective tissue fibers arising from the intervertebral ligaments and fusing with the epineurium. Occasionally, it has been noted in dissecting these peridural spaces that a median fenestrated fibrous raphe is produced by prolongation of the dura along the minute nerve fibers extending upward between the spines and to the periosteum of the vertebral arches. In one instance, clinical evidence of adherence of the dura to the promontory of the sacrum was found.

Thus, the dural sac with its contents of spinal cord and cerebrospinal fluid almost completely fills the vertebral canal, allowing only 3 to 6 mm. between the ligaments and the sac itself. Approximately nine tenths of the space lies lateral and posterior to the dura and is filled with adipose tissue in a solid and semisolid state and with a rich plexus of blood vessels consisting of the veins of the internal vertebral plexus.

There are 58 lateral openings into the peridural space: namely, 8 anterior and posterior sacral foramina, 10 lumbar intervertebral foramina, 24 thoracic intervertebral foramina, 14 cervical intervertebral foramina, and the 2 grooves between the atlas and the occiput. Superiorly, the space is limited by the foramen magnum; inferiorly, by the sacral hiatus.

Through each of the lateral openings

* Southworth, J. L., and Hingson, R. A.: Continuous caudal analgesia in surgery, Ann. Surg. **118**:945-970, 1943.

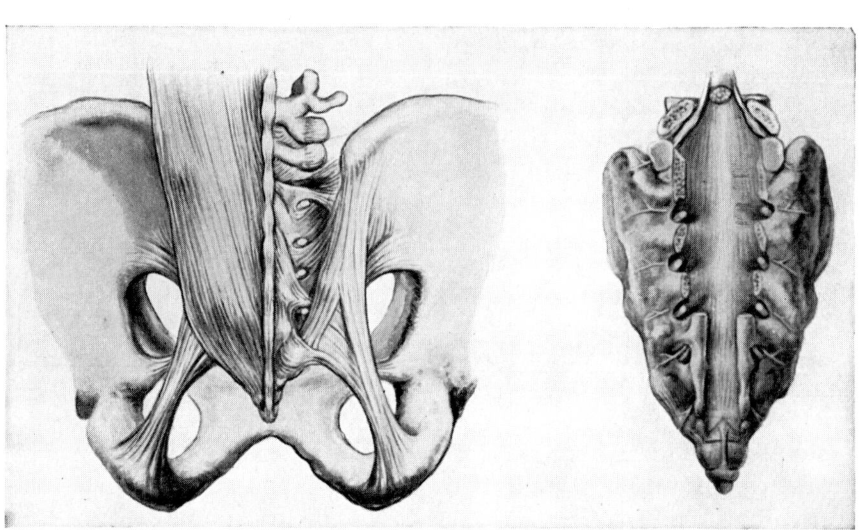

Fig. 25. Posterior sacral ligaments and sacral canal with posterior surface of sacrum removed. (Southworth & Hingson: Ann. Surg. **118**:945-970)

there emerges a spinal nerve. The efferent and the afferent roots arise separately and segmentally from the spinal cord and run laterally and inferiorly until they unite at the intervertebral foramen. The formed spinal nerve divides shortly after its formation into anterior and posterior primary rami which supply the body more or less segmentally. The anterior ramus of each nerve receives connections from the sympathetic trunk. The roots and the formed spinal nerves are comparatively small in the thoracic area and are large in the lumbar and the cervical segments. The epineurium of each nerve blends with the dura which has extended with the root. The sympathetic fibers are fine and nonmyelinated.

Inferiorly, the sacral prolongation of the peridural space is the sacral canal. In the normal subject the dura ends within the canal between the bodies of the first and the second sacral vertebrae. It has been found clinically that in a few cases the dura extends below this level so that the subarachnoid space may be entered with the usual caudal needle.

TABLE 7. INCIDENCE OF THE DISTANCES BETWEEN THE APEX OF THE HIATUS AND THE LOWER EXTENT OF THE DURAL SAC

PERCENTAGE INCIDENCE OF THE MEAN AND OF THOSE DISTANCES SHORTER AND LONGER THAN THE MEAN*

Distance in mm.	*Number of Bodies*	*Per Cent*
16 to 20	1	
21 to 25	1	
26 to 30	5	42.0
31 to 35	5	
36 to 40	3	
41 to 45	7	
46 to 50	12	22.0
51 to 55	5	
56 to 60	5	
61 to 65	2	36.0
66 to 70	3	
71 to 75	4	
Totals	53	100.0

* Lanier, V. S., McKnight, H. E., and Trotter, Mildred: Caudal analgesia: An experiment and anatomical study, Am. J. Obst. & Gynec. **47**:633-641.

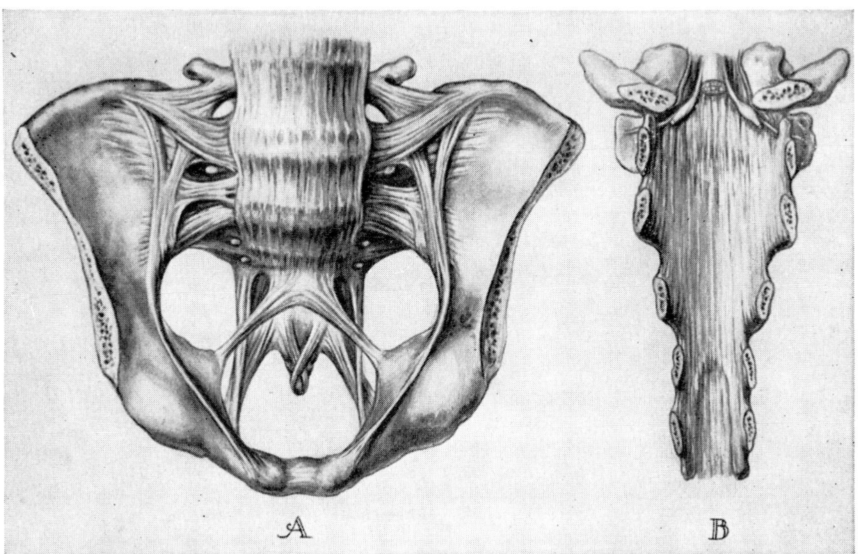

FIG. 26. Anterior sacral ligaments with roof of sacral canal exposed. Note spinal root ganglia in (B). (Southworth & Hingson: Ann. Surg. **118**:945-970)

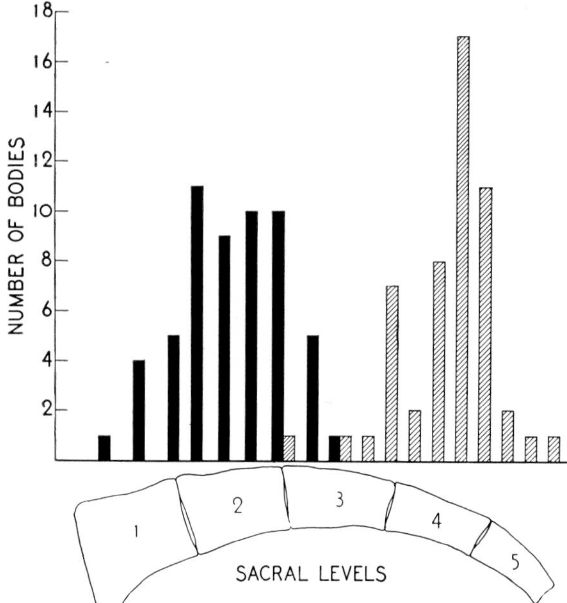

FIG. 27. Diagram representing the sacral level of the lowest extent of the dural sac (solid black) and the highest extent of the hiatus of the sacral canal (cross-hatched). The numbers across the bottom of the diagram indicate the segments of the sacrum; the numbers placed vertically indicate the incidence of observations on 56 cadavers. (After Lanier, McKnight & Trotter: Am. J. Obst. & Gynec. **47**:633-641)

In a study of fresh cadaver material, Lanier, McKnight and Trotter[2] determined that the point of termination of the dural sac occurred between the levels of the middle of the first and the middle of the third sacral vertebral bodies. The mean point was the middle third of the body of the second sacral vertebra. Of the 56 sacra studied, the termination of the dura was at a level cephalad to the mean in 37.5 per cent and caudad in 46.6 per cent. The dura in one of the bodies was quite tightly adherent to the dorsal bony wall of the canal in the sacrum. The same bodies used in determining the size of the hiatus (in the recent state) afforded measurements of the distance between the apex of the hiatus and the termination of the dural sac before and after skeletonization. There was no significant difference between the measurements made under these two conditions. The mean distance was 47.4 mm. on the cleaned bones with a range of 19 to 75 mm. A summary of the measurements is given in the table on page 81.

Thus, it may be seen that there were 42 per cent of the cases with a shorter distance between the apex of the hiatus and the dural sac than the mean distance.

A diagrammatic representation of the inferior limit of the dural sac and of the superior limit of the apex of the hiatus is given in Figure 27. A correlation between the level of the apex (the superior limit at which the needle might be passed into the sacral canal) and the distance from the apex to the dural sac is suggested as a warning.

The sacral canal varies in length from 3 to 4 in. Its direction is that of the sacrum, the axis of which is more sharply curved in the female than in the male. It contains the following structures:

Sacral and coccygeal nerves and dorsal root ganglia
Lower end of the dural sac
Loose areolar tissue
Solidified and partially liquid fat
Lymphatics and blood vessels

The blood vessels consist mostly of veins representing the lower end of the

[2] *Ibid.*

internal vertebral plexus. These veins are large and thin-walled and are most numerous anteriorly and laterally along the posterior aspects of the bodies of the fused sacral vertebrae. For this reason, in caudal puncture an effort is made to direct the needle along the roof or the posterior wall of the sacral canal in order to avoid venipuncture. In anomalous sacra, bony protuberances may extend into the canal, causing a needle in this region to traverse a devious course.

The peridural space ends inferiorly at the sacral hiatus. This is an oblique opening formed by failure of fusion of the fifth and sometimes the fourth sacral vertebral laminae. It lies about 2 in. above the tip of the coccyx, usually in the mid-line, and in about 90 per cent of subjects directly beneath the superior-posterior limit of the intergluteal crease of skin. However, it must be pointed out that the gluteal cleft may deviate with the position of the patient and, therefore, it serves only as a general guide to the location of the hiatus. For inserting the needle, only bony landmarks may be relied upon.

The plane of the hiatus is oblique. It is bounded above by the fused lamina of the third or the fourth sacral vertebra, the arch of which supports a sacral spinous process. Inferiorly, it is bounded by the posterior surface of the body of the fifth sacral vertebra. Laterally, the margins are formed by the edges of the deficient lamina of the fifth and sometimes the fourth sacral vertebra. At the inferior portions of the lateral boundaries two bony prominences, one on each side, are present. These form the sacral cornua which are valuable topographic landmarks. The hiatus is closed by a fibrous expansion 1 to 3 mm. thick, the superficial posterior sacrococcygeal ligament (of Cathelin) which transmits the primary rami of the coccygeal and the fifth sacral nerves, and the filum terminale. It is covered also by skin and subcutaneous fat in addition to the fibrous ligament. The thickness of the fat layer is variable, being greater in the obese and in women. This is of considerable practical importance, as thicker layers of fat interfere with palpation of bony structures and sometimes make successful caudal injection difficult or impossible.

Therefore, the sacral hiatus lies at a level superior to the sacrococcygeal junction, and it is well to determine the lower limits of the sacrum in each patient before attempting caudal analgesia. This simple precaution will prevent inadvertent insertion of a needle into the rectum.

In about 15 per cent of subjects the hiatus is clinically anomalous. These anomalies may be of location, of extent or of the related structures. The shape of the opening is triangular, the apex of the triangle being superior. The apical angle varies from 20° to 60° and its extent is determined by the width of the hiatus. Due to failure of fusion of the third and perhaps the higher sacral laminae, in addition to the fourth or the fifth, the hiatus may extend a great distance upward. In some instances it may be placed entirely at a high level so that the floor is formed by the body of the second or the third sacral vertebra rather than the fourth or the fifth. Due to intermittent failure of fusion additional openings into the sacral canal may exist together with a more or less normally placed hiatus. In some sacra no roof is present over the canal, in which case the hiatus may be said to extend from the usual location to the beginning of the lumbar peridural space. Bony overgrowths of adjacent structures may entirely obscure the hiatus, a flattened fourth sacral spinous process being the usual offender.

The practical importance of these facts

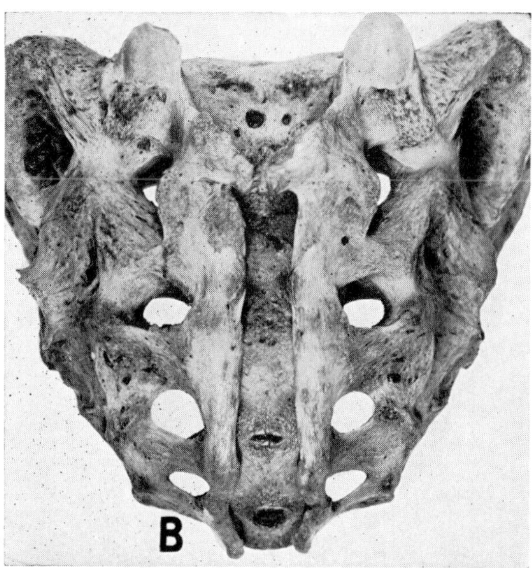

FIG. 28. Sacral canal with open dorsal bony wall of the female sacrum.

is evident. A knowledge of the variations of the sacral hiatus is necessary in order to introduce the needle into the sacral canal of all subjects. Lack of this knowledge is an obstacle to the beginner and is the cause of early failures.

Trotter and Letterman,* after a study of 328 female sacra from the Terry Anatomical Collection of Washington University, and of 346 from the Todd Anatomical Collection of Western Reserve University, made careful caliper measurements of the sacral hiatuses. They reported that:

Certain dimensions obtained served to provide a concept of the general configuration of the hiatus. The mean width of the base of the hiatus of the sacral canal was 16 mm. There was a range from 7 mm. to 28 mm. or a total variation of 21 mm. The length of the hiatus from the base to the apex had a mean of 19 mm. and varied from 0 to 66 mm.

On the average, the anteroposterior diameter of the sacral canal at the level of the apex of the hiatus was 5.3 mm. with a range from 0 to 16 mm. In 5.5 per cent of the series this diameter was 2 mm. or less.

The apex of the hiatus is described classically as occurring at the level of the lower third of the body of the fourth sacral vertebra. In this series, however, it was located at this level in only 35 per cent of cases. In 20 per cent of the cases the apex was found at various points below this region and in the extreme cases extended as far caudally as the lower border of the body of the fifth sacral vertebra. In the remaining 45 per cent, the apex lay at planes cephalad to the lower third of the body of the fourth sacral vertebra, the highest level was at the lower third of the body of the second sacral vertebra or at the union of the bodies of the second and the third sacral vertebrae (Fig. 29 E).

Variations in the structure of the dorsal wall of the sacral canal are numerous. It may be open throughout its entire length (Fig. 28); two examples of this type were found in the Western Reserve series. However, sacra are seen frequently in which the superior extent of the dorsal wall of the canal does not extend cephalad as far as the level of the inferior border of the body of the first sacral vertebra. This results in an increased distance between the laminae of the fifth lumbar and the bony dorsal wall of the sacral canal and a reduced distance between the superior limit of the dorsal wall of the canal and its hiatus. Such a condition may be the result of low-lying lamina of the first sacral vertebra (Fig. 29 E) or of a deficient development of the laminae of the first or even of several of the superior sacral vertebrae (Fig. 29 A). In some cases the dorsal wall of the sacral canal presents a deficiency somewhere between

* Trotter, Mildred, and Letterman, G. S.: Variations of the female sacrum: Their significance in continuous caudal anesthesia, Surg., Gynec. & Obst. **78**:419-424.

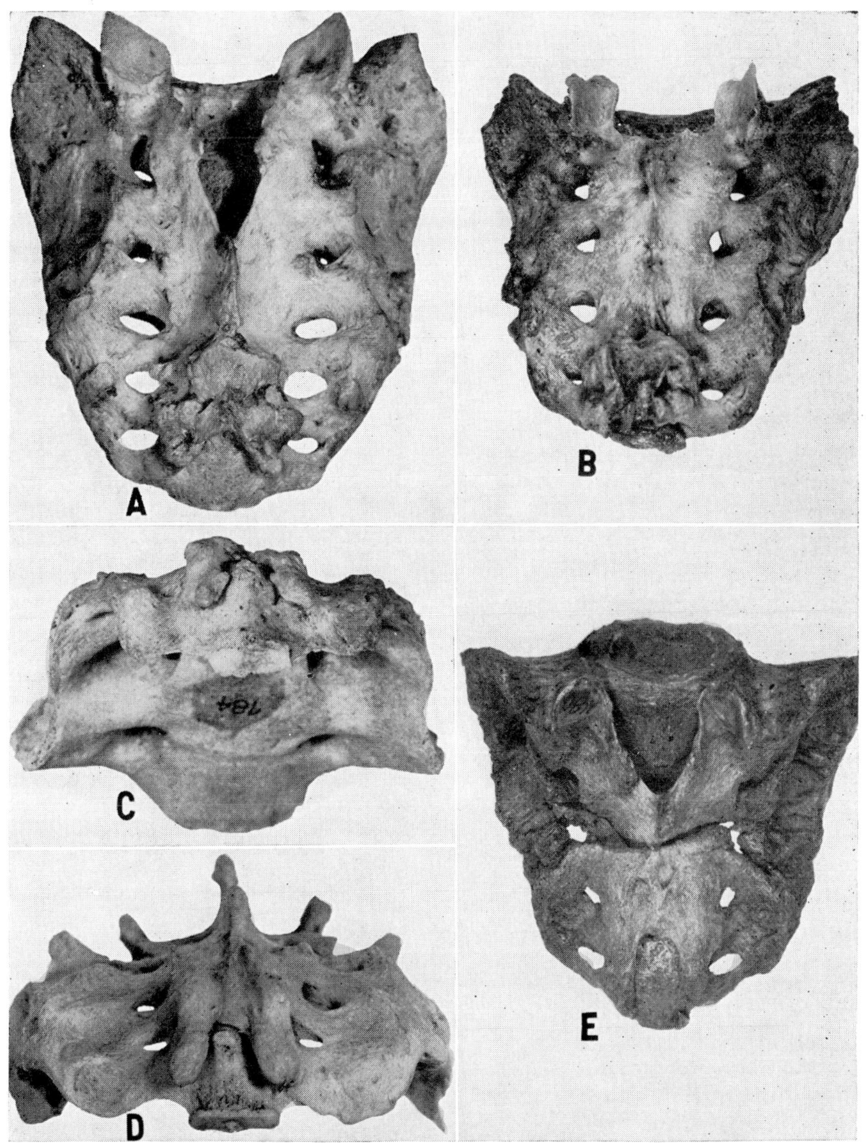

FIG. 29. Anomalies of interference in the female. (A) Overgrowth and coalescence of bony landmarks used in palpating hiatus. (B) Extensive overgrowth masking the apex of the hiatus. (C and D) Nodules of bone projecting into hiatus from posterior surface of sacral body. (E) Transverse sacral fold which obliterates the lumen of the sacral canal at the level of its occurrence; flattened sacral cornua.

its superior and inferior limits; this deficiency may be unilateral, bilateral or found in the mid-line, or it may be seriated as a result of a deficiency of development and subsequent union of the laminae and the spines of adjacent vertebrae. The distance from the apex of the hiatus to such apertures or to low-lying laminae was observed. The distance was 70 mm. or less in 22 per cent (148 sacra) of the series, 50 mm. or less in 10 per cent (69) and 20 mm. or less in 2 per cent (13 sacra).

The lumen of the sacral canal or the hiatus itself may be obliterated or partially blocked by at least 2 types of variations which are of opposite character. One type gives the appearance of a transverse fold in the dorsal wall of the canal and is accompanied by a forward projection of the body of the vertebra just cephalad to the level of the compression. This condition in the dorsal wall may and usually does obliterate completely the lumen of the canal where it occurs. Ten sacra of this series presented such a fold or compression; in 7 it extended between the second pair of posterior sacral foramina, and in the remainder it lay between the third pair of posterior sacral foramina. The second type of variation is the result of a backward or dorsalward projection of the body of a vertebra into the sacral hiatus or canal. Usually it occurs either in a markedly curved sacrum, and the projection is a constituent of the curve, or in a straight sacrum with the first coccygeal vertebra fused at an angle approaching 90°.

Lastly, there may be present an overgrowth of bone obliterating the hiatus and extending the dorsal wall of the sacral canal inferiorly (Fig. 29). The lumen is unaffected (Fig. 29), but the landmarks normally palpable are masked. This variation was pronounced in only 1 bone of the series.

Letterman and Trotter also observed that anomalies of the male sacrum are many times more common than in the female.[1] From the obstetric point of view this is a fortunate circumstance. The most common anomaly of the sacrum is a failure of fusion of the first and the second sacral dorsal arches. This anomaly has been estimated to constitute from 3 to 12.7 per cent of the cases. The second most frequent anomaly of the sacrum is a failure of closing of the second, the third and the fourth arches at the inferior pole of the sacrum. This anomaly is present in about 6 per cent of cases. The third most frequent anomaly is a failure of fusion of all the sacral dorsal arches, or a complete absence of a bony roof of the sacral canal. Wheeler reported that this defect occurred in 1.7 to 5 per cent or five studies of 2,300 specimens.[2] Trotter and Letterman reported this condition to be present in 2 per cent of 553 male sacra and in 3 per cent of 674 female sacra.

From this latter study, they found that in 45 per cent of female bones and in 50 per cent of the male bones the apex of the hiatus extended above the level of the lower third of the body of the fourth sacral vertebra, the level which has been described as normal. Increases in the cephalad extent of the hiatus, of course, decrease the distance between the hiatus and the lower limit of the dura and increase the chance of puncturing the dura with the caudal needle.

In 22 per cent of the female sacra and 26 per cent of the male, deficiencies existed in the dorsal wall of the sacral canal that might permit an exit of the needle and its subcutaneous injection.

[1] Letterman, G. S., and Trotter, Mildred: Variations in the male sacrum: Their significance in caudal analgesia, Surg., Gynec. & Obst. **78**:551-555.

[2] Wheeler, Theodora: Variability of the sacral canal as regards defective neural arches: Rudimentary spina bifida, Contrib. Embryol. **9**:95-107, 1920.

In 5.5 per cent of the female specimens and 4 per cent of the male, the anteroposterior diameter of the canal at the level of the apex of the hiatus was 2 mm. or less. It would be difficult, if not impossible, to introduce a 19-gauge needle into such a canal. Uncommonly, the lumen of the canal was found to be obliterated at one level or other, and sometimes the sacral cornua and other landmarks were so ill-defined as to make difficult the recognition of the sacral hiatus. Of course, the possibility of all these variations must be kept in mind when attempting location of the hiatus and insertion of the needle.

Other less frequent anomalies of the sacrum are:

Complete osseous obliteration of the sacral hiatus

Sacralization of the fifth lumbar vertebra with a great increase in size of the sacral canal

Anterior or posterior flattening of the lower portion of the sacral canal, often more pronounced on one side than on the other

Excessive curvature

Greatly enlarged anterior and posterior foramina. This condition sometimes permits a rapid escape of fluid from the sacral canal and accounts for the difficulty of establishing a high level of analgesia.

Formation of osseous projections in the sacral canal from the roof or the floor to cause partial or complete obstructions for insertion of needles and diffusion of the injected solution

Congenital absence of one half of sacrum with associated anterior sacral meningoceles. This condition has been reported 26 times in the literature. Some of these individuals are mothers of several children. This anomaly was found more often in females than in males in a ratio of 20 to 3. It should be emphasized that these cases were associated with low-lying dural sacs. An attempt at caudal analgesia in any of these probably would have resulted in subarachnoid injection.*

From the standpoint of technic, certain topographic landmarks should be emphasized in aiding one to identify the sacral hiatus and to prevent the hazard of inserting the needle into the rectum or pararectal structures through bypassing the coccyx:

1. The tip of the coccyx can be palpated through the skin in the anogenital crease.

2. The sacrococcygeal junction can be palpated as a bony knuckle from 1 or 2 in. superior to the tip of the coccyx.

3. The sacral hiatus itself, in the overwhelming majority of cases, lies immediately under the superior-posterior pole of the intergluteal crease. This sacral hiatus is bounded by the sacral cornua and is formed by the failure of the fourth and the fifth dorsal arches to close.

4. In the average obstetric patient, the hiatus is covered by ¾ in. of skin, subcutaneous fat and ligaments. In the very thin individual sometimes only ¼ in. of skin lies above the sacrococcygeal ligament (*the membrane of Cathelin*) covering the aperture of the hiatus. *In*

TABLE 8. FETAL HEAD MEASUREMENTS (SCAMMON AND CALKINS†)

DIAMETER	45-CM. INFANT	50-CM. INFANT
Occipitofrontal	10.98	12.15
Biparietal	8.75	9.70
Suboccipitobregmatic	9.60	10.60
Occipitomental	10.78	11.95

* Shidler, F. B., and Richards, Victor: Anterior sacral meningocele, Ann. Surg. **118**:913-918.

† The Development and Growth of the External Dimensions of the Human Body in the Fetal Period, Univ. of Minnesota Press, 1929.

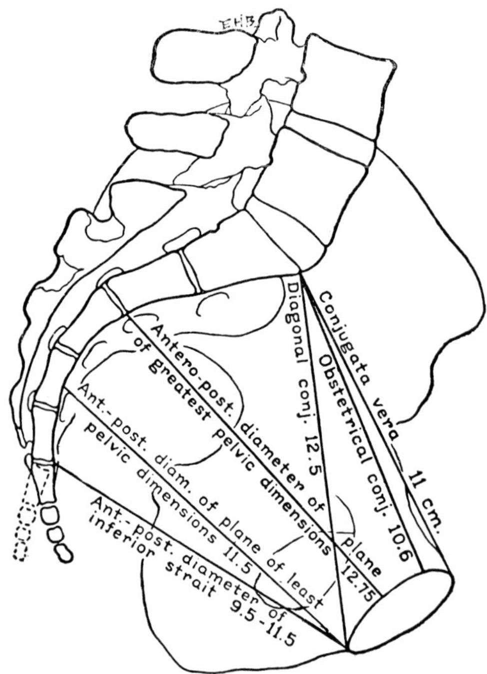

Fig. 30. Diagram showing various pelvic planes and diameters. (Eastman, N. J.: Williams Obstetrics, ed. 11, New York, Appleton)

the insertion of the needle it is imperative that one always insert the point of the needle superior to the sacrococcygeal junction. In the average case the hiatus is found to be ½ to 1 in. superior to this latter topographic landmark.

ANATOMY OF THE BIRTH PASSAGE

In essence, the process of labor consists of the passage of the infant through the bony canal. The various diameters of the fetal head are shown in Table 8.

The figures are based on the measurement of a large number of heads of term infants at birth. These diameters are shorter for Negro children, which is to be expected in view of their slightly lesser weight. Not only does the fetal head size vary from one individual to another, but also, there is some motility of the bones which enables the head to mold to the pelvis and may account for as much as 0.5 cm. shortening in any diameter. Whether the heads of Negro

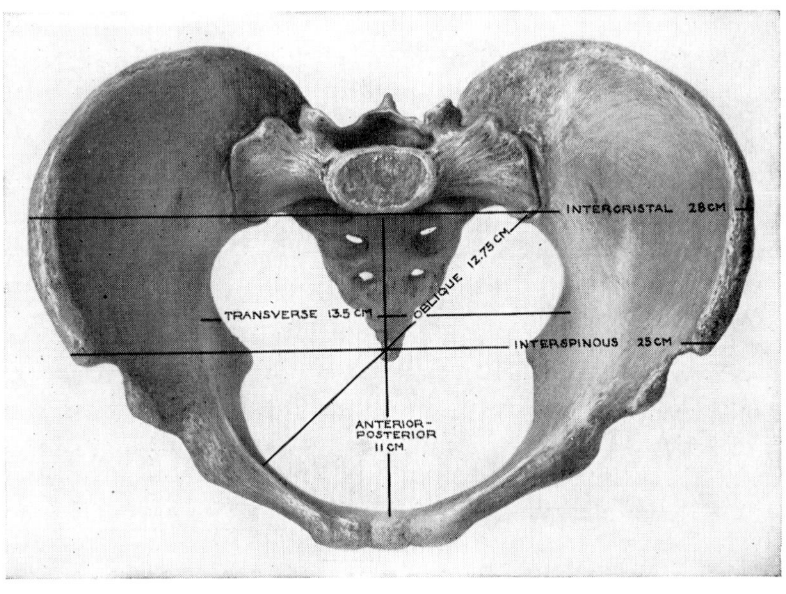

Fig. 31. Normal female pelvis showing diameters of the superior strait. (Zabriskie & Eastman: Nurses Handbook of Obstetrics, ed. 9, Philadelphia, Lippincott)

children are more compressible than those of white, as has been said so often, is a view that needs to be proved. There is unpublished evidence by Kohl, derived from the measurement of heads of Negro and white children after birth, that there is no more molding in the former than in the latter.

The normal diameters of the pelvis are shown in Figures 30 and 31. It can be seen readily that any material decrease in pelvic size may interfere with egress and may possibly jeopardize the infant's life, if not the mother's. Such contractions of the pelvis furnish problems not only for the obstetrician but also for the anesthesiologist as well.

The question of pelvic measurement is one of intriguing historical interest. Even today, the problems presented are not fully solved. It may seem a little astonishing, but the fact of the matter is that no clinical measurements of the pelvis that can be taken on living unanesthetized women have much accurate bearing on the crucial diameters through which the fetal head must pass.

The external diameters of the pelvis, that is, the spines, the crests, the bitrochanteric and the distance from the rhomboid of Michaelis to the anterior border of the symphysis (Baudelocque's diameter) not only are unrelated to the size of the cavity but also often may give entirely false impressions. Unfortunately, this applies also to the measurement of the outlet. Here, although one is close to the bony prominences of the tuberischi, the fat of the buttocks and the inability to define the inner borders of the tubers make for untrustworthy measurements.

In many contracted pelves there is a shortening of the anteroposterior diameter of the inlet. It is customary to estimate the obstetric conjugate by measur-

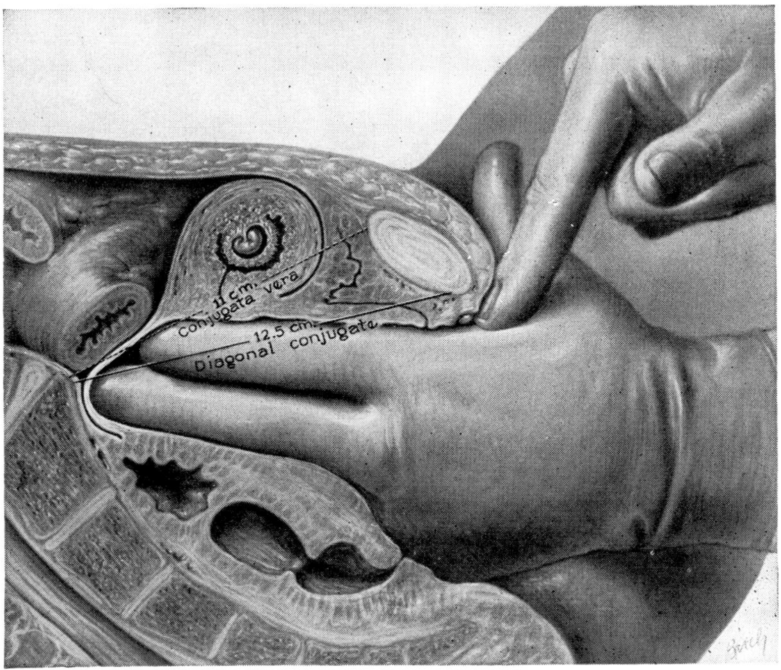

FIG. 32. Method of obtaining diagonal conjugate diameter. (Zabriskie & Eastman: Nurses Handbook of Obstetrics, ed. 9, Philadelphia, Lippincott)

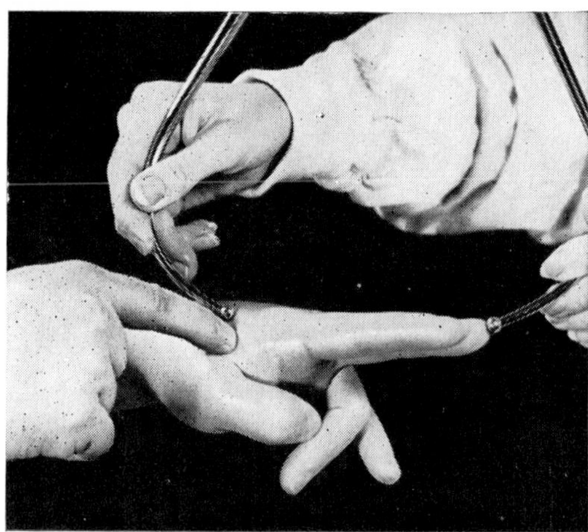

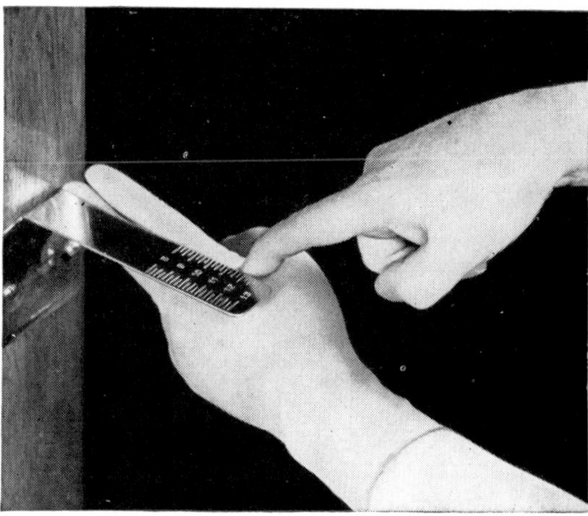

FIG. 33. Methods of measuring diagonal conjugate diameter as obtained in Figure 32. (*Left*) Using pelvimeter. (*Right*) Using wall bracket. (Zabriskie & Eastman: Nurses Handbook of Obstetrics, ed. 9, Philadelphia, Lippincott)

ing the distance from the sacral promontory to the inferior border of the symphysis and subtract 1.5 to 2 cm. (Figs. 32 and 33). This distance, the diagonal conjugate, is the most important clinical measurement of the pelvis. For practical purposes, if it measures greater than 11.5 cm., the anteroposterior diameter of the pelvis can be said to be ample. On the other hand, a diagonal conjugate of less than 11.5 cm. is not always an index of pelvic contraction since the difference between this diameter and the obstetric conjugate may vary from 0.1 to 3.1 cm. (Fig. 34).

In most instances, the highly trained obstetrician learns to gauge the size of the pelvis not only by whatever measurements are available to him but also by the feel of its bony structure and the architecture of its walls. Also, to this he adds the "fit-ability" of the baby's head and the progress of labor. So, through integration of all this information he arrives at remarkably correct judgments concerning the prognosis of labor. In recent years, we have begun to see fewer pelves with anteroposterior contraction, and more with diminution in the transverse diameters. This may be due to the gradual disappearance of clinical rickets and the advent of some congenital or racial change. However the case may be, this latter type of contraction is unmeasurable clinically and may be extremely deceptive during labor, if the midpelvis is involved.

Highly accurate methods of x-ray pelvimetry have been developed. These not only furnish precise measurements of the anteroposterior diameters but also those mentioned above which are clinically unobtainable. In addition, these methods furnish information regarding the configuration of the pelvis. In experienced hands, especially when the measurements are borderline, this type of information is invaluable to both the obstetrician and the anesthesiologist.

Unfortunately, while x-ray pelvimetry is gaining recognition slowly, all too frequently its misuse has given it a bad name. The reasons for this are manifold, among which two stand foremost: (1) the technics are somewhat demanding; and (2) the interpretation of the plates requires more than casual knowledge. Some information regarding pelvic architecture is obtained fairly easily, but a thorough insight into the limitations of the methods comes only with long experience. Too often, definite prognostications are made from a casual glance at a roentgenogram only to be controverted completely once labor has begun. The x-ray picture cannot define the force of uterine contractions, measure accurately the size of the fetal head or predict its malleability. It is a tool, albeit a valuable one, measuring accurately only one of the several important variables upon which the obstetrician and the anesthesiologist must base their ultimate decisions. It is no more and no less than this and is similar to the chest roentgenogram in tuberculosis or the urea nitrogen determination in nephritis, furnishing only a part of the information necessary for formulation of the patient's response to his disease.

The anesthesiologist should have some knowledge of this subject. In borderline situations—and these are most frequent—it is important that maximum use be made of the powers of the uterus and that these not be inhibited by too much, or wrongly directed, pain relief. However, it is equally important that the patient's morale be maintained and not shaken by long hours of unrelieved pain. Also, it is of extreme importance for the anesthesiologist to realize that once the trial of labor through a borderline pelvis has failed, his technics of pain relief should be such that they can be shifted easily from those suitable for vaginal delivery to those adequate for abdominal delivery. Furthermore, long labors or those that cause the fetus to pass through borderline pelves often jeopardize the infant and subject it to decreased oxygen flow. The anesthesiologist who is igno-

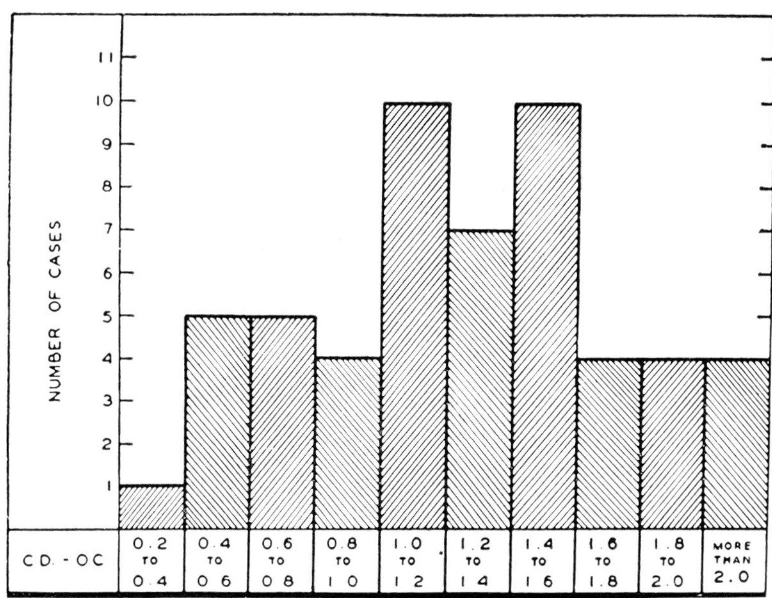

Fig. 34. The distribution of the difference between the diagonal conjugate and the obstetric conjugate (roentgenogram) in 54 cases in which the diagonal conjugate measured 11.5 cm. or less. The mean difference is 1.3 cm., the greatest difference is 3.1 cm., and the least difference is 0.1 cm. (Dippel, A. L.: Surg., Gynec. & Obst. **68**:642)

rant of or disregards these principles is incapable of making a proper choice of anesthesia for delivery.

There are three planes of the pelvis as commonly measured:

1. The plane of the inlet is bound posteriorly by the promontory of the sacrum, laterally by the linea terminalis and anteriorly by the rami of the pelvic bones and the superior border of the symphysis.

2. The plane of the mid-pelvis passes through the lower border of the symphysis and the ischial spines.

3. The plane of the outlet is not a true plane in the strict sense of the word. It consists of 2 triangular planes that meet at a line drawn through the ischial tuberosities. These are bounded by the tip of the coccyx posteriorly, the sacrosciatic ligaments laterally and the lower margins of the pubic arch, anteriorly.

Certain diameters in these planes are commonly considered. Critical measurements appear in Table 9. In general, pelves with measurements above these are considered to be normal, while pelves with diameters below these are contracted. Diminution of any of these diameters is not necessarily an indication for cesarean section.

Perhaps a few words should be said here regarding the soft parts of the pelvic floor. These consist of muscle, fascia and loose areolar tissue. The structures, particularly those of the fascial planes, are

TABLE 9. CRITICAL PELVIC MEASUREMENTS IN CENTIMETERS AS SHOWN BY ROENTGENOGRAM

PLANE	ANTERO-POSTERIOR	TRANS-VERSE	POSTERO-SAGITAL
Inlet.	10.0	12.0	—
Midpelvis. . .	11.5	9.5	4.0
Outlet.	11.0	10.0	7.5

complicated somewhat and need not be approached here in detail. In essence, the pelvic floor is a sling that maintains the abdominal organs—in particular, the uterus, the vagina, the rectum and the bladder, in proper position. In the female, this sling is weakened somewhat by the configuration of the pelvis and by the presence of the hollow tube of the vagina. The weakening of these structures is accentuated further by stretching at delivery. If this be traumatic, or if the structures be unsound fundamentally, relaxations of the vaginal wall and, in particular, of the urethra and the base of the bladder, may lead to difficulties later in life.

One meets successively the peritoneal connective tissue, the internal pelvic fascia, the levator ani and the coccygeal muscles, the external pelvic fascia, the superficial muscles of the perineum, the perineal fascia and subcutaneous tissue and skin.

The most important of these structures is the levator ani muscle and the fascia covering its upper and lower surfaces. For practical purposes, this constitutes the pelvic floor. Seen internally, it is concave while externally it constitutes the pelvic diaphragm (Plates 21 and 22). It will be seen readily from the figures that at full dilatation, with the head crowning, there is remarkable stretching of these structures. It has been maintained that some biochemical change takes place, making them stretchable to this degree without injury. However the case may be, it can be seen that perineal lacerations, either obvious or hidden, can cause considerable damage to the levator ani muscle. Of particular importance is the pubococcygeal division which not only helps to support the rectum and the vagina but also forms the main supporting structure of the base of the bladder and plays an important role in micturition and continence of urine.

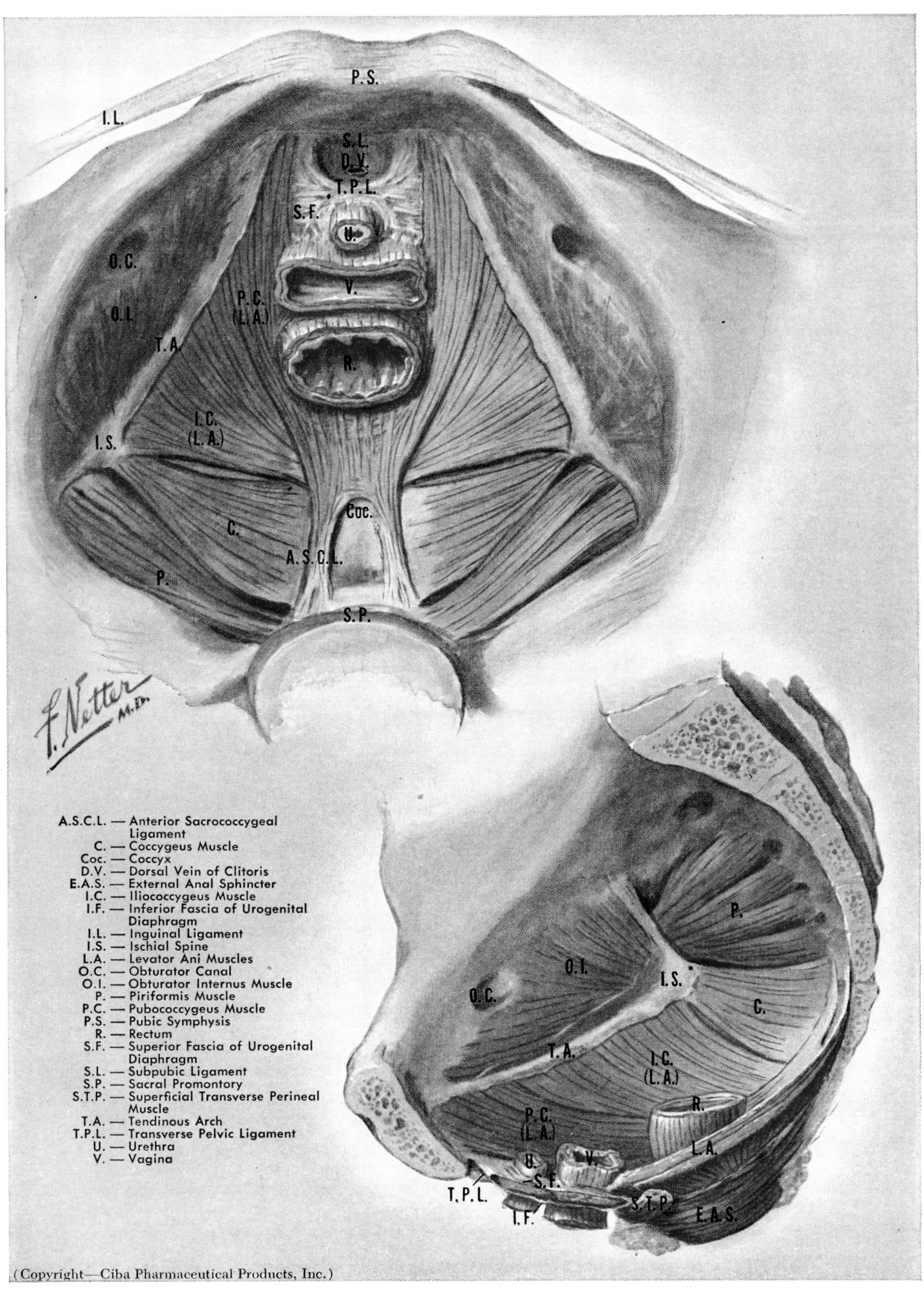

A.S.C.L. — Anterior Sacrococcygeal Ligament
C. — Coccygeus Muscle
Coc. — Coccyx
D.V. — Dorsal Vein of Clitoris
E.A.S. — External Anal Sphincter
I.C. — Iliococcygeus Muscle
I.F. — Inferior Fascia of Urogenital Diaphragm
I.L. — Inguinal Ligament
I.S. — Ischial Spine
L.A. — Levator Ani Muscles
O.C. — Obturator Canal
O.I. — Obturator Internus Muscle
P. — Piriformis Muscle
P.C. — Pubococcygeus Muscle
P.S. — Pubic Symphysis
R. — Rectum
S.F. — Superior Fascia of Urogenital Diaphragm
S.L. — Subpubic Ligament
S.P. — Sacral Promontory
S.T.P. — Superficial Transverse Perineal Muscle
T.A. — Tendinous Arch
T.P.L. — Transverse Pelvic Ligament
U. — Urethra
V. — Vagina

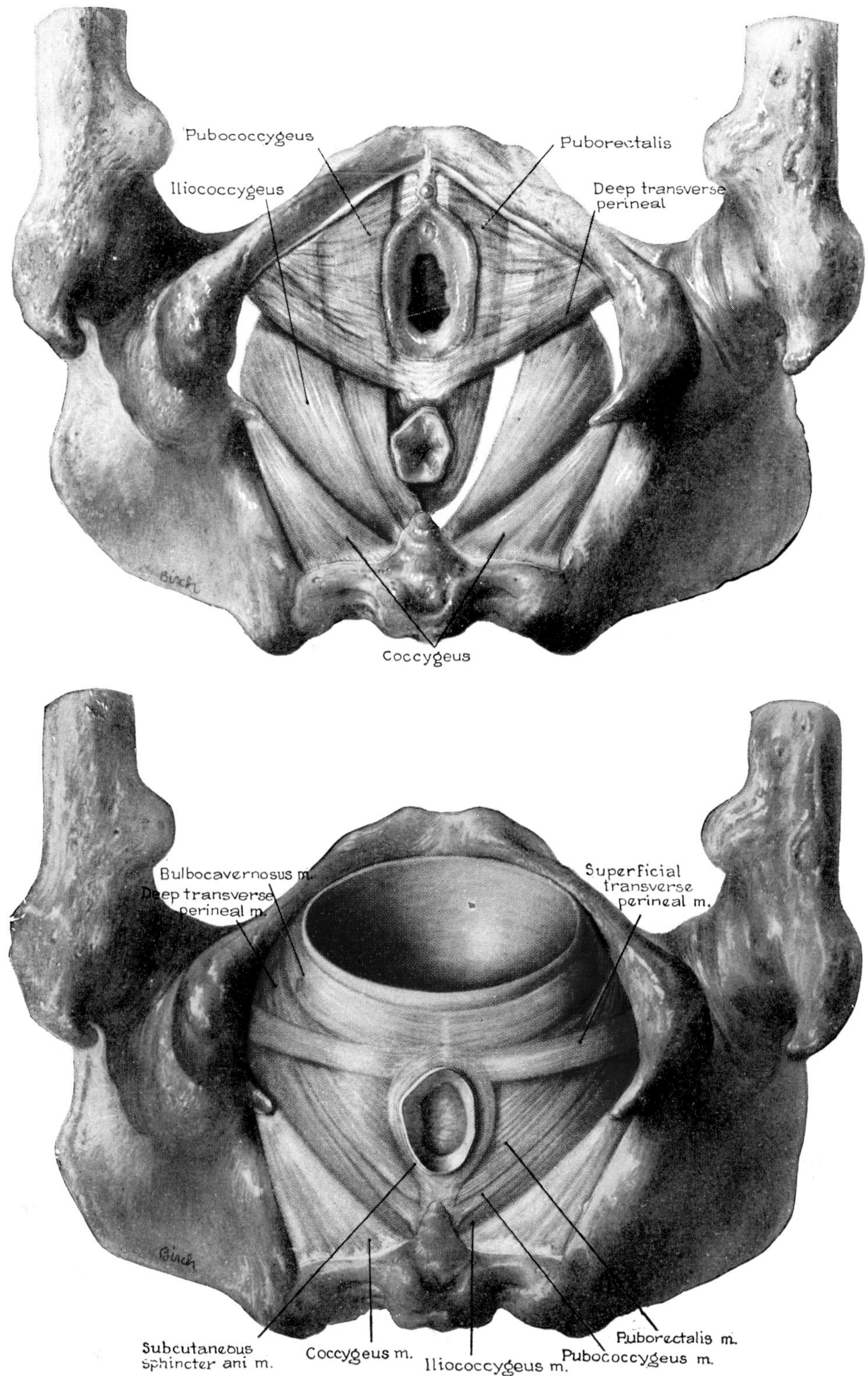

(Top) Deep muscles of the pelvic floor. *(Bottom)* Muscles of the pelvic floor when head is "crowning." (Eastman, N. J.: Williams Obstetrics, ed. 11, New York, Appleton)

This portion of the levator ani being most medial is most liable to damage. It is torn when any significant perineal tears take place and cut if a mediolateral episiotomy is performed. Its protection and adequate care in case of injury may prevent many urinary difficulties later. In certain types of conduction anesthesia, in particular spinal and caudal, very marked relaxation of all of these structures takes place. It is possible that through this type of relaxation they may be protected from damage. Conversely, an inexpertly given general anesthetic, offering poor relaxation and permitting explosive delivery or violent retching, can defeat the most careful obstetric finesse in operative delivery. The associated damage to these structures may cause both permanent impairment of perineal tone and fetal injury.

CONCEPTS OF ETIOLOGY OF ONSET AND CHARACTERISTICS OF LABOR

Avicenna, as quoted in Kurzrok, said that "at the end of 9 months, labor occurs by the grace of God." Four centuries before the Christian era, Hippocrates attributed the onset of labor to a decline in the nutritional status of the fetus (Findley). At that time he said: "When there is no more food for the young one in the egg and it has nothing on which to live, it makes violent movements, searches for food, and breaks the membranes. The mother, perceiving that the embryo is vigorously moving, smashes the shell."

Reynolds has done more than any other individual to illuminate the previously confused field of uterine physiology. He believes that the onset of labor is the result of the gradual, accelerating co-operation of a number of factors—anatomic, physiologic, humeral, nervous, nutritional and circulatory—which, at a time characteristic of the species, are so associated as to lead to the evacuation of the uterus.

The studies of Morrow indicate that there is a synergistic co-operation of the sex steroids, causing increasing uterine activity during gestation. At optimal uterine distention, with uterine muscle irritability at its highest point and aided by increased calcium ionization, blood concentration of the posterior pituitary secretion reaches threshold levels and brings about the onset of uterine labor contractions. Labor contractions are characterized by: (1) appropriate magnitude, (2) rhythmicity, (3) similarity, (4) high tonus, (5) co-ordination and (6) effectiveness. Retraction of the uterine muscle, the cervix and the lower uterine segment is inherent in the labor mechanism.

Likewise, it is probable that posterior pituitary secretion is continually present in the blood during pregnancy but reaches uterine threshold concentration only at term. Labor ensues beyond the physiologic threshold of uterine muscle. If distention is close to the optimum, the blood progesterone and estrogen at a high level, the pituitary secretion at effective levels or any combination of these, the threshold may be exceeded before estimated chronologic term. Normally, both Pitressin and Pitocin may be present and physiologically active in total posterior pituitary secretion concentration in the blood, so that artificial distinctions between them may be interesting experimentally but unimportant physiologically. It is possible that inherent physiologic rhythms (adrenal) provide a trigger mechanism after a certain multiple of the sex cycle has been exceeded. Theoretically, then, it should be possible to initiate labor in the pregnant primate at will, using synthetic sex steroids and posterior pituitary extract to duplicate physiologic endocrine relationships.

It is quite remarkable that whether one deals with a 2-Gm. fetus at the end of 21 days of pregnancy, as in the mouse, or a 200-lb. baby elephant, whose birth occurs at the end of 640 days, in most instances pregnancy terminates at the proper instant to secure a maximum number of extra-uterine survivals. Not only this, but there is considerable evidence that pregnancy in the mammal terminates at a time when fetal demands have begun to outstrip the supplies furnished by a senile placenta.

The question is not what causes the uterus to contract, for innocuous and ineffective Braxton Hicks contractions occur throughout pregnancy, but what factors cause this uterine activity to become painful and effective in cervical dilatation. In all probability, hormonal factors, possibly withdrawal of estrogen and progesterone, and mechanical factors, such as distention and irritation of the retrocervical ganglia by the stretching of the lower uterine segment, play a combined role. However this may be, there is an inevitableness about the process that seems to defy not only the absence of crucial endocrine organs but also the severance of nerves as in traumatic paraplegia. Should man be able to control this process with any degree of assurance, a great advance would have been made. In instances such as toxemia, labor could be started when the moment was most propitious; on the other hand, premature labors could be halted with obvious saving of fetal lives. However, such is not the case. It is true that labor may be started in a certain percentage of cases by either rupture of the membranes or judicious use of pituitary extract or both. However, the chances of success are reduced directly in proportion to the distance from term and the length and the thickness of the cervix.

Similarly, it is most difficult to stop true labor once it has begun. Thus, in cases of premature labor, it is unwise, perhaps, to administer morphine or barbiturate in an attempt to halt the process, for even in the rare instance where such methods succeed, the halt is only momentary. On the other hand, there are labors that can be disrupted or even postponed by too early attempts to relieve pain or induce amnesia. The problem here is one of unpredictability, so while it is unwise to attempt the postponement of premature labor by means of drugs, lest the infant be depressed unduly, so it is equally unwise to administer pain-relieving drugs too early in labor lest abnormal or inefficient uterine contractions be produced.

Certain characteristics of normal labor are so well known that their definition would seem to be fruitless. Thus, labor can be defined as the occurrence of painful uterine contractions, occurring at regular intervals and accomplishing progressive and continuous dilatation of the cervix with eventual descent of the fetus and delivery. On closer analysis, it will be seen that in normal cases cervical dilatation is a continuous process but that it progresses at different rates. Thus, at the beginning of labor there is a prodromal period during which the cervix is effaced but no dilatation occurs. During the mid-portion of labor, dilatation is progressive and nearly linear, but toward full dilatation there is frequently a slowing, thus giving an "S"-shaped curve, so well defined by D'Esopo. While the above facts are well known, the underlying physiology of uterine contractions had been obscure until recently. Even with the recent advances in knowledge through strain-gauge tokodynamometers and various other electrical devices for taking and recording uterine contractions in various portions of the uterus, our knowledge of this subject is far from complete. Ivy, Hartman and Koff and Malpas believed that the uterus, like the heart, possessed a pacemaker that initiated uterine contractions and controlled their rhythmicity. In the monkey these were thought to be located near the insertion of each fallopian tube, and it was thought that the uterine contractions progressed rhythmically over the uterus somewhat in the nature of intestinal peristalsis. While this may be true for the monkey, investigations to date have failed to reveal peristalsis in normal human uterine contractions.

The most striking discovery of recent investigators concerning uterine contraction is that progressive labor is the result of an increasing gradient of work from the fundus to the lower uterine segment. This realization that gradients of activity were of physiologic importance for cervical dilatation clarified much, not only in regard to normal labor, but also to false and abnormal labor as well. The tracing shown in Figure 35 was obtained with three strain gauges: one placed upon the fundus, one in the neighborhood of the umbilicus or the mid-zone and one just above the symphysis or over the lower uterine segment. It is apparent at once that the activity in the fundus far exceeds that of the mid-zone, while the lower uterine segment remains relatively passive. This concept of fundal dominance is well illustrated in Figure 36 where the force of uterine contractions of the various segments is analyzed for 10 minutes. The black area superimposed over the checked area indicates the fundal dominance and, as can be seen, this fundal dominance increases as labor progresses. This same phenomena is shown in Figure 37, which compares the hourly rate of work between the fundus and the mid-uterus and the lower uterine segment during the first stage of labor. Not only is fundal dominance present early in labor, but the increment of this dominance increases as

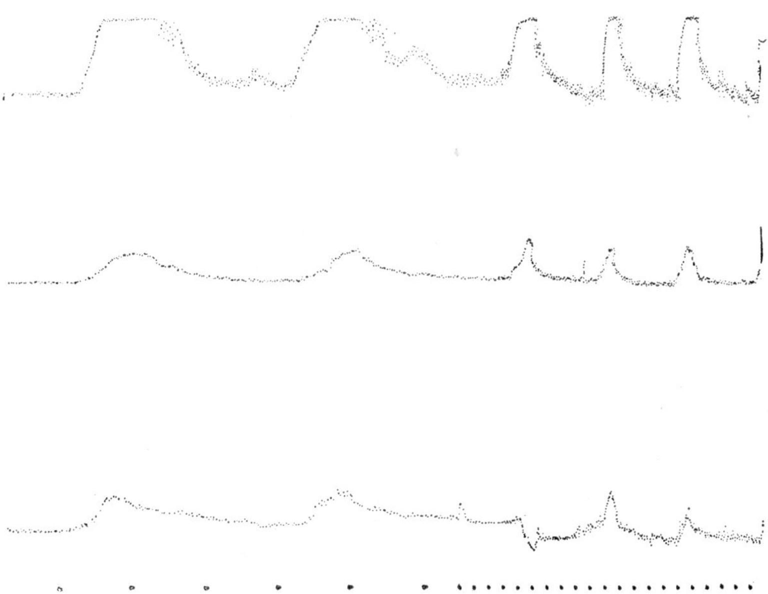

FIG. 35. A multichannel strain-gauge tokodynamometer, an instrument for studying patterns of uterine contractility in pregnant women. (Reynolds, Heard, Bruns & Hellman: Bull. Johns Hopkins Hosp. **82**:446)

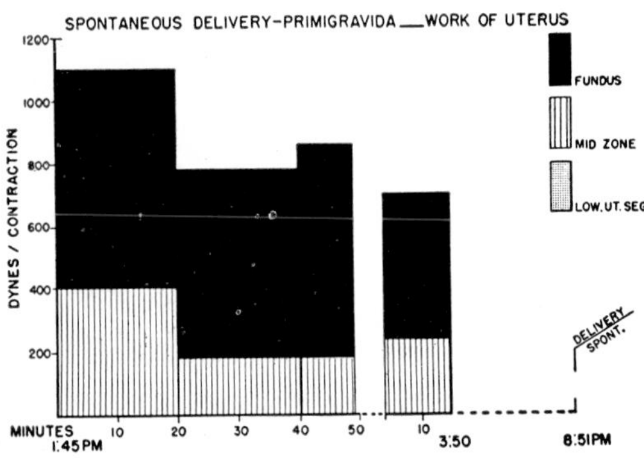

FIG. 36. Graph of normal labor showing the work of the fundus (base line to top of black) and work of the midzone (base line to lower portion of the black). (Hellman, L. M.: M. Clin. North America 35:792)

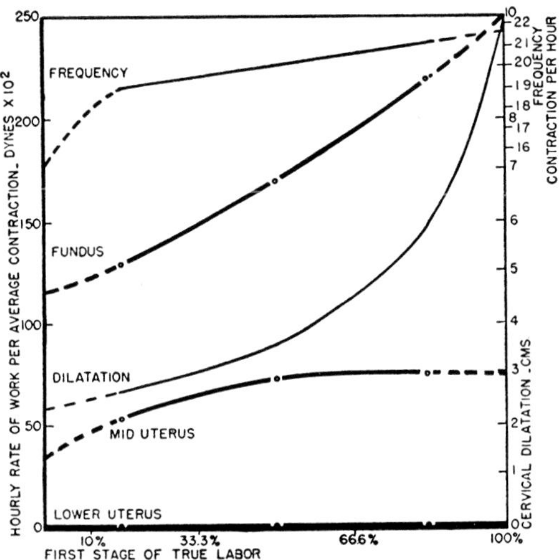

FIG. 37. Characteristics of the gradients of uterine contractility during the first stage of labor. (Hellman, Harris & Reynolds: Bull. Johns Hopkins Hosp. **86:**234–248)

labor progresses. This, then, is the second characteristic of normal labor.

Quite recently Reynolds and Caldeyro, combining simultaneous tracings, obtained from a multichannel external tokodynamometer and those from a needle passed into the uterine cavity, periabdominally, determined that at the height of a normal uterine contraction the amniotic fluid pressure exceeds 15 mm. of mercury, while during a period of relaxation it descends to a level of 10 mm. of mercury, which is the normal tonus of the noncontracted uterus. Also, it was determined by similar means that if the intra-uterine pressure falls below 15 mm. of mercury in the majority of the contractions, cervical dilatation will not occur. This is the third characteristic of normal labor.

Much also has been learned in recent times regarding the characteristics of abnormal labor. However, in spite of the increase in our knowledge, little, if anything, is known concerning the etiology of uterine dysfunction. Clinically, there seem to be two types. In many instances the onset of labor is desultory with pains occurring at more or less infrequent intervals and with great irregularity. While these contractions are painful out of proportion to their force, cervical dilatation does not ensue. Labor in these instances has been known to last for several days. On other occasions, labor begins normally, and cervical dilatation progresses, only to have the pains die out, and the labor, which has been progressing in an orderly fashion, comes to an abrupt halt. These two clinical types have been named *primary* and *secondary* uterine inertia, respectively. While the terms defy exact definition, and there exists some confusion regarding their meaning, they do serve in the main to differentiate two clinical entities whose treatment and physiologic basis seems to be different. Nothing is known in regard to the etiology of primary uterine inertia. It may be associated with developmental defects of the uterus, malposition of the fetus, cephalopelvic disproportion or some types of psychosomatic disorder. It is not particularly predisposed to occur in specific body types, for it appears both in the short and the tall, the lean and the obese, with about equal frequency. There can be little doubt that premature use of sedatives or block analgesics can and does cause many cases of primary uterine inertia. Endocrine imbalance and particularly insufficient estrogen may be a causative factor, although efforts to counteract it with large dosage of this hormone have not produced uniformly satisfactory results.

As has been stated previously, the patient with primary uterine inertia frequently complains of pains that are out of proportion to their severity. At the height of the contractions the uterus still can be indented readily on abdominal palpation. Furthermore, in most instances the cervix does not dilate, although some effacement may take place after many hours; nor does the head descend into the pelvis. Only the continuation of this process over a long period of time serves to differentiate it from false labor.

Tracings with the multichannel strain gauge tokodynamometer do not serve to differentiate primary inertia from false labor. The contraction patterns in false labor have no rule as to regularity, either in frequency or force. The fundal waves are sharp in both ascent and descent, and no plateau exists. Frequently, the mid-zone equals or is of greater intensity than the fundus, and there is no absolute dominance. Often, also, the uterine pressure will fall below 15 mm. of mercury in some or all of the contractions.

Equally difficult to define is secondary uterine inertia. In general, it includes labor that has started normally but has faltered midway, regardless of cause. Naturally, this would imply not only prolongation of labor but also a period of delay in cervical dilatation. Inasmuch as it is common practice to accept labors of 20 hours or more as being prolonged, these, too, are included in secondary uterine inertia. However, the length of time of cervical delay has not been defined and is the subject of some argument. Regardless of the time accepted for any definition, it must be admitted that if the cervix could be observed carefully during labor, particularly during the middle portion, progressive dilatation would be noted, and there should be no delay. Therefore, any delay, no matter how short, may be abnormal. One thing is fairly obvious, namely, that the more prolonged the delay in therapy, the more refractory this condition becomes.

Tracings with the multichannel tokodynamometer have delineated 3 types of abnormality in secondary uterine inertia.

1. The uterine contractions are few, irregular and far apart. The intrauterine pressure is less than 15 mm. of mercury, and fundal dominance is not absolute. The patient feels few if any pains, and the uterus is not firmly contracted to palpation.

2. Contractions are more or less regular, rather firm and extremely painful. While the intra-uterine pressure is adequate, there is a reversal of the contraction pattern, the mid-segment doing more work than the fundus. In other words, fundal dominance has been abolished.

3. Rarely, there is asynchronism between the left and the right side of the fundus or between the upper and the lower segments. When this persists, cervical dilatation does not occur.

While these 3 highly different patterns exist in uterine inertia, frequently combinations of all 3 are present. It is obvious that any therapy should be directed toward correction or at least amelioration of these pattern abnormalities and toward the resumption of strong and effective uterine contractions.

The question can be raised as to how frequently drugs, of both the analgesic and the amnesic types and those used with the conduction methods, contribute to uterine inertia. There can be no doubt that too early administration of pain relief of any type may cause abnormal labor. However, once labor has become firmly established, analgesia, by and large, causes only momentary delay. If the levels are too high, the drugs used in the anatomic approach to pain relief, particularly spinal, peridural and caudal, may delay early labor and render mild contractions ineffective. However, if the level remains at or below thoracic 10, major vertebral blocks appear to have little effect on the progress of well-established labor. During the second stage of labor, they do cause a significant delay in descent of the head and reduce the incidence of spontaneous delivery.

We believe that it is necessary to document thousands of labors before the above impressions can be proved statistically. In the Baltimore obstetric anesthesia study, where such documentation was available over a 3-year period on 5,489 mothers as shown in Table 10, we determined that once the cervix was 5 cm. or more dilated there was no significant retardation of labor. However, it did appear that when conduction blocks were begun before 3 cm. of cervical dila-

TABLE 10. MEAN HOURS OF ANALGESIA IN RELATION TO DILATATION OF CERVIX IN CENTIMETERS AT ONSET OF ANALGESIA*

TYPE OF ANALGESIA	*Primipara*					*Multipara*				
	DILATATION IN CENTIMETERS									
	1–3	*4–5*	*6–7*	*8–9*	*10*	*1–3*	*4–5*	*6–7*	*8–9*	*10*
	MEAN HOURS OF ANALGESIA									
Johns Hopkins Hospital										
1. Sedation—inhalation	4.95	4.35	3.93	2.57	1.07	2.84	2.39	1.62	1.19	.53
2. Sedation—intravenous	5.67	4.29	3.98	1.82	2.08	3.10	2.06	1.55	1.19	.56
3. Sedation—terminal block	5.81	4.17	3.12	4.26	1.57	4.21	2.31	2.37	1.46	.88
4. Continuous conduction	6.03	4.34	3.80	3.71	2.16	3.18	2.50	2.24	2.43	.93
Sinai Hospital										
1. Sedation—terminal block	6.03	3.91	2.55	1.61	1.37	3.37	1.94	1.44	1.27	.70
2. Continuous conduction	4.48	3.83	3.45	2.48	1.00	3.03	2.32	1.67	.63	1.65
3. Sedation—inhalation and/or intravenous	6.66	3.87	3.00	1.00	.75	3.39	1.95	1.08	.93	.85
	NUMBER OF MOTHERS									
Johns Hopkins Hospital										
1. Sedation—inhalation	107	81	48	41	30	258	302	112	60	101
2. Sedation—intravenous	47	57	33	14	4	68	86	47	16	30
3. Sedation—terminal block	71	92	42	19	15	62	84	50	23	16
4. Continuous conduction	50	116	80	38	26	101	171	90	48	18
Sinai Hospital										
1. Sedation—terminal block	382	185	53	31	13	473	321	119	59	41
2. Continuous conduction	86	63	20	9	2	173	130	44	6	2
3. Sedation—inhalation and/or intravenous	57	38	13	7	3	184	133	43	23	22

* Includes all deliveries in the two hospitals except prematures, cesarean sections, breech presentations and infants who died before labor.

tation, there was at least an hour's average delay in the Johns Hopkins group. The Sinai figures are difficult to interpret in this respect because of the frequent use of intravenous oxytocic drip.

PAIN IN LABOR AND DELIVERY

The pregnant uterus at term, because of its enlargement, is lifted up out of the pelvis. However, when "lightening" occurs, the presenting part often descends into the pelvis to cause a pressure on the lower bladder and the rectum that is interpreted frequently as discomfort or pain. These sensations are transmitted across the lower back along the distribution of the second, the third and the fourth sacral nerves. Sometimes this low "backache" is felt by the parturient as early as several weeks to several days before labor begins. With the onset of the uterine contractions of established labor, intra-uterine pressure is increased with a focus on the lower uterine segment and the cervical os. As a rule, when labor pains are present, they are felt as a dragging or aching in the back low down in the lumbar region. In some, there is present a sensation as though the back were breaking. At this time in the first stage of labor, the pain corresponds to the early stages of cervical dilatation. Later, when the uterus commences to contract more vigorously, its smooth muscle fibers pull and stretch the nerve fibers in the body of the uterus to initiate the uterine cramps. These increase in intensity as labor progresses. They are felt within the abdomen, deep in the groin and occasionally down the legs. By actual count in patients delivered without anesthesia or analgesia, the average primipara suffers with from 85 to 400 of these cramps in giving birth. However, it is possible for the occasional normal multipara to deliver a baby with as few as 4 to 6 of these uterine contractions. Later, when the cervix begins to dilate, pain is felt over the sacrum and the coccyx and the second, the third and the fourth sacral areas (Head). When the cervix has dilated and the contractions are forcing the head through the pelvis, there are many causes of pain:

1. Traction upon adjacent and associated organs, such as the tubes or the ovaries
2. Drag upon ligaments attaching the uterus to the pelvis
3. Pressure on the bladder, the urethra, the rectum and the pelvic sling of musculature
4. In some cases, projection of a fetal part against uterine wall
5. Obstruction to one or both ureters may occur from pressure of the presenting part, thus hydro-ureter, with its consequent pain, may result.

As the perineum is distended by the presenting part, a stretch is placed upon the perineal musculature with its enveloping fascia. This causes the "tearing-apart" sensation that increases with crowning. This pain may be accentuated by actual submucosal and sulcal tears of the perineal musculature with sometimes first-, second-, or third-degree lacerations. All of these physical factors are summated into the *poena magna,* the chief or the "great pain" of the Romans, which is the most intense that the human organism endures.

FETAL PLACENTAL RELATIONSHIPS

The anesthetist has a primary concern for fetal oxygenation. However, there are many interdependent factors, such as the transfer of gasses and other substances across the placental barrier; the circulation of the fetus; the hemodynamics of the circulation; the peculiar properties of fetal hemoglobin; and, finally, the striking changes in the entire fetal mechanism that take place at birth and in the first few hours of life. Unless these are understood, oxygenation by itself stands somewhat meaningless.

The fetal circulation in utero is illustrated in Plate 23. The principal factors of this type of circulation, which normally do not operate after birth, are: (1) the ductus venosis, (2) the foramen ovale, (3) the ductus arteriosis and (4) an inactive pulmonary circulation. The venous blood from the placenta at time of birth may be 50 to 60 per cent saturated with oxygen. As it traverses the liver, it divides into 2 branches, the major portion of flow being directed toward the left lobe. The branch to the right lobe receives unsaturated venous blood from the portal system. This is of some importance in comprehending the basis of some other changes in the liver in intra-uterine anoxia. The oxygenated blood from the left branch proceeds via the ductus venosis to the inferior vena cava and thence to the right auricle. While there is some mixture with venous blood in this vessel, the blood is oxygenated vastly better than the stream coming to the auricle from the superior vena cava. Two questions regarding this fetal circulation loom large today. The first has to do with whether there is a mixing of these two streams in the auricle, and the second has to do with the magnitude of the pulmonary circulation in utero. Formerly, it was thought that the 2 streams mixed in the auricle and that a mixed venous arterial blood circulated throughout the heart. Now, from the data available, it is thought that the blood from the superior stream passes through the tricuspid valve into the right auricle while the blood from the inferior stream proceeds to the left auricle by the foramen ovale and then to the left ventricle. Most investigators have assumed because of the anatomic importance of the ductus arteriosis that there was relatively little pulmonary circulation in utero and that most of the blood that came from the right ventricle reached the aorta through this shunt. The question of the magnitude of the pulmonary circulation is more than one of academic interest. If this circulation prior to the first breath is relatively of the same volume as it is after breathing has commenced, as Patten and Windle believe, then neither the ductus arteriosis nor the foramen ovale are of great importance to intra-uterine circulation and there is relatively little shift in hemodynamics with the onset of breathing. However, if the first breath inaugurates an opening of a little-used pulmonary circulatory bed and subsequent closure of the prenatal circulatory shunts, as Reynolds and Everett claim, then a very real burden is placed on the heart and the circulation at this period. Everett has shown that the amount of blood in the lungs of newborn guinea pigs increases 125 per cent in the first 24 hours of life. If this same phenomena occurs in humans, most normal infants' blood volume is sufficient to cover the burden. However, in some prematures, the sudden shift could induce a shocklike episode. It is possible that hyaline membrane disease is not so much one of a respiratory character as it is one of circulatory disturbance.

Another point of interest to the anesthesiologist is the extraordinary oxygen environment of the fetus. Because of the structure of the hemochorial placenta, fetal tissues necessarily must exist under much lower partial pressures of oxygen than do maternal tissues. Blood in the intervillous space, being a mixture of both the arterial and the venous systems, has a partial pressure of about 70 mm. of mercury or about two thirds that of arterial blood. This partial pressure is reduced further by transfer across the various layers making up the villi. Therefore, in the umbilical vein, which

PLATE 23

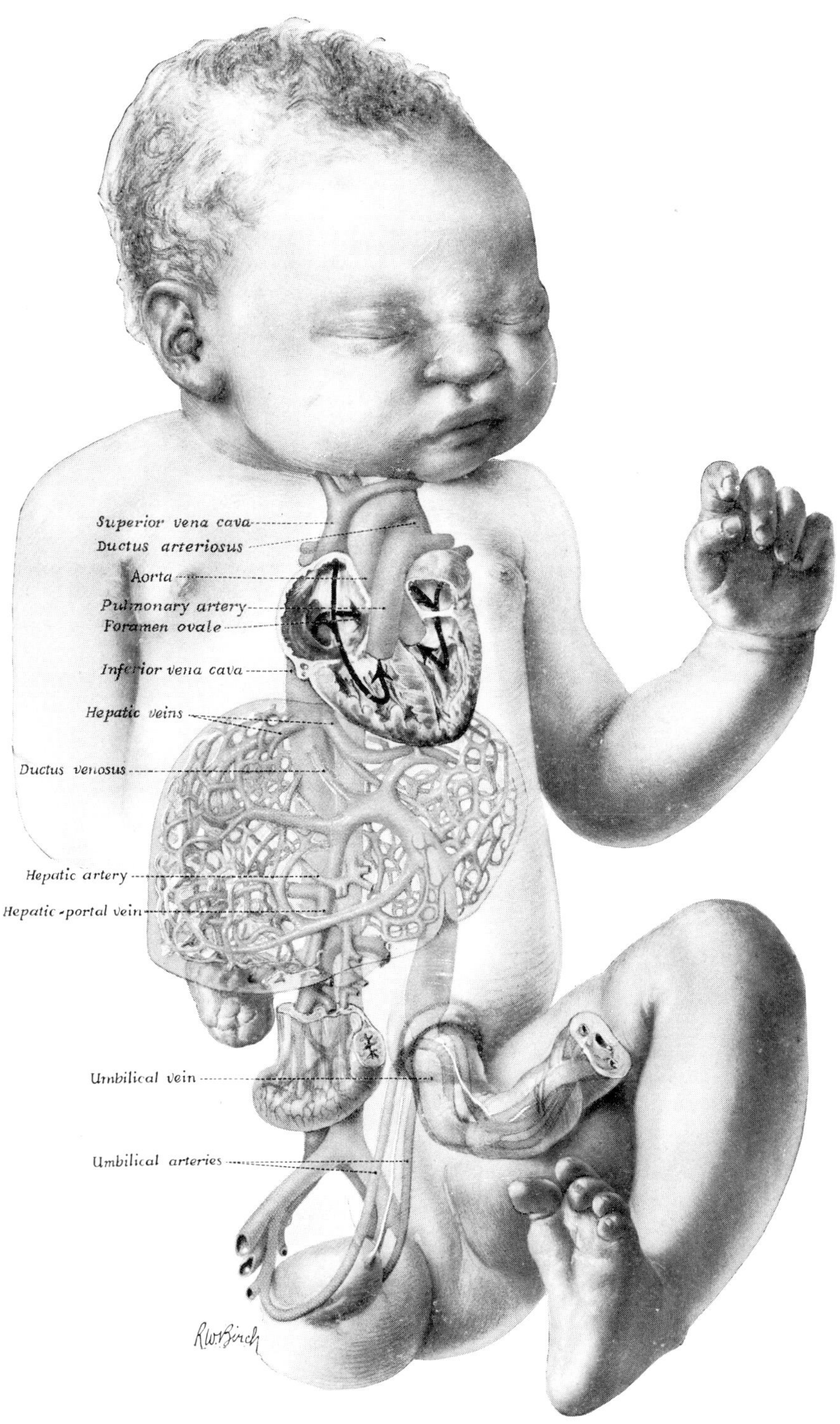

Cardiovascular system of fetus *in utero.* (Eastman, N. J.: Williams Obstetrics, ed. 11, New York, Appleton)

is the most oxygenated blood that the fetus receives, the partial pressure is only 40 mm. of mercury. These low pressures are responsible for the extremely low oxygen saturation of the fetus, amounting to 50 to 60 per cent. Not only is the fetus extremely cyanotic at these low pressures, but also it lives and grows in an environment in which no adult could live for more than a few minutes without additional oxygen support.

Exactly how the fetus manages this has been an intriguing question for scientists for several generations. It does so by adaptive mechanisms, some of which are known, but most of them are still unrevealed. Thus, fetal hemoglobin at birth is approximately 17 Gm., or about 20 per cent higher than in the adult. This is the same type of acclimatization as seen in peoples living at high altitudes. Then again, the fetal hemoglobin has peculiar properties in that its oxygen dissociation curve is shifted to the left, giving it a higher oxygen saturation for any given pressure. Interestingly enough, the fetal carbon-dioxide dissociation behaves in a reverse fashion, so that its affinity for this gas is less at any given pressure. Furthermore, the fetal carbonic anhydrase is considerably less than that shown in the adult. The reasons for these changes are not clearly understood. It is probable that the central nervous system of the fetus exists in a healthy state, not only by utilization of whatever oxygen it can get, but also by a system of anaerobic metabolism which it ceases to use shortly after birth.

It is peculiar that the human placenta, which transfers many, many times the amount of certain ions and water to the fetus than is required for its nutrition and development, fails to transfer oxygen in anything more than the barest minimum amounts necessary for survival. This point is of importance for the anesthesiologist. When the fetus begins to show signs of anoxia in utero, as demonstrated by bradycardia and passage of meconium, it already may be seriously damaged because of the low oxygen environment in which it exists. Certainly, remedial steps, if they are to be effective, should be quickly taken. The oxygenation to the fetus can be increased by the administration of certain drugs, that relax the uterus. Sometimes, this is accomplished with sedation or with block anesthetics. The oxygenation of the fetus also can be improved by administration of oxygen to the mother. While it is impossible to increase the saturation of oxygen in the intervillous space by breathing 100 per cent oxygen the mother can get rid of a certain amount of nitrogen in her blood and thus materially increase the partial pressure of oxygen in the intervillous space, thereby bettering the gradient across the placental villi.

RESPIRATION AND OXYGENATION

In obstetrics, as in surgery, there must be a thorough understanding of the physiology of respiration and the standard methods of oxygenation of the parturient during analgesia and anesthesia. Likewise, full attention must be given to carbon dioxide elimination. Resuscitative procedures for both mother and infant must be mastered.

Physiology of Respiration

The medullary respiratory center, acutely sensitive to humoral and pH changes, is a governor of both rate and depth of respiration. A rise in carbon dioxide concentrations in the arterial blood immediately stimulates this center, whereas a drop in carbon dioxide concentration or profound chemical or toxic narcosis of obstetric analgesia and/or anesthesia depresses the center's func-

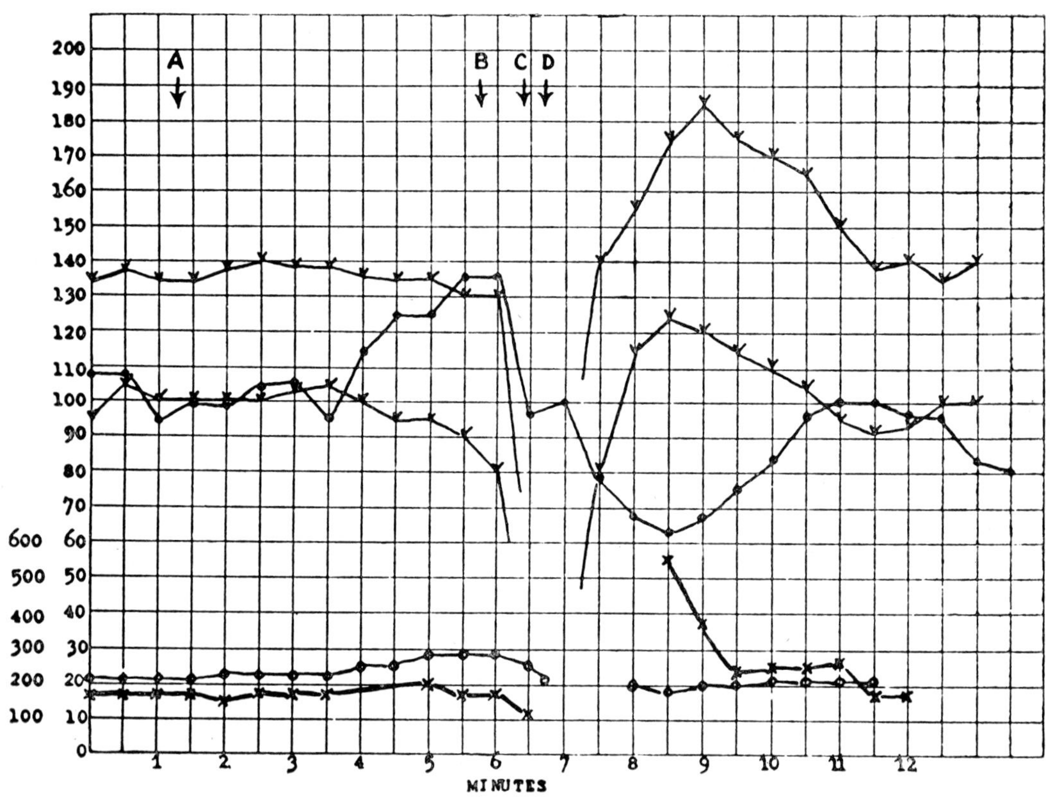

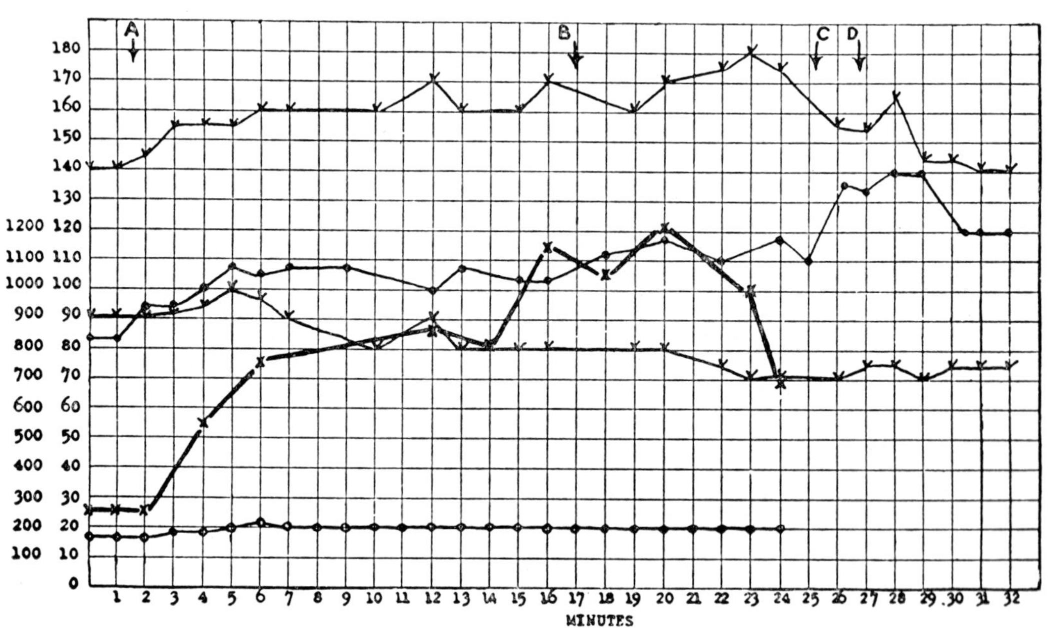

FIG. 38. (*Top*) The effect of experimentally induced hypoxia is shown at B. (*Bottom*) The effect of carbon dioxide retention is shown at A. (A.M.A. Fundamentals of Anesthesia, ed. 3, Philadelphia, Saunders)

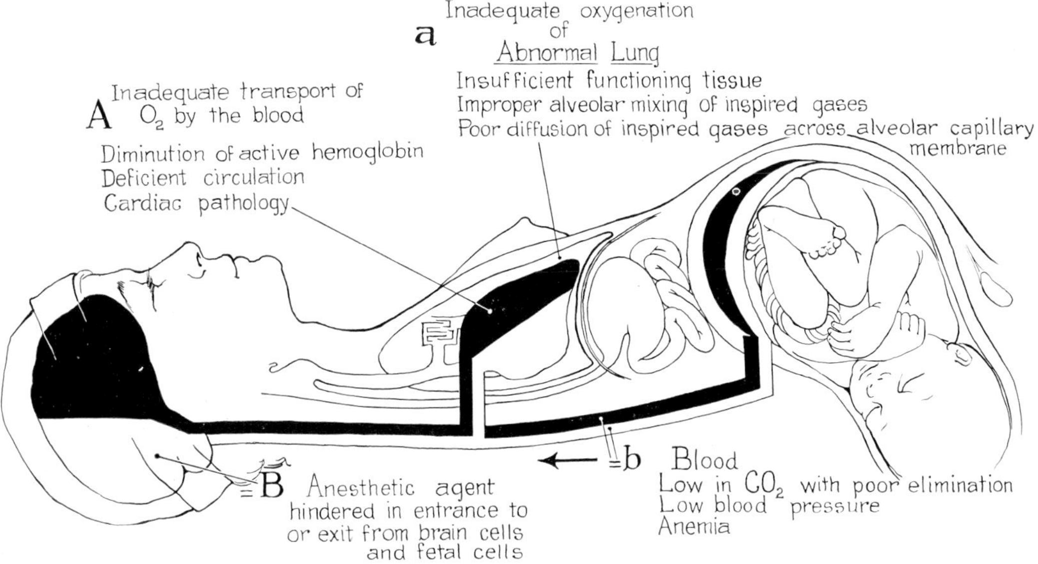

Fig. 39. Inadequate fetal and maternal oxygenation.

tion. The lung receptors constitute a peripheral checking mechanism, preventing overdistention through the Hering-Breuer reflex. The receptors of the carotid and the aortic bodies (chemoreceptors) are extremely sensitive to changes in oxygen tension of the arterial blood. In hypoxemia these receptors transmit stimulating impulses to the respiratory center, initiating deeper and more rapid respiration. Conversely, inhalation of gas mixtures containing high concentrations of oxygen depress these chemoreceptors slightly, resulting in a slight temporary respiratory depression. In the physiologic state, this dual control mechanism provides adequate intake of oxygen and adequate carbon dioxide elimination. The anesthetist and the obstetrician should be keenly aware of the pharmacologic and toxicologic effect of analgesia and anesthesia upon this vital mechanism. Likewise, the processes of disease in the mother's respiratory and circulatory systems must be assayed and corrected carefully, or at least compensated for, by auxiliary measures when there is gross interference with this vital mechanism.

Mechanics of Ventilation of the Lungs

Tidal Volume. In the obstetric patient, this measures from 350 to 500 cc. per breath.

Respiratory Minute Volume. At a respiratory rate of 15 to 20 times per minute, this amounts to 7.5 to 10 L. Thus, in semiclosed technics it is necessary to provide the patient with this volume of gas mixtures containing at least 20 per cent oxygen to eliminate entirely the hazard of carbon dioxide accumulation.

Total Air Capacity. At term, the total air capacity of the lungs is somewhat reduced by the abdominal enlargement of the uterus. This total air capacity may be reduced from 6,000 to 3,500 cc.

Dead Space. The 150 cc. in the mouth, the pharynx, the larynx, the trachea and the bronchi, not in intimate contact with the alveolar spaces, or involved in gas exchange, is called the *dead space*. This amount must be subtracted

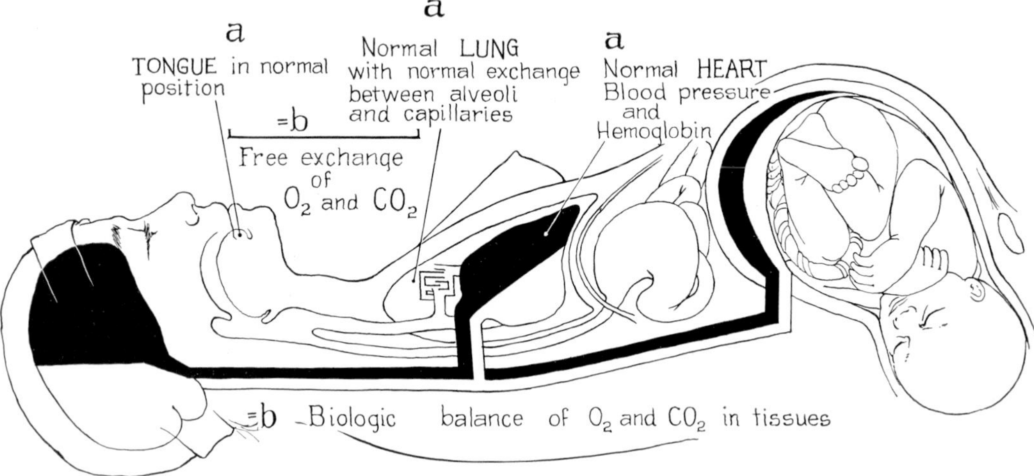

FIG. 40. Normal maternal and fetal oxygenation.

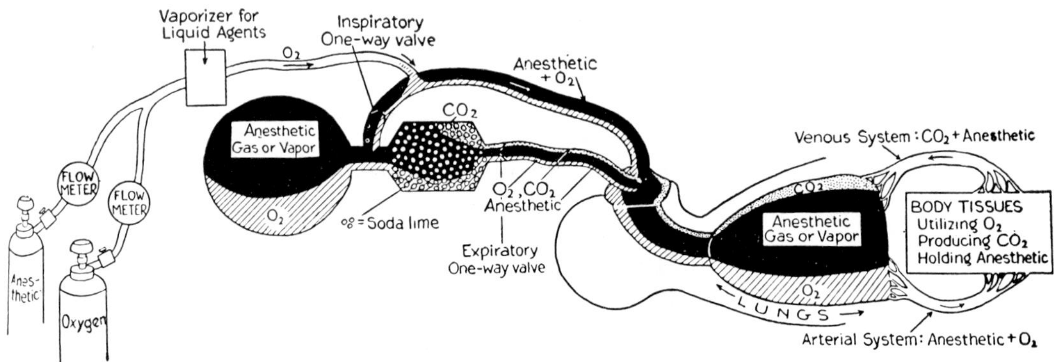

FIG. 41. The transport of gases and vaporized agents to the lungs and the body tissues by the closed system. (A.M.A. Fundamentals of Anesthesia, ed. 3, Philadelphia, Saunders)

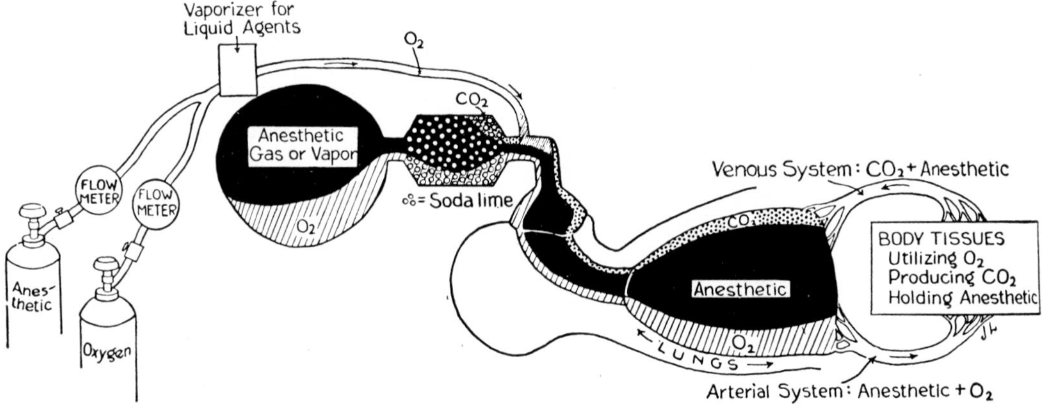

FIG. 42. The semiclosed system of transport of gases and vaporized agents to the lungs and the body tissues. (A.M.A. Fundamentals of Anesthesia, ed. 3, Philadelphia, Saunders)

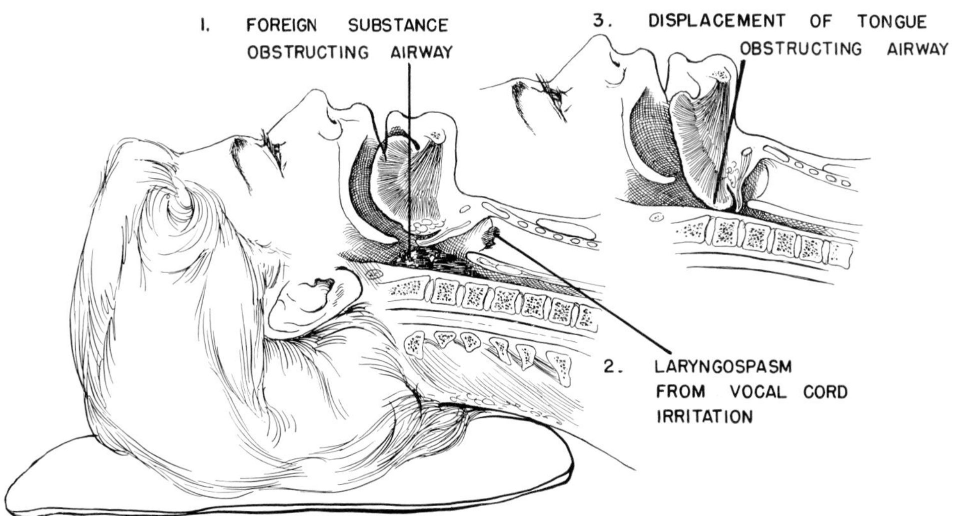

Fig. 43. Obstructions to the air passages: (1) by foreign substances, (2) by laryngospasm or bronchospasm, (3) by the tongue's blocking the pharynx.

from the tidal volume to yield the effective alveolar ventilation.

In view of the facts that the obstetric patient at term has an increased metabolic rate, has less tidal volume, less total air capacity and the added responsibility of oxygenating the fetus across the placental barrier, both the anesthetist and the obstetrician have increased responsibilities in maintaining adequate maternal oxygenation and carbon dioxide elimination of two patients at the same time.

In respiratory disease, major depression of the respiratory center and reduction in hemoglobin, interference with normal circulatory dynamics has a much greater significance in obstetrics than in general surgery.

This transport system is well described in the diagrams in Figures 39 to 42.

The diagrams in Figures 43 and 44 illustrate the most common causes and results from respiration obstruction. The danger from aspiration of vomitus in obstetrics has been documented already in increasing numbers of maternal deaths caused thereby and has been reported in the literature. From recent surveys the authors have collected data on 161 maternal deaths caused by this hazard. This is probably one of the most frequent causes of anesthetic deaths in ob-

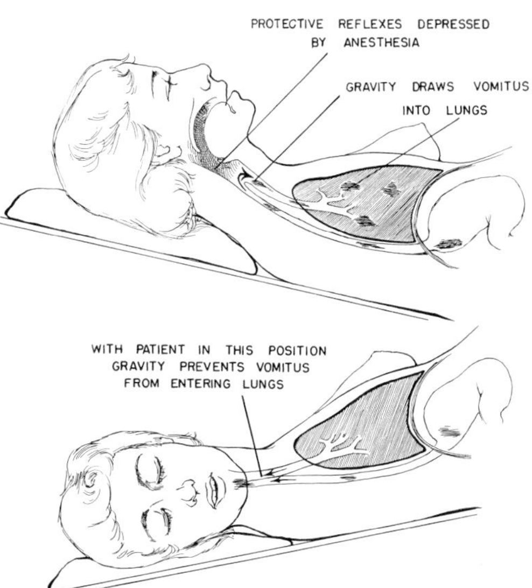

Fig. 44. (*Top*) Obstructed air passage caused by vomitus or blood. (*Bottom*) Prevention of obstruction by tilting the patient so that her head is lower than her body.

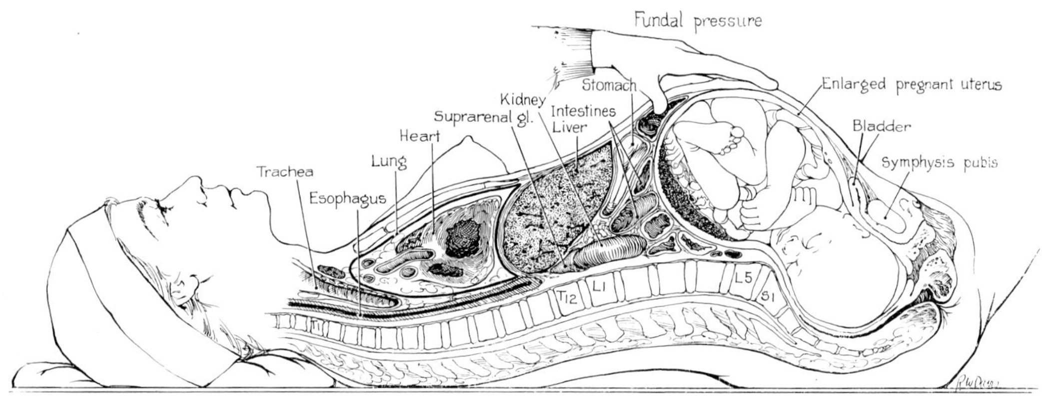

FIG. 45. Factors inhibiting normal chest expansion during obstetric anesthesia for vaginal delivery.

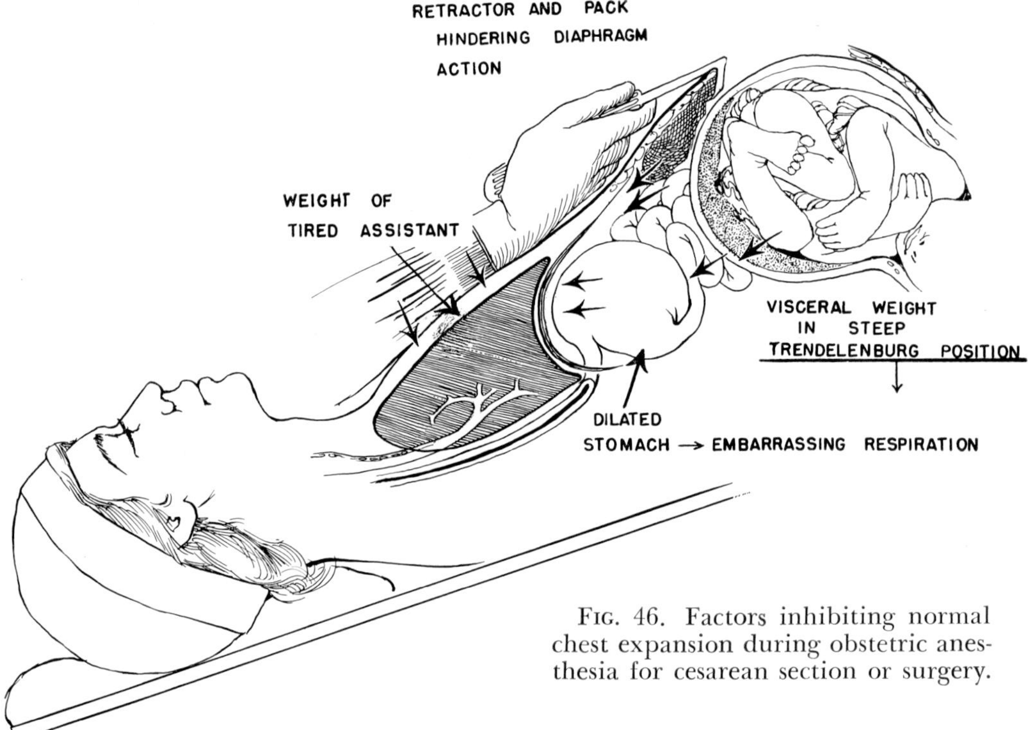

FIG. 46. Factors inhibiting normal chest expansion during obstetric anesthesia for cesarean section or surgery.

stetrics. Merrill and Hingson analyzed this subject in a paper in *Current Researches in Anesthesia and Analgesia,** as follows:

Furthermore, such aspiration may be both fatal to the fetus and a cause of anxiety to the anesthesiologist and obstetrician. The following are predisposing factors that are of particular significance in pregnant women:

1. By unfortunate coincidence labor frequently begins within an hour or two after ingestion of food.

2. Gastric motility is seriously impaired in labor, with the result that food ingested shortly

* Merrill, R. B., and Hingson, R. A.: Study of incidence of maternal mortality from aspiration of vomitus during anesthesia occurring in major obstetric hospitals in United States, Anesth. & Analg. **30**:121-135.

before the beginning of labor may be retained in the stomach for a long period.

3. Planned anesthetic premedication in many cases is impossible.

4. Certain obstetric emergencies, such as hemorrhage and fetal distress, might dictate immediate operative intervention without proper preparation.

5. Limitation of respiratory exchange by subdiaphragmatic encroachment of the enlarged uterus predisposes the obstetric patient and the fetus to dangers of anoxia as illustrated in Figures 45 and 46.

6. Light anesthesia is required more frequently in obstetrics in order to maintain uterine contractility and co-operation of the patient.

VOMITING DURING ANESTHESIA AND DELIVERY

Emptying time of the stomach, according to Best and Taylor, after an ordinary mixed meal is from 3 to 4½ hours. The fluid leaves the stomach more rapidly than the solids. For most women in labor this would provide ample time to ensure an empty stomach before delivery, if no food were given. However, some women in labor have decreased gastric motility and retention of food as shown by the type and amount of vomitus during anesthesia and delivery. Guedel* states, "Too much emphasis cannot be placed upon the danger from aspiration of vomitus. . . . Accident cases and women in labor, when brought to the hospital as emergencies, are the worst offenders. Unless there is positive evidence that no food has been taken within the past eight hours, their stomachs must be assumed to be full." Multiparas may eat a full meal just before going into labor and then have short labors. Since most women seem to bolt their food and many feel it necessary to take a sustaining morsel just before entering the hospital, there are apt to be large pieces of undigested food in the stomach.

Hirscheimer *et al.* found that in gastro-intestinal serial roentgenograms on 10 primigravidas in labor, 2 of the 10 women showed delayed gastric emptying time, and the rest had normal gastric evacuation. From this small series, they stated that there was no constant or characteristic alteration of gastric evacuation in primiparas during labor and that delay apparently occurs in some patients as an individual disturbance.

Chase studied the gastric emptying time of mongrel dogs under treatment with analgesic or amnesic agents or combinations of agents commonly used in obstetrics. He utilized serial roentgenograms. He found that barbiturates, Amytal, Seconal, or pentobarbital seemed scarcely to delay the gastric emptying time at all, despite the production of pronounced ataxia. Meperidine (Demerol) and methadone (AN 148) in average doses delayed the gastric emptying time slightly, except in particularly sensitive animals. Morphine and methadone in large doses produced a decided delay in passage of a test meal, as shown by roentgen ray. Scopolamine in 5 doses over a 5-hour period greatly prolonged emptying time and in combination with other medications added to their effects. The doses and the combination of drugs employed were designed to simulate those used in obstetric practice. Delayed gastric emptying time varied from 1 to 9 hours. Chase states that delay in emptying the stomach of food may be brought about by the emotional and physical strain of labor in synergism with the pharmacologically depressed activity of the smooth muscle of the gastro-intestinal tract. Often such residual food is augmented by fluids and gas. At the time of delivery, when there is pressure on the fundus of the uterus to aid in expulsion of the fetus, some of the force may be exerted against a distended stomach. With the patient under anesthesia the reflex that prevents regurgitation is abolished. The anesthetist likewise has no warning from the usual reflex signs of vomiting. Such patients may awake with pain in the chest, blood tinged sputum, cyanosis, tachycardia and hyperpnea.

Hartzell and Mininger state that out of 20 cases of bronchopneumonia from aspiration of gastric contents following ether anesthesia in obstetrics, only 2 patients had eaten within 6 hours and 16 patients had not eaten 6 hours or more before anesthesia.

W. A. Weiss reported that the three main factors that favored regurgitation and aspiration into the lungs were:

1. Complicated induction of anesthesia including swallowing and vomiting during this phase

2. Light anesthesia during operation with coughing, swallowing or vomiting

3. Surgical manipulation and position of patient on operating table. When the anesthetist is experienced, incidence of regurgitation tends to be lower.

Hall has reported 15 cases of aspiration pneumonitis with 5 deaths. Of the 15 cases, 14 were women in labor and 1 was undergoing a surgical operation. Three of these cases died of respiratory obstruction on the delivery or operating table, and 2 resulted in delayed deaths from bronchopneumonia with secondary bacterial in-

* Guedel, A. E.: Inhalation Anesthesia, ed. 2, pp. 89, 90, New York, Macmillan.

vasion. One died 22 hours and another 13 days postpartum.

DeLee and Greenhill have reported that incidence of dilatation of stomach of women in labor occurs more often than usually realized. This atony predisposes to eructation of massive amounts of vomitus as soon as the protective pharyngeal reflex is lost during general anesthesia. Light in-and-out anesthesia also is conducive to vomiting.

Gordon, of Brooklyn, who reports 15 deaths from this cause, states that if delivery impends within 12 hours after admission to hospital it should be assumed that the stomach is not empty.

With induction of anesthesia, the patient passes from Stage I with loss of consciousness into Stage II just lighter than surgical anesthesia when the vomiting center is hypersensitive. At this level pharyngeal reflexes are present and active. If the stomach is full or induction is slow in passing through this "area of danger," vomiting is apt to occur (Fig. 47). During recovery, according to Lundy, with emergence from the third stage, vomiting appears immediately after swallowing. Swallowing occurs during the lightest anesthesia of the third stage, and vomiting occurs during the deepest of the second stage. Warning signs of vomiting are shallow respiration, pale color, weak pulse and contracted pupils.

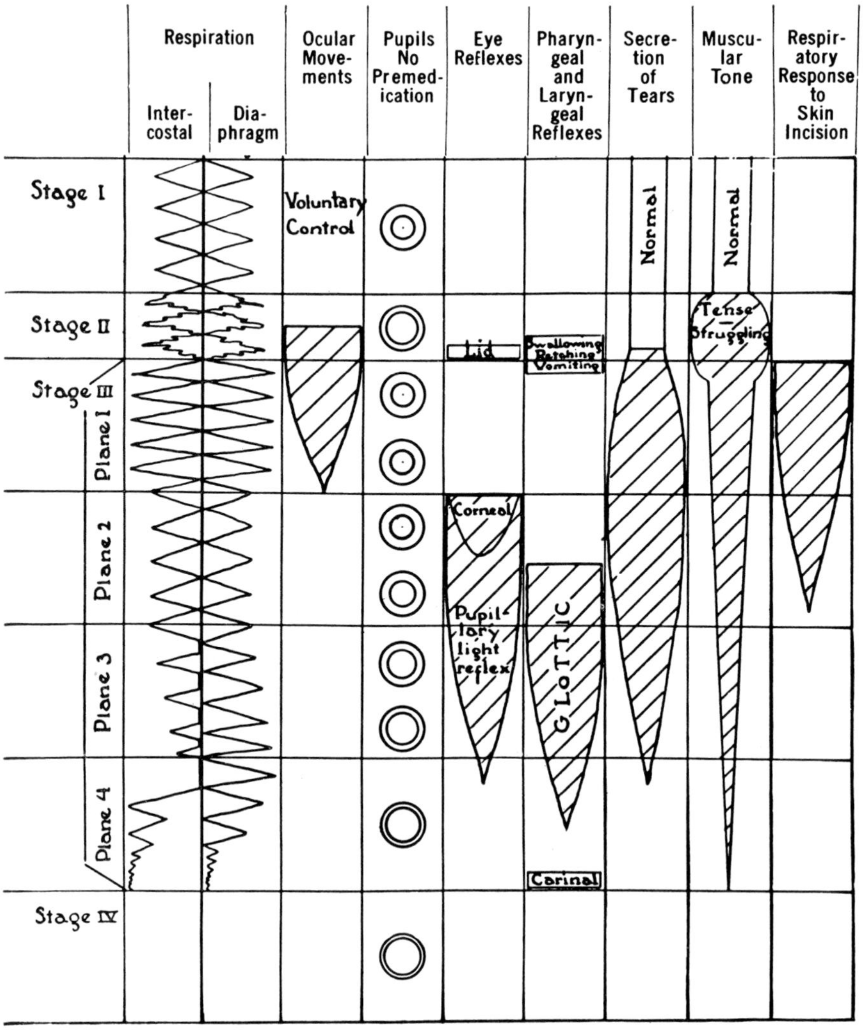

Fig. 47. Variations in the physiologic responses according to the stage of anesthesia. (A.M.A. Fundamentals of Anesthesia, ed. 3, Philadelphia, Saunders)

The act of vomiting is governed by the vomiting center in the medulla near the dorsal nucleus of the vagus close to the respiratory center. Efferent innervation which controls co-ordinated action of the muscles of esophagus, stomach and abdominal wall courses through the phrenic nerve, the vagi and the sympathetic nerves. Afferent stimulation from any part of the body can cause reflex vomiting.

Mendelson, in an excellent experimental work on rabbits, introduced into the lungs of rabbits, by laryngoscopy or tracheotomy 7 different materials as follows:

Distilled water
Normal saline solution
20 cc. of 0.1 normal hydrochloric acid
Unneutralized liquid vomitus from a patient
Neutralized liquid vomitus from a patient
Vomitus with solid undigested food from a patient
Neutralized vomitus with solid undigested food from a patient

From this study, Mendelson found two major types of reaction as cause of death: First vomitus with solid undigested food produced the classical picture of death from laryngeal or bronchial obstruction as seen in man. The pH of the fluid made no difference. When the rabbits were relieved of the obstruction, they recovered completely; with incomplete obstruction, the picture was one of massive atelectasis. The second reaction was an asthmatic type of chemical pneu-

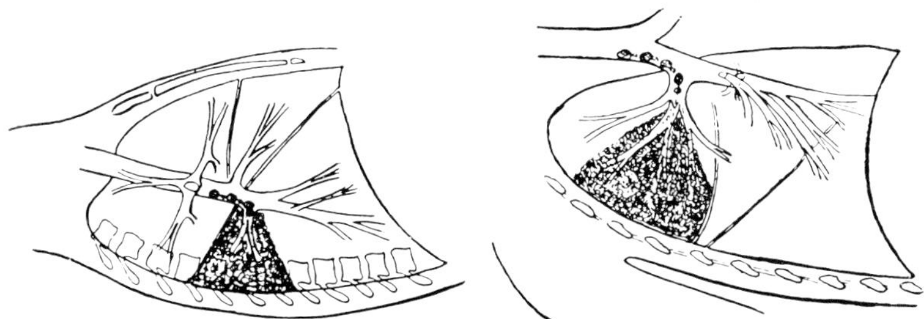

Fig. 48. The suggested relationship between posture and focal incidence of lung abscess. When the patient is lying on his back (*left*), the apical part of the lower lobe is vulnerable. (*Right*) When he is lying on his side, the "axillary" and posterior part of the upper lobe is affected. (Brock, R. C.: The Anatomy of the Bronchial Tree, ed. 1, London, Oxford)

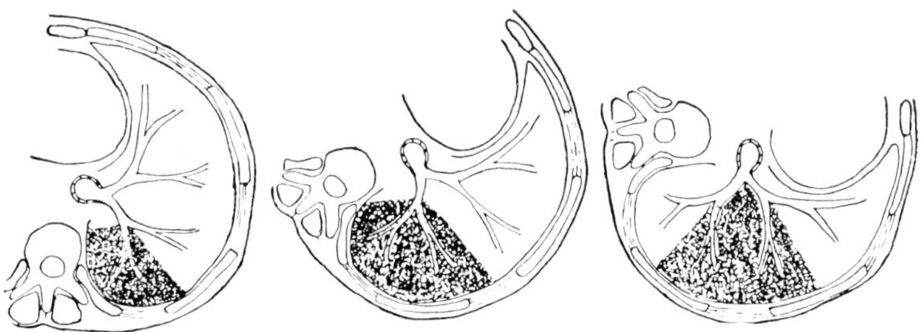

Fig. 49. The varying effect of an inhalation lesion in the right upper lobe, depending upon how much the patient is on his back or on his side. The segment of the bronchial tree shown is made up of the anterolateral and the posterolateral (pectoral and subapical) branches of the right upper lobe bronchus and is drawn accurately from an actual metal cast. (*Left*) Only the posterior branches of the subapical are affected. (*Right*) The "axillary" area is affected, i.e., axillary branches of the pectoral and the subapical bronchi. (Brock, R. C.: The Anatomy of the Bronchial Tree, ed. 1, London, Oxford)

monitis, found with unneutralized liquid vomitus and 0.1 normal hydrochloric acid.

The clinical signs and symptoms were cyanosis, tachycardia, dyspnea, wheezing with rales and rhonchi. Roentgenograms showed irregular, soft, mottled densities in the involved area. Death was due to cardiac failure and pulmonary edema with obstruction to the passage of oxygen through the alveolar membrane.

Brock, in a study of lung abscesses, has shown that bronchial configuration favors right-sided aspiration. In 12 months he had 35 cases of lung abscess in the right lung compared with 15 cases in the left lung. Hartzell and Mininger found that 15 of 20 cases of aspiration bronchopneumonia were on the right side, 3 cases were bilateral and only 2 were on the left side. The upper lobe was involved most often in their series.

With patient lying on the back, the most frequent site is the apical branch of the lower lobe. When the patient is lying wholly or partly on the side, the most likely site for a small amount of inhaled material is the subapical posterior and axillary portion of the upper lobes, especially the right. With a large amount of aspiration, both sides of the lungs will be involved. This is in accord with *Gray's Anatomy,* which states that "the right bronchus is wider, shorter and less abrupt in its divergence from the trachea than the left. On looking through a bronchoscope the carina is to the left of midline and the right bronchus appears as a more direct continuation of the trachea."* Figures 48 to 50 are reproduced from Brock.

Anoxia and Autopsy Observations

The central nervous system is especially sensitive to anoxia, and there is a gradient reaction in the different parts. Barach has shown selective vulnerability of the brain to be as follows:

1. Smaller pyramidal cells of the cortex
2. Purkinje cells in the cerebellar area
3. Medulla, retina and spinal cord
4. Spinal root ganglia

The length of time the brain can withstand anoxia varies from 2 to 20 minutes.

Irons and Apfelbach in a series of 1,074 autopsies found 160 cases of aspiration of stomach contents into the lungs with resultant bronchopneumonia and death. It is important that necropsy be done within 1 to 2 hours after death so that alterations do not confuse the picture. The pathologic picture shows lungs overdistended with air and not collapsed because of presence of aspirated material, exudate in the bronchial tree, hemorrhage and edema.

* Gray's Anatomy, vol. 26, p. 1217, Philadelphia, Lea & Febiger, 1954.

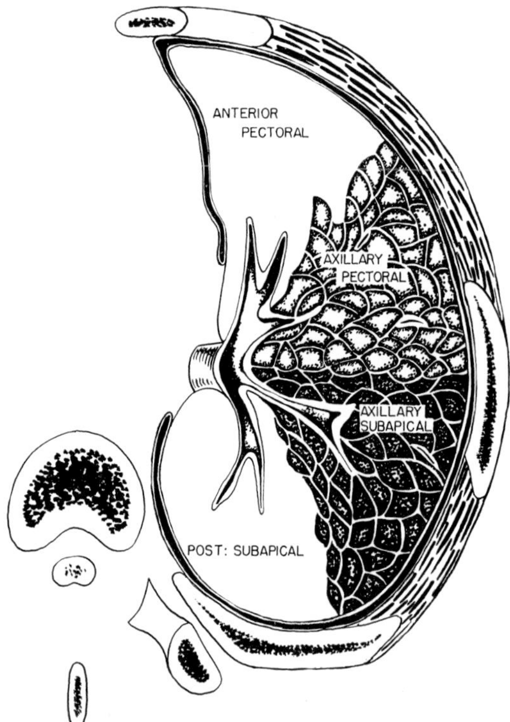

Fig. 50. Drawing of a slanting transverse section of the right upper lobe in which the axillary branches have been injected separately with gelatin to show the typical arrangement. The section is viewed from above. The drawing of the lung is from an actual specimen; the ribs and the vertebrae have been added to indicate their relationship. (Brock, R. C.: The Anatomy of the Bronchial Tree, ed. 1, London, Oxford)

The lungs are increased in weight unless death results from immediate suffocation. Blood in the lung is much darker due to chemical changes caused by aspirated gastric contents. The lung tissue is stained by hemolyzed blood. This is not characteristic of death by bacterial pneumonia. Examination of the bronchial tree shows intense hyperemia with material in the larger and the smaller bronchioles that resembles those found in the gastro-intestinal tract. Hemorrhage and hyperemic areas are unevenly distributed. Usually, there is dilatation of the stomach. To confirm their observations bacterial cultures were taken from lung, bronchial tree, stomach and right ventricle. These cultures showed the same organism, except that culture from the right ventricle was sterile and was used as control.

The microscopic picture shows intense engorgement of alveolar capillaries with erythrocytes and edema in alveolar spaces. There is extensive loss and desquamation of the lining of the bronchial tree with the desquamated cells found in the alveolar spaces. Particles of undigested food may be found in alveolar areas of hemorrhage and edema. Often, large masses of bacteria are present.

Treatment

1. Conservative for small amount of vomitus
   - A. Place patient immediately in deep Trendelenburg position.
   - B. Stop anesthesia to permit return of cough reflex and protective laryngeal reflex.
   - C. Establish suction under direct vision of airway down to larynx.
   - D. Administer 5 to 10 per cent carbon dioxide to produce hyperpnea.
   - E. Beat chest on each side, turning patient and urging cough.
   - F. Elevate foot of recovery bed.
   - G. Since the process is mainly irritative, direct therapy to bronchiolar spasm and cardiac embarrassment, with use of oxygen, atropine, adrenalin and aminophylline, together with antibiotics and chemotherapy to control infection.
2. Radical for complete obstruction or signs of suffocation
   - A. Tracheobronchial toilet must be accomplished by competent operator.
   - B. By direct bronchoscopic examination, aspiration is made, and any solid food removed immediately.
   - C. Above outline is continued.

Bronchoscopy is of little value in the asthmatic type of syndrome associated with chemical pneumonitis. It may only increase spasm or bleeding and may aid secondary invasion by bacteria.

Deaths from Aspiration of Vomitus Are Unnecessary

Prevention is more important than treatment.

1. Prenatal instruction by the physician should include warning of danger of eating at home after onset of labor.
2. In the hospital, all food should be withheld from patients in active labor; when indicated, parenteral administration of fluids and glucose and amino acids should be substituted.
3. In rapidly advancing labor of patients who have eaten within 6 hours, inhalation and intravenous anesthesia should be withheld unless the stomach is emptied artificially.
4. In such patients local, low-dose spinal and caudal analgesia should be substituted.
5. Competent administration of general anesthesia is required, with standard equipment by experienced anesthetists who are acutely aware of this danger during both induction and recovery.
6. Standard equipment in the delivery room for treatment of vomiting during anesthesia should include the following:
   - A. Adjustable table for Trendelenburg position
   - B. Efficient suction appartus
   - C. Laryngoscope and intratracheal tubes
   - D. Transparent face mask
   - E. Proper sizes of smooth airways of nasal and oropharyngeal type
   - F. Bronchoscope
7. Repeated and prolonged use of analgesic and amnesic drugs that delay gastric emptying time should be avoided.

Additional factors interfering with respiratory and circulatory physiology are presented in Figures 39 and 40. These emphasize clearly the importance of: (1) adequate airway; (2) respiratory exchange; (3) fluid balance; (4) adequate hemoglobin and (5) vasomotor tone. The anesthetist and the obstetrician must be equally conversant with this physiology and the correction of interfering pathologic processes in the mother that could jeopardize both the mother and the baby. There must be a complete understanding of such safeguards as: (1) available oxygen in efficient anesthetizing machines for every anesthetized patient; (2) workable suction apparatus; (3) intravenous fluid and vasopressor therapy; and (4) the elimination of synergistic incompatibilities resulting from unnecessary overdosage of the oxytocic drugs and the vasopressors. (Refer to p. 31, Chap. 2.) The obstetrician-anesthesiologist team that ignores or misinterprets anatomic fundamentals and physiologic basic principles in choosing and executing methods of management of labor and delivery endangers each mother and baby entrusted to it.

BIBLIOGRAPHY

Brock, Samuel: The Basis of Clinical Neurology, ed. 2, Baltimore, Williams & Wilkins, 1945.

The Ciba Collection of Medical Illustrations, vol. 2, Reproductive System, Summit, N. J., Ciba, 1954.

Cleland, J. G. .P: Paravertebral anesthesia in obstetrics: experimental and clinical basis, Surg., Gynec. & Obst. **57**:51, 1933.

Curtis, A. H., Anson, B. J., Ashley, F. L., and Jones, T.: The anatomy of the pelvic autonomic nerves in relation to gynecology, Surg., Gynec. & Obst. **75**:743, 1942.

DeLee, Joseph B., and Greenhill, J. P.: Principles and Practice of Obstetrics, ed. 8, Philadelphia, Saunders, 1943.

Dogliotti, A. M.: Anesthesia (English translation by C. S. Scuderi), Chicago, S. B. Debour, 1939.

Eastman, N. J.: Mount Everest in utero, Am. J. Obst. & Gynec. **67**:701, 1954.

Gruber, C. M.: The autonomic innervation of the genito-urinary system, Physiol. Rev. **13**:497, 1933.

Hare, Kendrick: The visceral functions of the nervous system, Ann. Rev. Physiol. **8**:375, 1946.

Hirsch, E. F., and Martin, M. E.: The distribution of nerves in the adult human myometrium, Surg., Gynec. & Obst. **76**: 697, 1943.

Lanier, Patricia Farnsworth, and Trotter, Mildred: The volume of the sacral canal, Am. J. Phys. Anthrop., N.S., **4**:—, 1946.

Lanier, Virginia Singleton, McKnight, Howard E., and Trotter, Mildred: Caudal analgesia: an experimental and anatomical study, Am. J. Obst. & Gynec. **47**: 633, 1944.

Learmonth, J. R.: A contribution to the neurophysiology of the urinary bladder in man, Brain **54**:147, 1931.

Letterman, Gordon S., and Trotter, Mildred: Variations of the male sacrum: their significance in caudal analgesia, Surg., Gynec. & Obst. **78**:551, 1944.

Maxson, Louis H.: Spinal Anesthesia, Philadelphia, Lippincott, 1938.

Moore, D., and D'Esopo, D. A.: The Friedman curve as adapted to study of uterine inertia, Am. J. Obst. & Gynec., 1955 (in press).

Morris' Human Anatomy, ed. 10, edited by J. Parsons Schaeffer, Philadelphia, Blakiston, 1932.

Needles, Joseph Herman: The caudal level of termination of the spinal cord in American whites and American Negroes, Anat. Rec. **63**:417, 1935.

Peham, H. v., and Amreich, J.: Operative Gynecology (translated by L. K. Ferguson), vol. 1, p. 60, Philadelphia, Lippincott, 1934.

Pitkin, George P.: Conduction Anesthesia, ed. 2, revised and edited by James L. Southworth and Robert A. Hingson, Philadelphia, Lippincott, 1953.

Ranson, S. W.: The Anatomy of the Nervous System, ed. 7, Philadelphia, Saunders, 1943.

Reynolds, S. R. M., Harris, J. S., and Kaiser, I. A.: Clinical Measurement of Uterine Forces in Labor, Springfield, Thomas, 1954.

Rutherford, R. N.: Presacral neurectomy: a gynecological and obstetrical follow up, West. J. Surg., Obst. & Gynec. **50**:597, 1942.

Shidler, Frederic B., and Richards, Victor: Anterior sacral meningocele, Ann. Surg. **118**:913, 1943.

Smith, C. A.: The Physiology of the Newborn Infant, ed. 2, Springfield, Thomas, 1951.

Southworth, J. L., and Hingson, R. A.: Continuous caudal analgesia in surgery, Ann. Surg. **118**:945, 1943.

Stander, Henricus, J.: Textbook of Obstetrics, New York, Appleton-Century, 1945.

Trotter, Mildred: The sacrum and sex, Am. J. Phys. Anthrop. **9**:445, 1926.

Trotter, Mildred, and Heath, Robert D.: Transverse sacral folds, J. Bone & Joint Surg. **28**:120, 1946.

Trotter, Mildred, and Lanier, Patricia F.: Hiatus canalis sacralis in American whites and Negroes, Human Biology, **17**: 368, 1945.

Trotter, Mildred, and Letterman, Gordon S.: Variations of the female sacrum: their significance in continuous caudal anesthesia, Surg., Gynec. & Obst. **78**:419, 1944.

Wheeler, Theodora: Variability in the spinal column as regards defective neural arches (rudimentary spina bifida), Carnegie Institution of Washington, Publication No. 272, Contributions to Embryology **9**:97, 1920.

Windle, W. F.: Physiology of the Fetus, Philadelphia, Saunders, 1940.

———: Respiratory conditions in the fetus and effects of their impairment, Harvey Lectures **40**:236, 1945.

»» 4 «« Technics in Obstetric Amnesia, Analgesia and Anesthesia

Frontal Lobe Block—Total Brain Block—Regional Nerve Block

Since the pharmacologic principles, the supportive therapy and the management of complications before, during and after labor and delivery are presented in detail in other chapters, the material in this chapter will be given in an arbitrary and didactic fashion for instantaneous reference and use. By no means do we wish to imply a separation from or a disregard of the initial physical and psychological preparation of the patient and the surrounding of parturient and her baby with every proved safeguard that a modern hospital should provide. Rather, we present herewith the sequential use of both tested and modern knowledge in the management of both labor and delivery.

In general, all technics used in obstetric analgesia and anesthesia can be grouped into 5 major categories, as listed below:

Group 1. Systemic sedation for labor and general inhalation anesthesia for delivery with agents nitrous oxide, ethylene, cyclopropane, trichlorethylene and ether.

Group 2. Systemic sedation for labor and intravenous barbiturate anesthesia for delivery with agents Pentothal Sodium, Surital Sodium, Seconal Sodium and Nembutal.

Group 3. No drugs other than 50 mg. Demerol during labor or delivery, but psychoanalgesia established with suggestion, comfortable air-conditioned environment, therapeutic music and interior decorating.

Group 4. Systemic sedation for labor with terminal conduction block of spinal, caudal or local for delivery.

Group 5. Continuous conduction block without systemic narcosis during labor and delivery. However, the following technics are described as uncombined methods of management and may be grouped together as synergistic supplements as indicated by the requirements of obstetrician, anesthesiologist and patient.

PHYSIOLOGIC RELAXATION THERAPY: PSYCHOLOGICAL LOBOTOMY

Most experienced normal multiparas and some primiparas can be managed by this method in a satisfactory manner. The success of the method is dependent upon:

1. The enthusiasm engendered and the faith fulfilled in the minds of parturients, obstetric nurses, obstetricians and anesthetists who practice it.
2. The total efficiency of the educational program.
3. The comfort and the decor of the labor and delivery environment.
4. The understanding and the support of the husband.
5. The elimination of unnecessary language suggestive of pain by all personnel; the soundproofing or quarantining of distracting noises of the average maternity from the patient.
6. The sympathetic and trained professional team's patience, desire and readiness to win with parturient this predominance of "mind over matter."

However, let none be deceived. There is less total relief from discomfort with this method practiced in its purest form than with the other methods. Yet when used as some of the basic philosophy of the obstetric art, it is of value in conjunction with all methods through:

1. Protecting both mother and baby from undesirable and excessive narcosis.

2. Reducing the duration and the degree of narcosis.

3. Permitting the parturient the privilege of belonging to the team concerned with her own baby's birth and of sharing the joy of accomplishment denied her in the total amnesia, analgesia and general anesthesia technics.

4. Interfering the least with the physiologic tempo of labor and delivery.

Yet, in our hospitals the parturient is made to know that her election to forego other forms of analgesia and anesthesia in no way removes from her the safeguards of oxygenation, airway management, control of hemorrhage, resuscitative measures for the baby and standard expensive equipment so often needed suddenly and unexpectedly in obstetrics and anesthesia. Nor does it reduce staff requirements commensurate with the daily case load. Wherever these total factors are ignored, anesthesia services become atrophic and inadequate, and thus would obstetrics itself return to the midwifery from which it sprang.

Requirements

1. Intelligent instruction of patient in processes of normal labor begun during prenatal visits to obstetrician

2. Comfortable and cheerful environment of labor room

3. Teaching patient to dissociate herself from uterine contractions and to relax as completely as possible during them

4. In case discomfort becomes extreme, use of 50 mg. of meperidine hydrochloride (Demerol Hydrochloride) every 3 or 4 hours during active labor is beneficial. The instructed multipara requires on the average 160 mg. during labor; the instructed primipara requires on the average 186 mg. during labor. Extreme care should be used to avoid maximum depression caused by the drug.

PSYCHOPROPHYLACTIC PAINLESS CHILDBIRTH

(The Technic Conducted by Dr. Lamaze at the Maternité des Metallurgistes in Paris, Based upon the Concepts of Conditioned Reflexes First Defined by Pavlov and Developed by Nikolaev, of Russia)

This method is based on 3 principles:

1. The parturient arrives in the delivery room after a psychic preparation that has built in her cerebral cortex a certain number of conditioned reflexes inhibiting the perception of uterine contractions as painful stimuli.

2. Childbirth must be an active process in which the parturient is thoroughly instructed and aware of the sequence of events surrounding parturition and personally takes an active part in following or, rather, mastering the successive episodes of her confinement.

3. The parturient has been taught certain reactions, built as conditioned reflexes, which she will practice actively during childbirth. These reactions contribute to the maintenance of the conditioned state necessary to painful confinement.

The 3 principles of the psychoprophylactic method of painless childbirth are described further:

1. Until now it has been admitted universally that painful contractions are the first symptoms of onset of labor. Every obstetrician points out this fact during the last weeks of pregnancy. Not every pregnant woman knows very much about confinement, but she is aware of the fact that the beginning of her par-

turition is induced by painful contractions. She knows that these pains are due to increase progressively until the very end. She is prepared to feel the uterine contractions as painful.

Credit must be given to the Psychoprophylactic Method of Painless Childbirth in helping to change this attitude. Now, pregnant women are taught that the former ideas were correct for *unprepared* parturients, for whom confinement was an unknown, mysterious and painful process. But the patient who *knows* exactly everything about the different phases of childbirth, who knows how to behave, what to do in every circumstance, who has confidence in her physicians and her nurses and has been trained and prepared psychically in conditioning her brain against pain, can consider with certainty the former assertions as obsolete and incorrect.

2. The psychic preparation is based on studies of the Physiology of Adaptation as described in the basic principles:

By birth we have a certain number of fundamental mechanisms of reacting. As soon as a baby is born, it cries. If a finger is put into its mouth, the child sucks. No one has taught it these actions. They are fundamental and are called *unconditioned reflexes,* phylogenetically acquired and strongly built into the nervous system. Because of these inherent mechanisms, a certain number of special exciting factors stimulating special zones of the body produce very precise reactions. For example, we know how salivation can be provoked by seeing food or thinking of one's favorite dish. If you show a piece of meat to a dog, he salivates; it is an *unconditioned reflex,* as described in the famous Pavlov experiment. If you simultaneously ring a bell, after a certain number of repetitions, say 20 or 30, the mere sound of the bell will produce salivation. You have built a conditioned reflex in the dog's brain. New and temporary nervous connections have been produced in the brain cortex between the point of excitation due to the bell and the center of the *unconditioned reflex* of salivation. The bell's sound has become a conditioning factor, a conditioning stimulus or signal.

Conditioned reflexes constitute a system of temporary connections between signals in the corresponding activities of the brain. Numerous signals strike our nervous system simultaneously. Some of these come from without and others from within, the latter being proprioceptive and interoceptive signals. But, fortunately, only a certain number of these signs have the capacity to produce a certain number of *specific dynamic stereotypes.*

This selection and concentration of our activity is realized by 2 fundamental nervous processes, namely, *positive excitation* and *negative excitation* or *inhibition.*

This negative or suppressive activity of the brain cortex can be conditioned in the same way as positive excitation. Inhibition is an active process and its biologic activity is not reduced. With a stimulus a conditioned inhibitory factor may be built up. Consider the following experiment:

A strong electric current burns the skin of a dog for a short time. A normal defense reaction is observed. A few seconds later a piece of meat is given to the dog. After a certain number of repetitions of these proceedings, the irritating factor is transformed into a conditioned excitator of the alimentary reflex, and after the passage of the electric current *no longer is a defense reaction noted.* The feeling of pain has been inhibited, and the alimentary reaction has taken its place. When the British physiologist

Sherrington witnessed this experiment, he said: "Now I understand the martyrs' psychology."

The question arises: "What relation is there between these experiments and painful uterine contractions?" Salivary secretion is no more a simple glandular phenomenon than labor is a pure uterine action. The essential variability from one woman to another makes it clear that an important psychic factor must be considered.

The feeling of pain is neither a simple mechanical phenomenon nor a mysterious psychic one. It is the result of processes happening in the cerebral cortex where excitation and inhibition are in constant conflict. Perception of pain depends on the general functional state of the cortex. Perception of pain, as well as other signals, can be stimulated or inhibited by conditioning.

In painless childbirth the conditioning is the result of an education, of a real rational psychotherapy, modifying the cortical nervous activity and inhibiting the notion of pain correlated to uterine contractions. This education needs an average of 8 hours. From the seventh month on, the pregnant women are invited to attend 8 lectures. Here is the program of these lectures as conducted in Paris:

1. Theory on the building of conditioned reflexes
2. Theory on respiration. The importance of good oxygenation during pregnancy and childbirth is stressed, and effective breathing methods are shown.
3. Neuromuscular education
4. Theory on the first 2 stages of labor —dilatation and expulsion
5. How to behave during dilatation
6. How to behave during expulsion
7. Painless childbirth from the point of view of cortical nervous activity
8. Revision of the acquired notions; visit to a delivery room and, if possible, contacts with a recently delivered patient. Practical repetition (dress rehearsal of delivery) on the delivery table to make patients familiar with it. Finally, a film on painless childbirth is shown.

A pleasant atmosphere in the delivery room and in the hospital is essential. Confidence developed in physicians and nurses, as well as moral support, is of great importance. Everything must be done by the staff to prevent a "deconditioning" of the patient. For example, the word *pain* must be banned and replaced by *contractions.*

Now the results: On December 4, 1954, Dr. Lamaze claimed 3,522 painless deliveries. The failure rate was between 10 and 20 per cent, but undoubtedly 80 per cent of his parturients had a really painless confinement without any drug or sedative. One can understand that when no chemical sedative or depressing agent of any kind is used, the babies cry practically immediately. The astonishing perineal relaxation due to a conditioned attitude maintained during the second stage made episiotomies very rare.

Finally, Dr. Lamaze, of Paris, and Dr. I. Bonstein, of Geneva, summarized the advantages:

1. It is the most harmless process for both mothers and babies available at present.
2. It brings the physician the highest degree of professional satisfaction for not only having helped his patients physically but also for having built in their cortex a new attitude, a new state of mind, for which, as experience has shown, they are highly grateful. They gain a feeling of achievement and of accomplishment that may be of value in the familial structure, and it increases the prestige of the delivering physician.
3. In the 10 or 20 per cent of failures,

one meets the most co-operative patients for any kind of anesthetic procedure such as caudal, spinal or general anesthesia.*

SEDATION FOR AMNESIA AND ANALGESIA

While it is necessary to individualize dosage schedules of sedation for most patients according to the progress of labor, the following schedules have been satisfactory in providing a good measure of amnesia and safe analgesia.

Schedule 1. Barbiturates and Scopolamine Hydrobromide (Applicable for Second Through Fourth Quarters of First Stage of Labor)

1. Barbiturate: pentobarbital sodium (Nembutal), secobarbital (Seconal), vinbarbital sodium (Delvinal Sodium): 0.1 to 0.3 Gm. at onset of established labor. Established labor is the occurrence of regular painful uterine contractions resulting in progressive dilatation of cervix, usually present in a primipara when strong pains occur at intervals of 5 minutes or less and the cervix is dilated 3 cm., and in a multipara when cervix is dilated 4 cm.
2. Scopolamine: 0.4 to 0.6 mg. given hypodermically within 20 minutes.
3. Supplementary scopolamine: at intervals of 30 minutes to 2 hours as required. (Do not exceed total of 1.5 mg. Do not give added dosage within 1 hour of expected delivery time.)
4. Barbiturate: repeated doses of 0.1 to 0.2 Gm. every 4 hours as needed, but not within 2 hours of expected delivery, or longer interval if previous dosage has been high.

* One of the authors visited the clinics in Paris, Geneva and Lisbon conducting labor with these technics and found patient enthusiasm for these methods waning after the fifth cm. of cervical dilatation. Late labor was characterized by outcries and birth screams. The good statistics were the assessments of midwives and obstetricians, who arrived frequently after the birth of the baby.

Schedule 2. Meperidine Hydrochloride (Demerol Hydrochloride) and Scopolamine Hydrobromide (Applicable for Second Through Fourth Quarters of First Stage of Labor)

1. Barbiturate: 0.2 mg. by mouth or rectum at onset of established labor.
2. Meperidine: 50 to 100 mg. and scopolamine: 0.4 mg. by intramuscular injection within 20 minutes.
3. Meperidine: 50 to 100 mg. doses repeated every 3 to 4 hours as needed.
4. Supplementary scopolamine: not to exceed a total of 1.5 mg. at intervals of 30 minutes to 2 hours as required.

CONTINUOUS CAUDAL AND PERIDURAL ANALGESIA AND ANESTHESIA IN PAINFUL DISORDERS

Introduction

Conduction anesthesia through peripheral axon block of nerve impulses with local anesthetic solutions is 50 years younger than general anesthesia, but no less significant in the alleviation of suffering. However, since conduction anesthesia is regional, somatic or segmental, it is used to eliminate pain at its source of origin rather than to obtund its central interpretation. With its application, those areas of the body and those organs with innervation not affected by its contingent nerve depolarization are spared a primary effect upon their metabolism and physiology. Both general and conduction anesthesia have been used primarily to control, to prevent or to obliterate the impulses of pain.

Erlanger and Gasser and Bishop and O'Leary have determined that the nerve axons that transmit pain, thermal, touch and pressure, vasomotor, proprioceptive and motor impulses, vary in size and in their quantitative protection afforded by myelin insulation. They have determined that the vulnerability of the non-

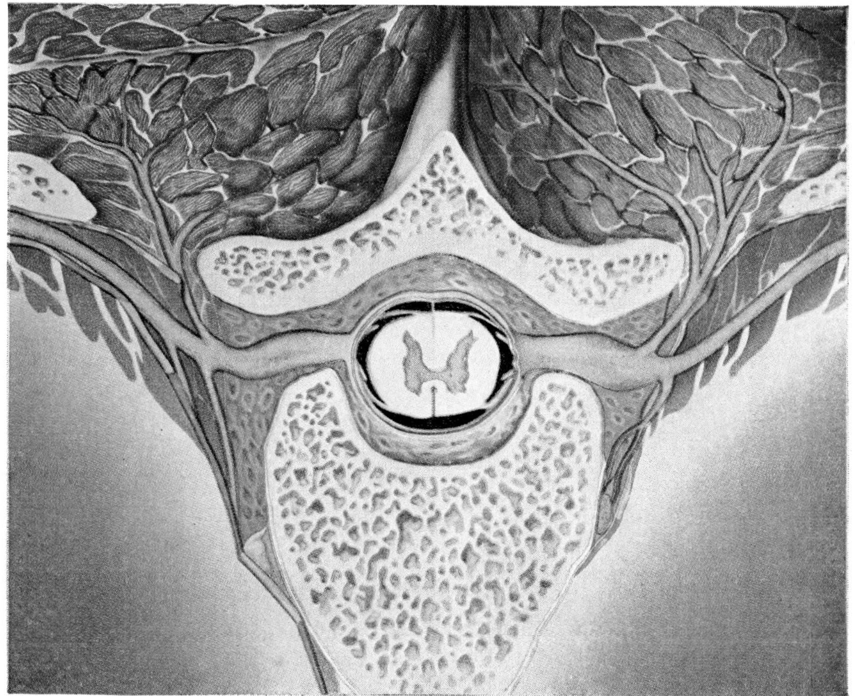

Cross section of vertebral column differentiating peridural and subarachnoid spaces.

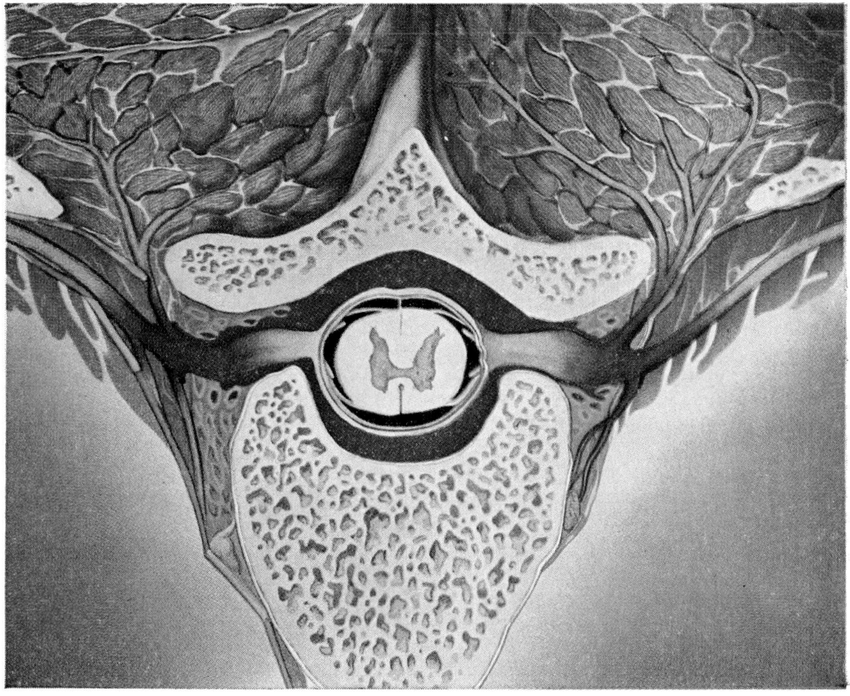

Cross section of vertebral column with injected anesthetic solution in peridural space emphasizing site of nerve block distal to merging of dura mater.

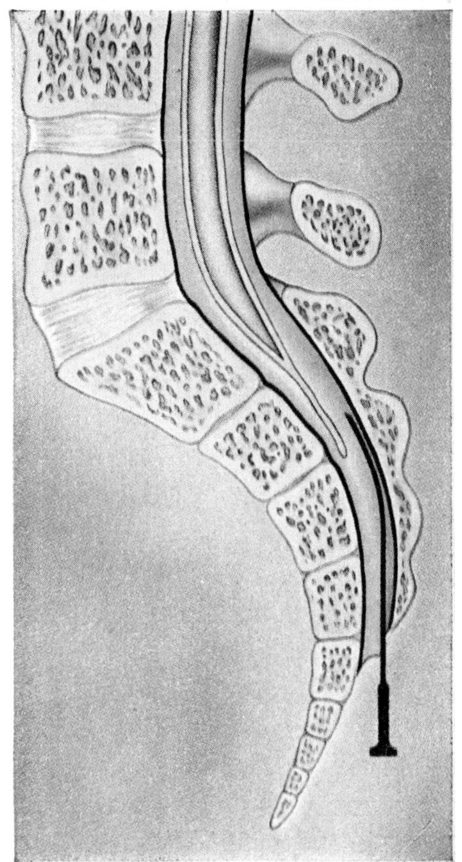

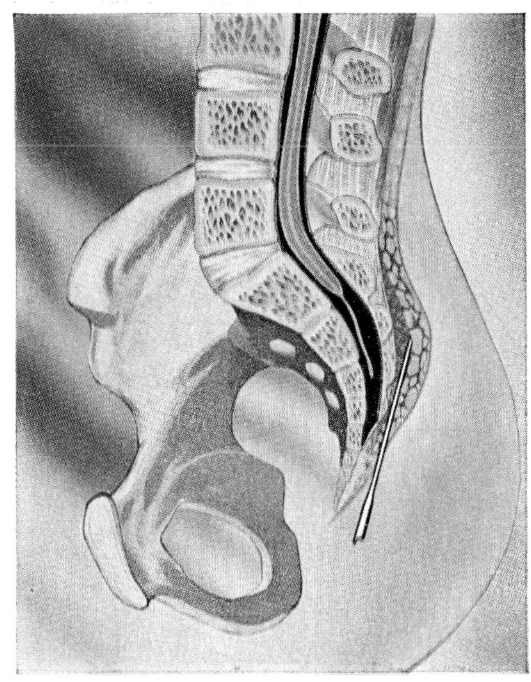

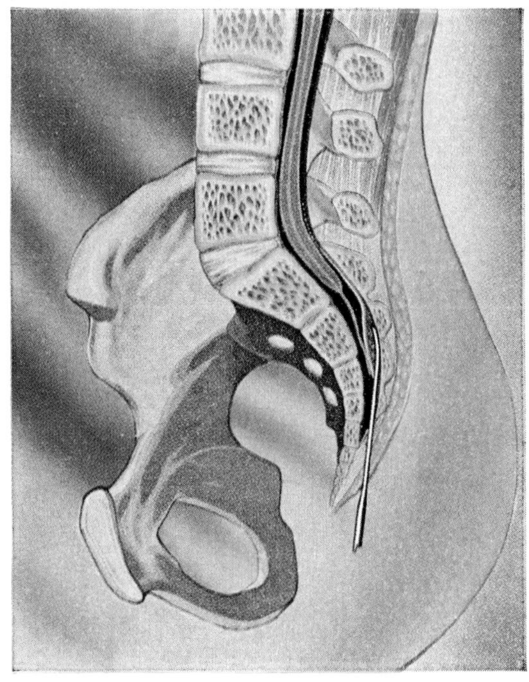

(Top, left) Sagittal section of sacral canal with caudal needle properly placed. *(Top, right)* Episacral injection. *(Bottom)* Subperiosteal injection. (The 2 figures at top, right, and bottom, right, are the most common errors of technic.)

myelinated pain and the vasomotor fibers (which are blocked earlier, more intensely and longer than the larger motor components) is the prime mechanism of therapeutic nerve block. We have substantiated their laboratory studies with an experience including observations on more than 15,000 patients under spinal, caudal, paravertebral, presacral, peridural and sympathetic ganglion anesthesia.

As the intensity of conduction anesthesia is accentuated with concentrations of anesthetic drugs more potent than is necessary to block out the small pain fiber, altered functions are produced in glands and viscera, blood vessels and heart, lungs and skin when the specific organ's nerve supply is affected.

The purpose of the authors in this section is: (1) to describe the development of continuous caudal and continuous peridural anesthesia in the prolonged control of pain; (2) to present the most effective technic with the safest and the most effective concentration of the anesthetic drug; (3) to emphasize the indications for these technics in specific disorders; (4) to delineate the hazards associated with faulty technic and with profound pharmacologic effect; (5) to provide the appropriate safeguard so that patient and physician may appreciate the application of the conduction anesthesia technic as a delightful experience. If the physician masters these stated criteria, these technics become tools in his hand with which he is able to unshackle the parturient from her pain for as long a period as may be necessary to achieve the desired therapeutic effect.

Definition

Caudal analgesia is a form of regional analgesia in which insensibility to pain is produced by injection of a local anesthetic drug into the sacral canal through the sacral hiatus. The drug within the sacral canal is confluent throughout the peridural space for as great a distance as the volume permits. Because the medication is distributed extradurally, caudal analgesia is to be distinguished sharply from spinal anesthesia, in which the agent is placed beneath the dura in the subarachnoid space.

Likewise, peridural analgesia is a form of regional analgesia in which insensibility to pain is produced by injection of an anesthetic drug between the vertebral spines and beneath the ligamentum flavum into this same extradural space. Thus, the two technics are kindred in that they provide the same pharmacologic effect from different anatomic approaches. Both technics are like local anesthesia peripheral axon blocks affecting their influence upon nerve trunks distal to the dura mater.

Historical Development

Caudal analgesia was first performed in the year 1901 simultaneously and independently by M. A. Sicard and M. F. Cathelin. Cathelin described this epidural injection and the penetration of the sacral canal as a "méthode nouvelle qui mérite d'être etudiée par les chirurgiens et par les médecins, comme procédé d'analgésie opératoire ou simplement comme procédé pour calmer les douleurs (accouchement douloureux, douleurs des cancers inopérables du rectum, fissures, hémorroïdaires)" [a new method which merits study both by surgeons and by physicians as a procedure of operative analgesia or simply as a procedure to relieve pain (the pains of labor, the pains of inoperable cancers of the rectum, fissures and hemorrhoids)].

This method was developed further by Stoeckel, who was the first to introduce it into Germany and to make use of it in obstetrics. Stoeckel later abandoned the technic because of the short duration of anesthesia, which was insufficient to effect comfortable labor or delivery. The work of Läwen and Gross, and of von Gaza and Schlimpert, of the Freiberg-Frauenklinik, stimulated anew the interest in this technic. Bergouignan, of France, promptly applied caudal analgesia in the treatment of tabetic crises.

However, it was not until 1917 that this method was used in the United States, first by Thompson, of Texas, in orthopedics, and later by Edwin Davis, of Omaha, in urology. In 1925, Pierce Rucker, of Richmond (Va.), reported on his wide experience with caudal analgesia in obstetrics. In 1926 Robert E. Farr, of Minneapolis, investigated extensively the use of caudal analgesia in therapeutic nerve block for sciatica and as an anesthesia for pelvic and perineal surgery. He concluded: "It is possible that the scope of epidural anesthesia may in the future be made to encompass regions far beyond those which are anesthetized by methods now in use." During the next 10 years, Lundy and his group at the Mayo Clinic studied and developed the use of caudal analgesia for rectal and perineal surgery. They were able to report 18,000 administrations without mortality.

Hoffman, of Florida, tried to extend the duration of action of caudal analgesia in obstetrics by adding quinine and urea hydrochloride to a 2 per cent procaine solution. In 1921, Pages, of Spain, introduced the related technic of epidural anesthesia through the approach to the peridural space by a needle inserted between the lumbar spines. In Italy a few years later, Dr. Dogliotti, of Turin, independently introduced the same technic. In 1932, Graffinino and Sayler, of New Orleans, reported the first successful series of epidural anesthesia for obstetrics. The use of these technics did not become widespread or well understood because of the short duration of anesthesia. Cleland, of Oregon (1933), Baptisti, of Maryland (1939), and Hopp, of California (1941), sought to extend the duration of action of single-injection caudal analgesia by repeating the block on indicated cases. It is not surprising that physicians who have contributed the most to the development of these technics should have used them to control the pain of childbirth. However, since the pains of labor and delivery extended over a period of hours, both single-injection caudal and single-injection peridural nerve block were inadequate and offered only a limited field of usefulness for the termination of labor or for the relief of pain.

CONTINUOUS TECHNICS

In 1930, Eugene Aburel, of Rumania, reported to the Society of Obstetrics and Gynecology, in Paris, that he had developed a technic for continuous local anesthesia in obstetrics. The firm of Maupiac developed with him a special combination of needle and catheter which he used in the following way: (1) the introduction of the needle into the spot of choice through the paravertebral approach to the region of the aortic plexus; (2) the injection of 30 cc. of 0.005 per cent percaine solution; (3) the introduction of an elastic silk catheter (similar to a urethral catheter) through the needle; (4) the withdrawal of the needle, leaving the catheter in position; (5) the strapping above the silk catheter. When repeated injections were needed they were made through a 25-gauge needle inserted into the catheter. This technic provided protracted local lumbo-aortic anesthesia. Thus, this technic antedated the continuous spinal technic of Lemmon by 8 years and the continuous caudal technic of Hingson and Edwards by 10 years. Also, it was the first record in medical literature of a ureteral catheter's being left in position for continuous local anesthesia injections.

In 1942, Hingson and Southworth reported their first series of surgical anesthesias with continuous caudal technic through an indwelling needle. With Edwards, one of the authors promptly adapted this technic for obstetrics, where it has received wide application.

Malleable Needle Technic for Continuous Caudal Analgesia

The patient for surgical and therapeutic nerve block anesthesia is placed in the prone position with a pillow under the pelvis. He is instructed to keep his toes together and his heels apart to provide the maximum of muscle relaxation about the sacral hiatus. The obstetric patient is placed in a modified lateral Sims position with the lower leg extended and the upper leg flexed at the hip and the knee joints toward the abdomen. The sacral and coccygeal area is cleansed with ether and prepared with one of the antiseptic tinctures or modern antiseptic detergents. Bony landmarks are used as identification. These are:

1. Inferior tip of coccyx
2. Sacrococcygeal junction recognized as a palpable or bony protuberance
3. Sacral cornua defining the U- or V-shaped hiatus

The tip of the coccyx is palpated with the middle finger of the left hand, and the thumb is used to find the U- or V-shaped notch indicating the sacral hiatus between the sacral cornua. This usually is about 1½ in. from the tip of the coccyx. In 90 per cent of patients, the sacral hiatus lies exactly beneath the superior pole of the posterior intergluteal cleft. In cases in which there was a failure of the inferior sacral arches to fuse into the bony roof of the sacrum. this hiatus may be 2½ to 4 in. from the inferior caudal tip. Experience with the standard single caudal injections is a desired prerequisite for the success in the use of the continuous method. The index or the middle finger of the left hand then changes place with the thumb and marks the spot for raising the initial skin wheal. A special apparatus has been developed for this procedure. The analgesic agent recommended by us is 1.5 per cent Metycaine or procaine, or 1 per cent Xylocaine, or 0.15 per cent Pontocaine, in isotonic solution of the 3 chlorides. Special ampule No. 404 (Lilly) contains this concentration of Metycaine in 200 cc. of sterile Ringer's solution in a reservoir bottle. When the physician makes up his own solution, we recommend that he use 2 of the No. 313 (Lilly) 1-Gm. ampules of the solution of Metycaine diluted in approximately 125 cc. of saline or the 3 chlorides. With a few cubic centimeters of this solution, skin anesthesia is obtained by raising a skin wheal with a 25-gauge needle, and deeper infiltration to the sacrococcygeal ligament with a 2-in. 22-gauge needle. Then the special malleable stainless-steel 19-gauge needle is inserted in the midline in the direction of the hiatus at about a 45° angle with the skin. As soon as the bevel of the needle pierces the sacrococcygeal ligament, its reinforced metal collar is depressed through an arc of 1 to 3 cm., and the needle is thrust slowly and evenly in the mid-line for 1 to 2 in. within the sacral canal, where its bevel should lie inferior to the lowest extent of the dural sac. This may be ascertained by measuring on the skin with the stilet the approximate extent of the needle. The point of the needle always should be below the level of the second sacral spine. Then the small section of tubing with special adapter is slipped over the collar of the needle. The Luer-Lok syringe is attached securely to the adapter. A careful aspiration is performed.

1. Should clear spinal fluid be obtained, the needle has pierced the dura and lies within the subarachnoid space.

In such event, the needle should be withdrawn immediately and the case ruled unsuited for caudal analgesia for fear of producing a massive spinal injection of the analgesic drug. Anatomic anomalies with such low-lying dura are rare. (In our experience this has happened only 15 times in 8,000 injections.) A failure to recognize this situation would be extremely hazardous, if not fatal.

2. The withdrawal of pure blood indicates that the needle has pierced a small blood vessel in the highly vascular peridural space or the sacral corporal bone marrow. In this event, the point of the needle should be moved until blood can no longer be obtained. Then the injection is continued cautiously.

The danger of intraspinal injection, with appearance of spinal fluid previously mentioned can be minimized if a trial dose of 5 to 8 cc. of the solution is injected and if further action is delayed for 10 minutes to see that a low spinal anesthesia does not ensue. Without relief of pain or diminution of motor power in the lower extremities in 10 minutes after injection, one can safely assume that the subarachnoid space has not been entered.

After these precautions have been carried out, the hose end of the special 4-ft. tubing is secured over the collar of the special caudal needle. The tubing should have been connected previously to the remainder of the apparatus, all air having been expelled by filling the entire system with anesthetic solution. With the palm of the left hand pressed firmly over the skin area against the dorsum of the sacrum, 30 cc. of 1.5 per cent solution is injected slowly, the penicillin or sulfathiazole or an antiseptic ointment is spread generously around the collar of the needle.

Indications That the Solution Is Being Injected into the Peridural Space Sacral Canal

1. The patients usually experience a sense of fullness, progressing to an uncomfortable sensation in one or both legs as the solution circumscribes the perineural components of the sciatic nerves. This sensation can be minimized by slower injections.

2. There will be a progressive analgesia in the areas supplied by the coccygeal, the hemorrhoidal, the perineal, the pudendal, the ilio-inguinal and the iliohypogastric nerves. Analgesia should be complete in 20 minutes.

3. There is relief of abdominal uterine cramps within 5 to 15 minutes after injection.

4. Pronounced vasodilatation, cessation of sweating and increase in temperature of the skin of the feet will ensue within 5 to 15 minutes after injection. Clinical experience indicates that the great toe and the ball of the foot are the first part of the feet to develop vasomotor block. Usually, the heels are the last part of the feet to become pink, warm and dry. Often this phenomenon is noticed on one side several minutes before it occurs on the other.

Indications That the Solution Is Being Injected Outside the Sacral Canal

1. Failure of the injection to relieve pain within 30 minutes.

2. The appearance of an "injection tumor" superficial to the dorsum of the sacrum.

Supplementary Injections

The time and the amount of the supplementary injection will depend on the rate of metabolism of the drug by the individual patient and upon the anatomic level of block desired. In our experience, 20 cc. of the short-acting local anesthetic solutions in 1½ per cent concentrations is sufficient to relieve pain from the umbilicus downward for 30 to 60 minutes per dose. When one uses the longer-acting local anesthetics such as 0.15 Pontocaine or 1 per cent Xylocaine, we were able to provide this pain relief for periods of 1½ to 5 hours when 1:200,000 Adrenalin is included in the mixture. We have continued pain relief with continuous caudal analgesia for a maximum of 8 days and for an average of 3 to 5 hours per patient.

Catheter Technic

When it is anticipated that the nerve injection will be continued for longer than 4 hours, we recommend the following alternate technic of continuous caudal analgesia by means of an indwelling ureteral or plastic catheter.

A 16- or 17-gauge specially adapted Love-Barker needle (distributed in the Becton, Dickinson Company's Irving Catheter Caudal Set) is passed into the sacral canal though the same maneuvers recommended in the malleable needle technic. The bevel of this large needle penetrates the canal a distance of only 1 to 3 cm. The stilet is removed. A test dose of 2 cc. of air is injected in an attempt to elicit the rebound of the plunger, which delineates an episacral placement. If the air goes in with no resistance, a No. 4 or a No. 3½ radiopaque ureteral catheter is passed through the needle a distance of from 6 to 9 cm. into the canal. Recently at the Johns Hopkins Hospital we substituted a small polyethylene catheter or a special divinyl translucent catheter (developed for the Becton, Dickinson Company). Either the ureteral catheter or the plastic catheter passes easily into the canal and beyond the bevel of the trocar needle if entry into the sacrum is correct. Then the trocar needle is slipped over the catheter as a sleeve, to leave the catheter in position. In more than 500 cases we have left all types of catheters in the extradural space for from several days to over 1 week without evidence of nerve irritation or residual neuropathy.

The dosages and the signs of correct and faulty insertions with the catheter technic are the same as those described in the needle technic.

The following conditions associated with pain have been treated by us with the schedule of doses indicated with all types of local anesthetic agents: (1) pruritus ani; (2) postoperative control of pain following rectal surgery; (3) control of pain in lower extremities (peripheral vascular disease with or without total occlusion, crushing trauma, severe burns); (4) ureteral and vesical calculi; (5) pains of labor; (6) postoperative abdominal pain; and (7) for surgery below the umbilicus, such as for cesarean section.

We began the use of these technics with plastic catheters in 1945. Simultaneously in March, 1946, at the University of Tennessee in Memphis and at the Johns Hopkins Hospital, we substituted the polyethylene and the vinylite (B-D vinyl tubing) plastic catheters for the costlier larger and more traumatic shellacked nylon ureteral catheters for the technics of continuous caudal, continuous peridural and continuous spinal analgesia and anesthesia. Since that time we have utilized these technics in obstetrics, surgery and therapeutics in more than 5,000 cases.

We studied the use of these plastic catheters for the continuous administration of anesthetics and therapeutic medicaments in the Johns Hopkins Hospital and allied institutions from July 1, 1948, to June 1, 1950. We used 4 types of catheters during this period: polyethylene, vinyl, radiopaque nylon ureteral and nonradiopaque ureteral.

The polyethylene catheter has been used in the majority of cases. Kirchof and Boals (West. J. Surg. **57**:88, 1949) found this tubing to be excellent for continuous spinal anesthesia, and we have found it equally efficacious for the other technics. The tubing is flexible and relatively inelastic but will stretch markedly without breaking. It is inexpensive, and it has been our policy to discard it after each use. It is easily introduced through a 17-gauge needle and admits a 25-gauge hypodermic needle.

There are possibly 2 disadvantages to the polyethylene catheter. One lies in the fact that it must be prepared for use by chemical sterilization. The tubing is perfused with a solution of Zephiran chloride (1:1,000), then coiled and immersed in the same solution for 24 hours. This method of sterilization has been most satisfac-

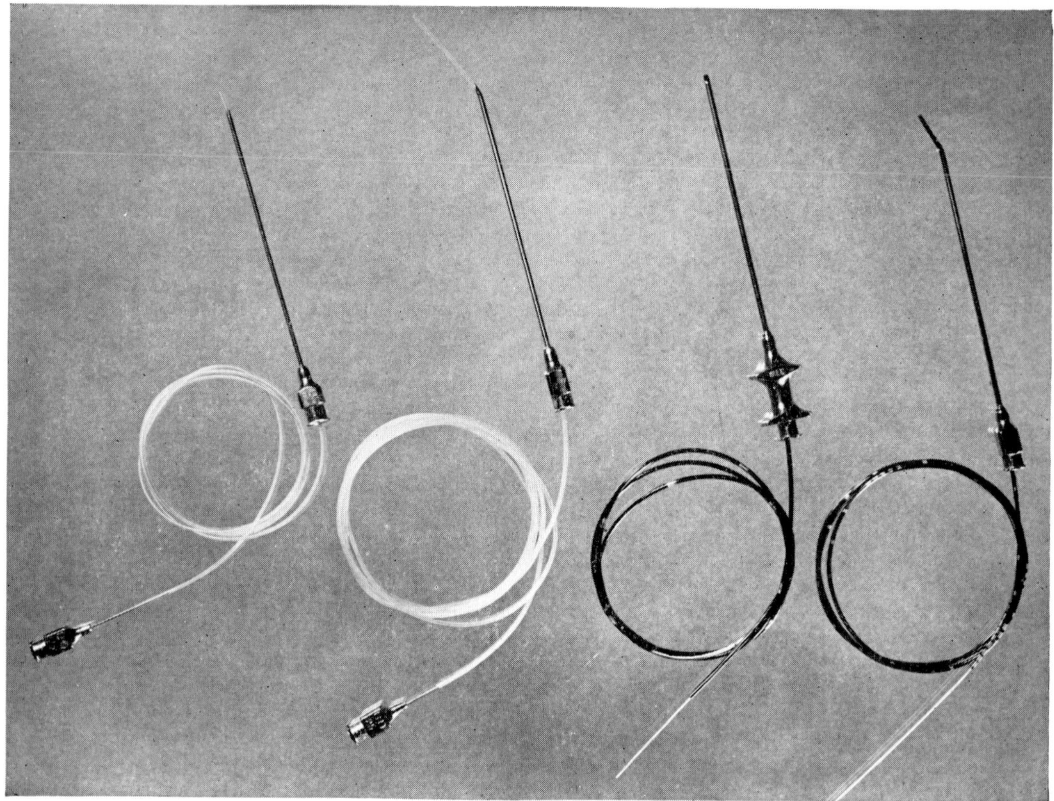

Fig. 51. Needles, ureteral catheters and plastic tubes used for continuous conduction anesthesia. (Southworth, Hingson & Pitkin: Pitkin's Conduction Anesthesia, ed. 2, Philadelphia, Lippincott)

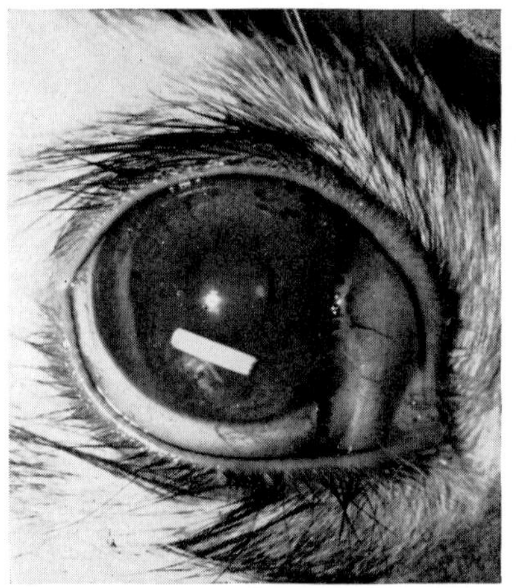

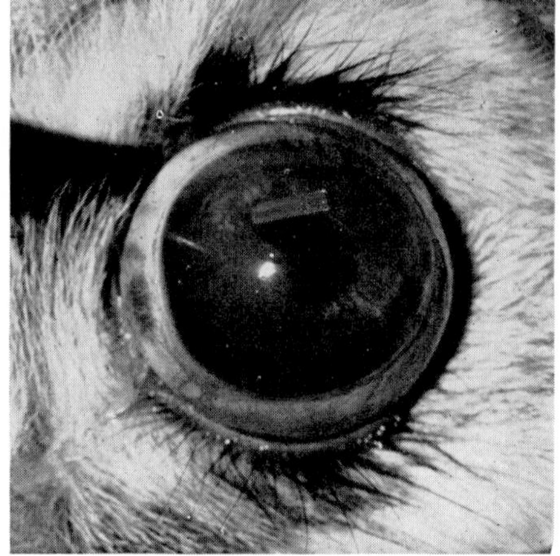

Fig. 52. Catheter material inserted into rabbit's eye. (Davidson, Hingson & Hellman: A.M.A. Arch. Surg. **62**:540–545)

tory for us, and we have encountered no reactions that we could attribute to the method of sterilization. Occasionally some difficulty is encountered because of the flexibility of the polyethylene catheter. We have noted this occasionally in attempting to place the catheter in the peridural space through the Tuohy needle and have found it advisable to substitute the more rigid vinyl catheter or the ureteral catheter with the stilet in place.

The B-D vinyl tubing catheters have proved to be satisfactory. This catheter is slightly less flexible than the polyethylene one and offers 2 distinct advantages. It may be sterilized by autoclaving and is of smaller diameter, but it has a larger lumen than the polyethylene tubing. It is easily introduced through an 18-gauge needle and will admit a 23-gauge hypodermic needle. We have found it of particular value in the subarachnoid space, where repeated withdrawal of spinal fluid may be desired. We have used the vinyl catheters from 2 to 10 times each without difficulty.

Occasionally we have used the No. 3.5 French shellacked nylon ureteral catheter. Its chief disadvantage lies in its expense, and we prefer the nonradiopaque catheter for routine use, as the cost is 50 per cent less. These catheters are sheathed in long test tubes with the stilet in place and sterilized by autoclaving. We have found them to be particularly valuable when difficulty is encountered in introducing a more flexible catheter into the peridural space through the Tuohy needle. The 3.5 ureteral catheter is introduced through a 16-gauge needle and admits a 25-gauge hypodermic needle.

Each batch of catheter material that we have obtained has been first tested for irritative properties by inserting a small segment of it into the anterior chamber of the rabbit's eye. This method places the material where it is easily observed and also in a sensitive medium. The rabbit is observed for 7 days, and if there is no evidence of reaction at the end of that time the tubing is prepared for clinical use.*

Continuous Caudal Analgesia for Labor

Advantages

1. When properly performed at appropriate time during progressive labor, this technic approaches ideal. It is more satisfactory for the last half or quarter of labor than for the first quarter, when a minimum of pain relief is required.

2. On the Hardy-Javert dolorimeter scale it provides complete analgesia for labor and intense anesthesia for delivery.

3. It has provided great protection from stress and strain of labor to patients handicapped with severe heart disease, pulmonary tuberculosis, acute respiratory infections, metabolic disease, severe toxemia and nephritis, and it protects the premature baby.

4. Its greatest usefulness is in delivery of the occiput posterior, the large baby from transverse arrest, in multiple births and for the premature baby.

5. It is recommended in breech delivery, but prerequisites are good descent of the presenting part and a forceful type of labor before induction.

Disadvantages

1. It demands hospital facilities and more time and skill in administration, which limits its use to a small percentage of cases.

2. It increases forceps delivery rate.

3. Hypotension, infection and inadvertent spinal injection are dangers.

4. Uterine tone maintenance makes the breaking up of a frank breech more difficult. Superimposition of suitable relaxing anesthetic may be necessary.

5. It may prolong labor.

Requirements for Use

1. Multipara: Cervix should be dilated 3 cm. or more; presenting part in pelvis; uterine contractions at 3-minute intervals or less and lasting for 40 seconds or more.

2. Primipara: Cervix should be dilated 5 cm. or more; presenting part in pelvis; uterine contractions occuring 3 minutes apart or less and lasting for 40 seconds or more.

---

* Davidson, Harold H., Hingson, Robert A., and Hellman, Louis M.: Use of various plastic catheters in the subarachnoid and peridural spaces, A.M.A. Arch. Surg. **62**:540-545, 1951.

Technic of Administration

1. Position: Obstetric patient is most comfortable in the lateral modified Sims position, lying on left side for right-handed anesthetist and on right side for left-handed anesthetist. Leg on which patient is lying should be extended, and opposite thigh and leg flexed.

2. A wide area of skin over the sacrum, the ilia and the buttocks should be prepared surgically.

3. The sacral hiatus is found by palpating the sacral cornua. It lies in the mid-line above the distal tip of the sacrum in the form of an inverted V. When this point is related to the posterior sacral cornua, it forms an equilateral triangle with its base cephalad.

4. An intradermal wheal is raised in the middle of this space, somewhat distal to the mid-point.

5. A 50-mm. needle is passed through the skin, the subcutaneous tissue and the sacrococcygeal ligament and finally into the caudal canal. From 3 to 5 cc. of anesthetic solution can be injected just before the needle enters the membrane to block coccygeal nerves.

6. Imminence of delivery or intensity of pain may demand that the test dose and the later anesthetic dose be administered through the fascia needle.

7. Total obstetric dose of 20 to 30 cc. of anesthetic solution is required to block the afferent nerve supply from uterus and provide anesthesia to tenth thoracic dermatome. Above T-10 uterine atony increases proportionately.

8. Height of anesthesia or analgesia may be raised or lowered by timing and quantity of injected doses. Upon obstetric indication, caudal procedure may be abandoned entirely with catheter left in place and begun several hours later through the same undisturbed catheter. With this technic it is possible to provide perineal anesthesia only and/or control of sacral backache pain of labor and/or control of abdominal contraction pain.

Continuous Caudal Anesthesia for Delivery

Technic

Spontaneous deliveries can be accomplished in most multiparas and in one third of primiparas by this management.

1. Carefully recheck intensity and somatic level of anesthesia by:

A. Pin prick

B. Observation of motor power of lower extremities

2. If patient has not had supplementary injection within 20 minutes, and if level of nerve block is not above umbilicus, inject one of the following:

A. 20 cc. of 1.5 per cent piperocaine hydrochloride

B. 20 cc. of 0.15 per cent tetracaine hydrochloride

C. 20 cc. of 1 per cent lidocaine hydrochloride

D. 20 cc. of 2 per cent procaine hydrochloride

3. Prepare patient in usual manner for delivery.

4. Administer 100 per cent oxygen inhalations with patient holding mask.

5. Comfort is achieved by elevating head on 1 or 2 pillows. Patient can cooperate and bear down when desired or instructed.

6. Use of intravenous fluids with 5 per cent glucose is beneficial as a supportive measure in extremely hot weather.

Disadvantages

1. Increased incidence of necessary outlet forceps

2. Hypotension. If blood pressure falls below 100 mm. systolic, administer intravenous doses of 5 mg. of methamphetamine hydrochloride or 15 mg. of ephedrine.

The Trendelenburg position favors

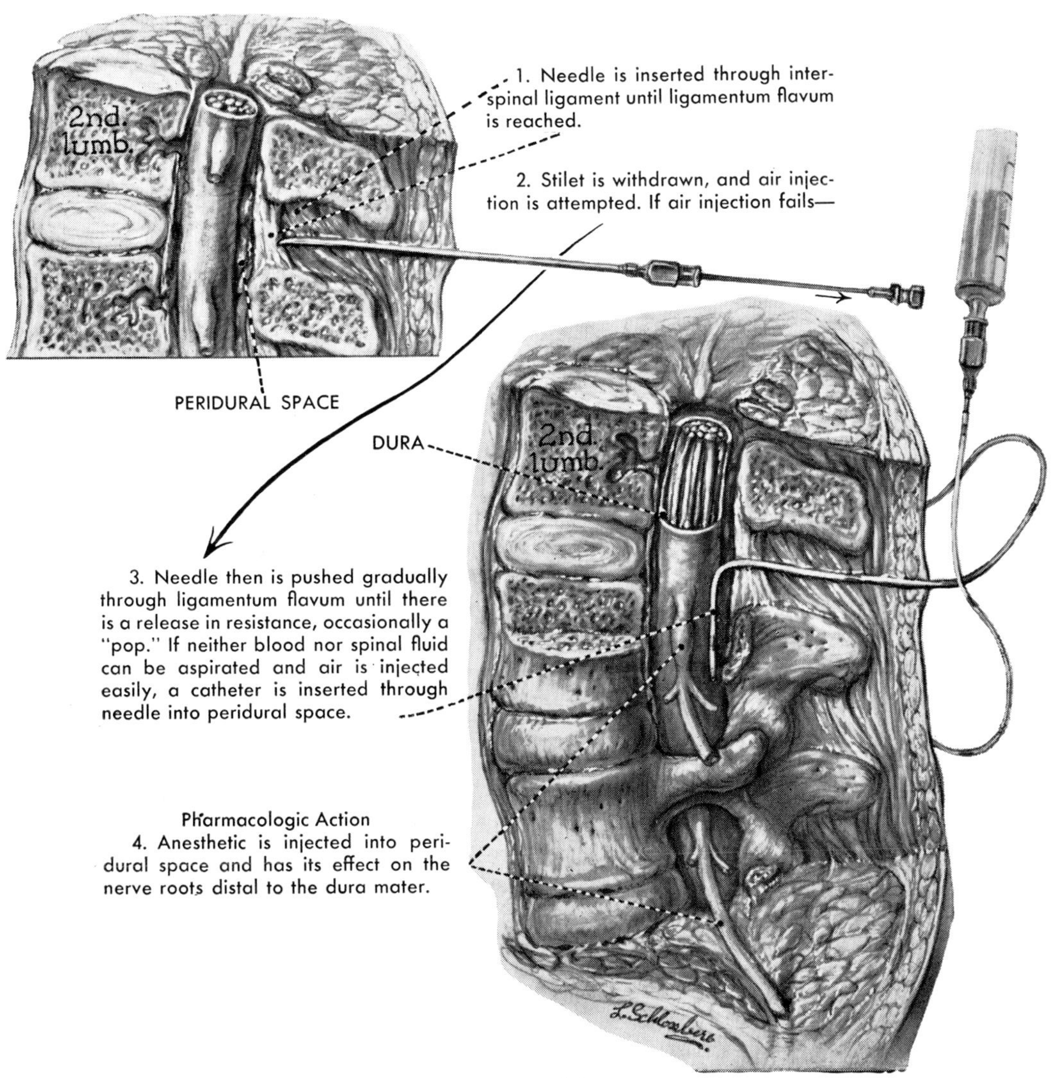

FIGURE 53

dissemination cephalad, and the sitting position favors a caudal flow of the injected fluid. Thus, through the peridural space, one is able to block the 16 nerves transmitting the pain of labor and delivery, namely, to the visceral afferents of thoracic 11 and 12, the second, the third and the fourth sacral posterior nerves carrying pelvic afferents, and the hemorrhoidal, the perineal and the pudendal branches of the anterior divisions of the sacral nerves.

TECHNIC OF CONTINUOUS PERIDURAL ANESTHESIA

The technic employed here is no more difficult than the method used for continuous caudal analgesia. The patient is placed on her left side, the shoulders parallel and the legs partially flexed. No attempt is made to have the spinal column convex, as this would reduce the peridural space and also stretch the dura and make it more liable for puncture. If the interspaces of the patient are small, the sitting position is most efficacious.

The back is cleaned and draped as for a spinal puncture. The skin, the interspinous ligament and the ligamentum flavum are infiltrated with the same anesthetic solution that is used for the continuous block. A 16-gauge Tuohy spinal needle, which has been blunted but has a sharp stilet in place to facilitate piercing the skin, the subcutaneous tissue and the interspinous ligament, is introduced into any of the lumbar interspaces. Frequently, the site of election is lumbar, as this is the largest peridural space in the lumbar area. The needle should be placed directly into the center of the interspace without anterior or posterior deviation. The needle should engage the ligamentum flavum. This ligament is the most important demarcating structure in marking a peridural injection, for unless the needle pierces the middle of the ligamentum flavum, the center of the peridural space will not be entered, and a catheter cannot be passed with ease. When the dense ligamentum flavum has been entered, one pauses and tests the ease with which 2 cc. of air can be introduced into the ligament with a small syringe. When an attempt is made to inject air into the ligamentum flavum, the plunger of the syringe rebounds quickly.* However, when air is injected into the peridural space, the plunger of the syringe literally falls into place. As the needle is advanced through the ligamentum flavum, frequent minute air tests are made with a small syringe to determine when the area of negative pressure in the peridural space is entered. Often this entrance is evident by the release of resistance that is felt when the blunt 16-gauge Tuohy needle passes through the dense ligamentum flavum and enters the peridural space.

When the Tuohy needle has been placed properly and there is no aspiration of spinal fluid, a plastic tube is introduced through the needle into the peridural space. The tubing is placed either cephalad or caudad, depending upon the somatic neurologic segments involved in transmitting the painful impulses. The plastic catheter passes as easily into the peridural space as it does into the caudal canal. On one occasion, using a radiopaque catheter, we have passed it in a cephalad direction from the entry into the space in the last thoracic interspace to the level of thoracic 3. Its passage sometimes elicits a distinct hyperesthetic response in a leg, a hip or a back, if the soft nose of the catheter touches a nerve in the peridural space. This was positive in 60 per cent of the patients in our series. We have the following indications of a properly placed catheter in the peridural space:

1. The ease with which air can be injected through the Tuohy needle after the ligamentum flavum has been passed

2. Hyperesthesia upon the passage of the catheter in the peridural space, in the absence of spinal fluid

3. The easy passage of the catheter either up or down the peridural space in the absence of spinal fluid

4. Absence of somatic anesthesia following test dose of 2 cc. of anesthetic agent to rule out spinal anesthesia

5. Prompt somatic anesthesia after one 10-cc. dose of anesthetic agent main-

* This "air-rebound" method for determining the depth of needle insertion for peridural anesthesia is preferred by some anesthetists as the most reliable sign. The essential features are illustrated in Figures 48 and 49. The needle is inserted by feel into an interspace until the blunt bevel impinges on the ligamentum flavum. Then this location is verified by injection of a small amount of air. If the needle is situated properly on the ligament, as shown in the figures, a rebound of the plunger of the syringe is obtained. Once this rebound has been obtained, the depth of the needle at the ligament is reasonably certain, and its insertion to another millimeter or so will result in extradural tap. When the extradural space has been entered properly, air may be injected with ease (Figs. 51 and 52), and no cerebrospinal fluid can be aspirated.

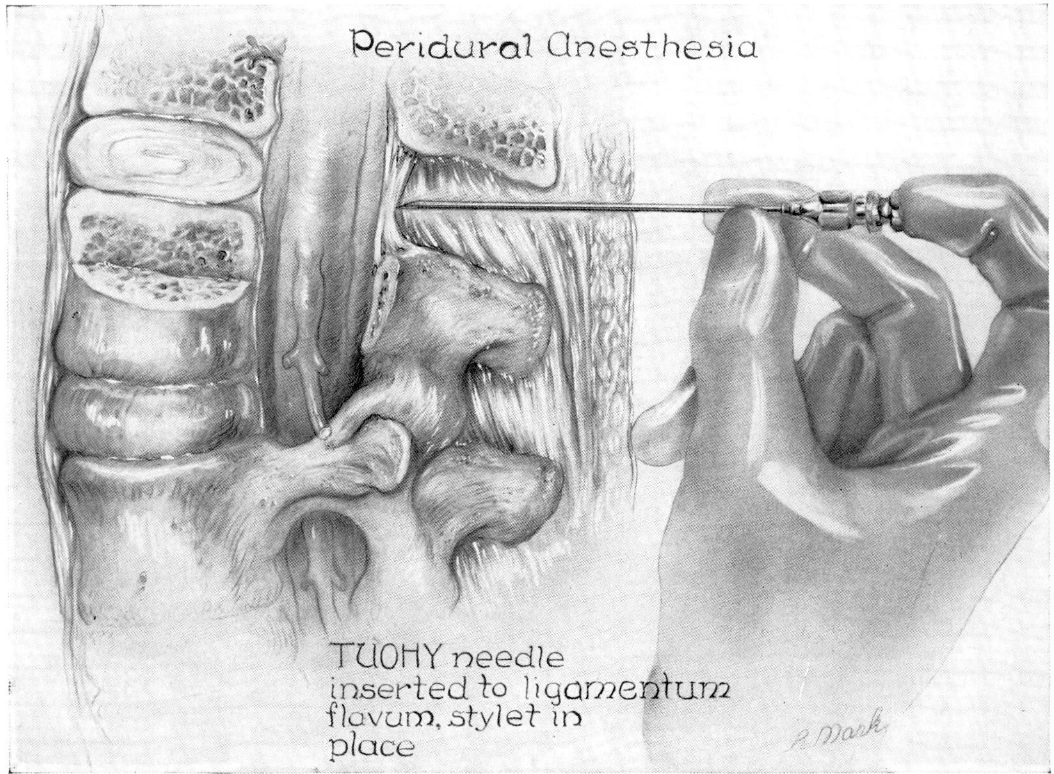

FIG. 54. Peridural anesthesia. Insertion of needle to ligamentum flavum. (Pitkin's Conduction Anesthesia)

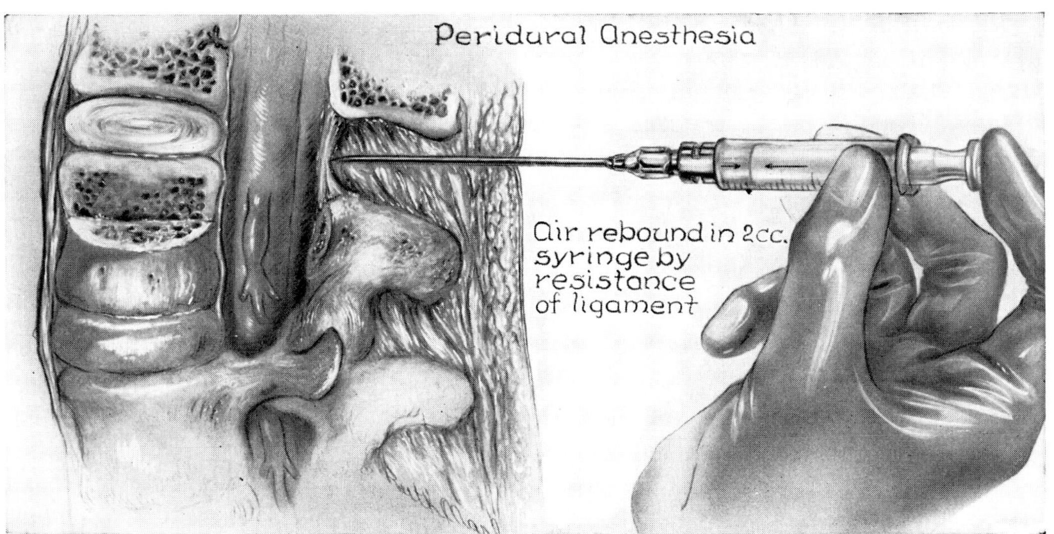

FIG. 55. Peridural anesthesia: air-rebound technic. When the bevel of the needle rests against the ligamentum flavum, air cannot be injected with ease. (Pitkin's Conduction Anesthesia)

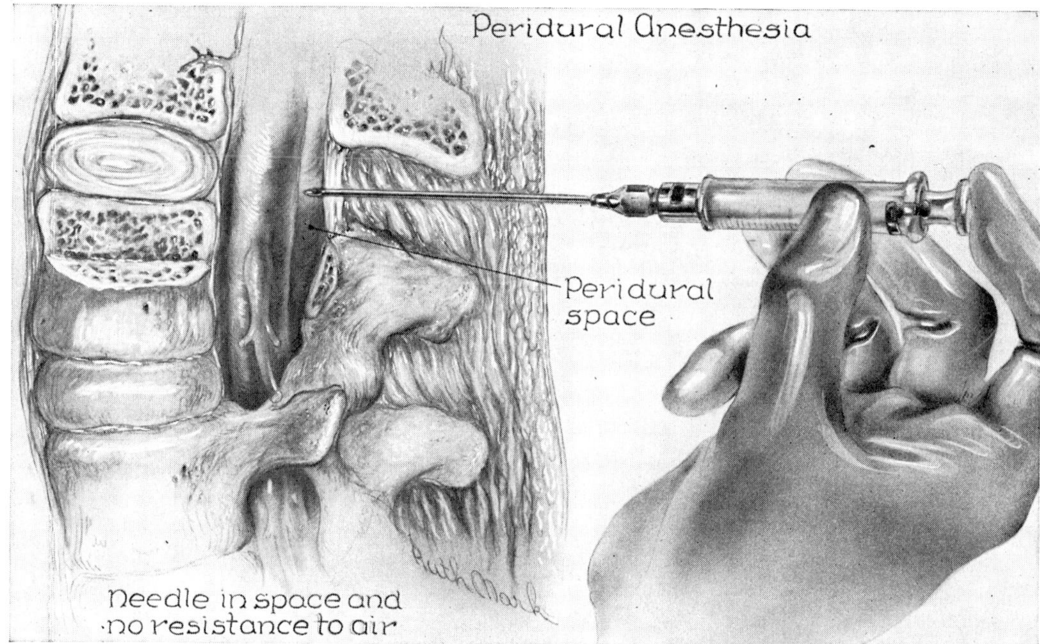

FIG. 56. Peridural anesthesia: air-rebound technic. When the needle has entered the extradural space, air can be injected with ease. (Pitkin's Conduction Anesthesia)

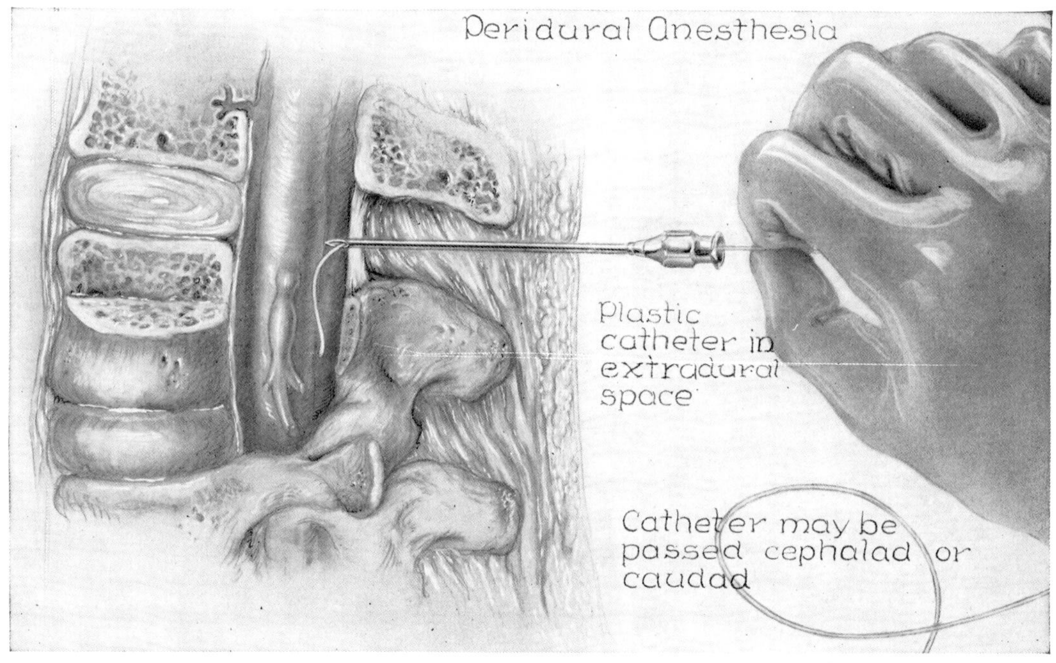

FIG. 57. Continuous peridural anesthesia: plastic-tube method. The plastic tube is passed through the needle and advanced into the extradural space. (Pitkin's Conduction Anesthesia)

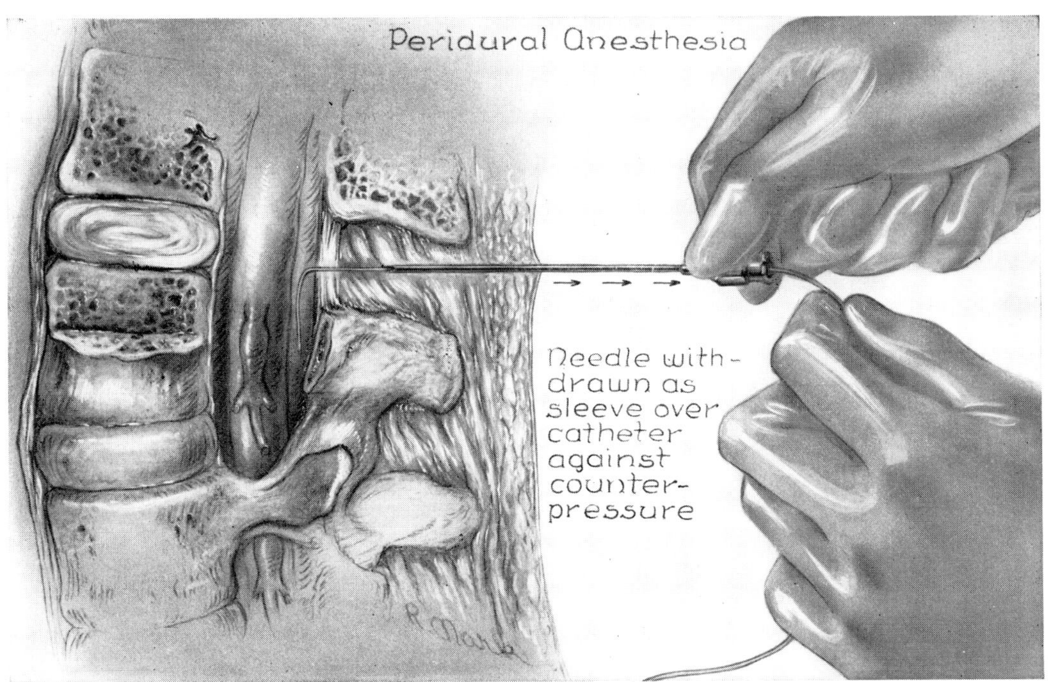

Fig. 58. Continuous peridural anesthesia: plastic-tube method. The needle is withdrawn carefully, the plastic tube being left in place in the extradural space. The plastic tube never should be pulled out of the needle, as the sharp bevel of the needle may shear off a piece of tubing within the extradural space. (Pitkin's Conduction Anesthesia)

tained 1 to 2 hours with short-acting agents.

Notwithstanding these signs of a properly placed catheter and needle, there are two safeguards of the utmost importance. The first is the use of 2 test doses of 2 cc. of 1.5 per cent Metycaine, 1 per cent Xylocaine, 2 per cent procaine, 0.15 per cent Pontocaine or 2 per cent Intracaine 5 minutes apart to ensure absolutely the absence of spinal anesthesia. Either of these 2 test doses will produce a safe low spinal anesthetic but cause no somatic anesthesia if the solution is placed properly in the peridural space. The second safeguard is the ready availability of oxygen, vasopressors and fluids (Figs. 53 and 54). (See Figs. 55 and 56.)

We have been able to carry out continuous peridural block by the technic outlined below. This method overcomes the disadvantage of comparatively short duration of anesthesia encountered with single injections. While it is possible to extend the length of block by the single-injection method by use of a 2 per cent Metycaine-epinephrine-ephedrine solution, we have preferred the continuous technic because either a short or a long anesthesia can be administered. In addition, if the block is not placed at the proper level from the first injection, one can extend the effect up or down by additional doses combined with manipulation of the table.

Plastic Tubing Method

Some of the precautions and objections with regard to continuous peridural anesthesia cited above are not so important when the ureteral catheter (Curbello, 1949) or the plastic tubing method (Flowers, Hellman and Hingson, 1949) is used (Figs. 55 and 56).

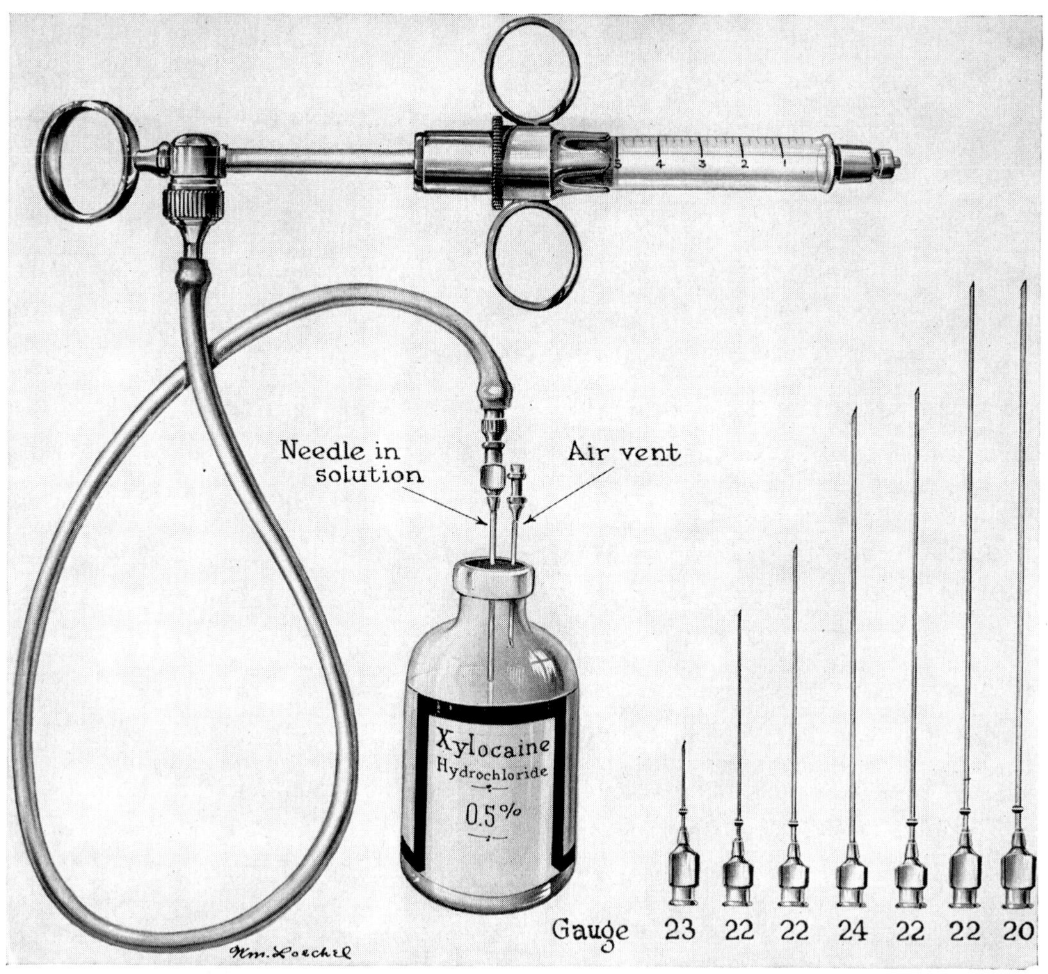

FIG. 59. A representative collection of needles for local anesthesia. The Pitkin continuous flow syringe shown here is preferred by a number of anesthetists when large amounts of solution are to be injected. Xylocaine ½ per cent, as shown, is used for local infiltration when the area is large; however, often the 1 per cent solution is used, since with this agent the total amount or volume of solution can be reduced greatly as compared with procaine or Metycaine. (Pitkin's Conduction Anesthesia)

There is little danger that a properly situated plastic tube will penetrate the dura after it is placed, and the precaution against supplementing continuous peridural anesthesia for surgical operations is not pertinent. In addition, when the rigid needle is not used, the necessity for frequent retesting against accidental spinal anesthesia is not necessary. In Curbello's method, the patient is placed in the sitting position, and a 16-gauge Huber-point Tuohy spinal needle is inserted at the appropriate interspace down to the ligamentum flavum. A small syringe containing from 2 to 3 cc. of anesthetic solution is attached to the needle, and the needle and the syringe are advanced inward together. As the point of the Tuohy spinal needle pierces the anterior surface of the ligamentum flavum and enters the extradural space, the solution is forced into the space, pushing the dura forward. Aspiration is carried out, and, if no spinal fluid is obtained, a No. 3½ ureteral catheter is inserted into the extradural space and advanced cephalad for high anesthesia or caudad for obstetric or urologic operations. An appropriate test dose of medication is given, and, if spinal anesthesia does not result, the ureteral catheter is taped in place along the patient's spine so that its end with attached syringe lies near the left ear. After the patient is turned to position, an additional 10 to 50 cc. of anesthetic solution is injected. Curbello does not use more than 5 cc. at a time. His solution contains procaine (2%), tetracaine (0.1%) and Adrenalin (0.0005 Gm.) in isotonic saline. The peridural puncture is made at any interspace that is appropriate for ease of anesthetizing the operative area.

Improvements in continuous peridural anesthesia have been made by Flowers, Hellman and Hingson (1949) and by Flowers (1950). A modification of the Huber-point Tuohy spinal needle assists in making the extradural puncture without entering the subdural space. The Huber point of a 16-gauge Tuohy spinal needle is made slightly longer and then blunted in such a manner that the terminal portion lies flat, as shown in Figure 62. The stilet is made slightly longer, broader and sharper to facilitate piercing the skin and the subcutaneous tissues.

Continuous Peridural Anesthesia for Labor, Delivery and Cesarean Section

Flowers, Hellman and Hingson (1949) have described the application of the continuous plastic-tube peridural block

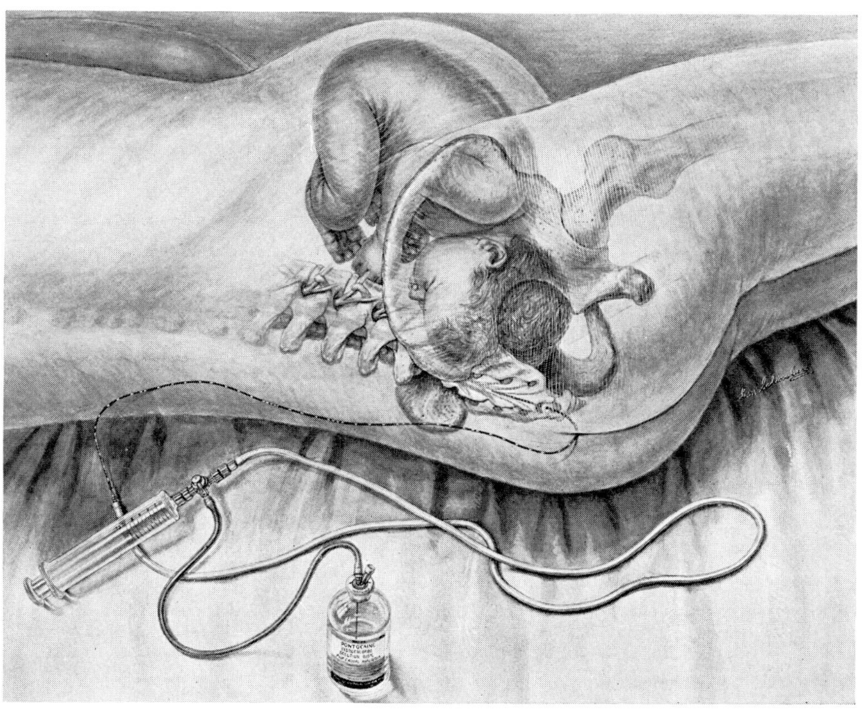

Fig. 60. Apparatus in position recommended for ureteral catheter continuous caudal analgesia with a .15 per cent Pontocaine in a vehicle of Ringer's solution with 1 to 200,000 Adrenalin for vasoconstrictive purposes. (Winthrop Laboratories, Inc.)

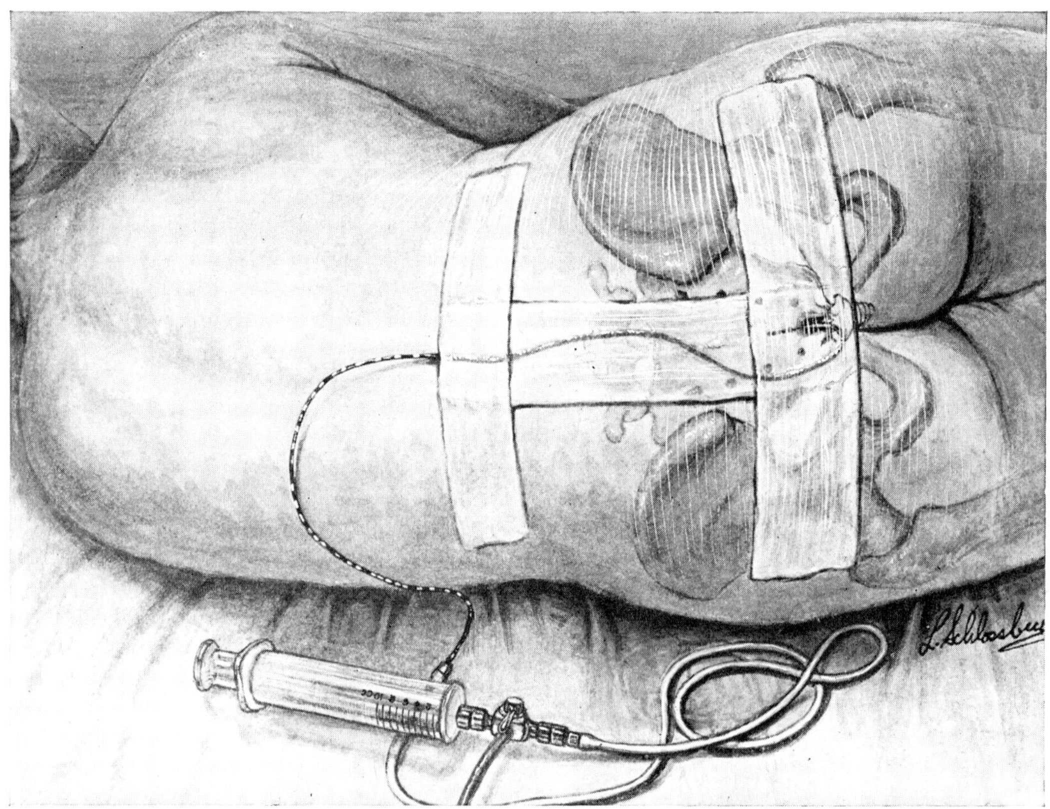

FIG. 61. Continuous caudal analgesia: catheter method. The apparatus for continuous technic is shown attached to the ureteral catheter in place in the sacral canal. Note method of taping the catheter in place. (Pitkin's Conduction Anesthesia)

for obstetric cases. In general, this form of block is indicated in the same obstetric conditions in which continuous caudal analgesia is useful, and sometimes it is employed in preference to caudal when the sacral hiatus or canal is anomalous, making caudal tap difficult or impossible. According to Flowers, Hellman and Hingson:

Patients who are to receive peridural analgesia should be in the last 5 to 6 hours of labor; the labor should be adequate and effective. Patients with slow, irregular and ineffectual uterine contractions are not suitable for conduction block. There should be no obstructive factors to the labor, either fetal or maternal. Severe hemorrhage is a contraindication.

During the first 30 to 45 minutes of peridural block the sacral plexus is not anesthetized completely, and patients may walk with support, sit in a chair, urinate or defecate. These actions should be encouraged. Liquid refreshment, reading material and a radio are good adjuncts of conduction analgesia. After the test dose as described, or after 2 test doses to be more certain that subarachnoid injection has not been made, the maintenance and therapeutic dose of the selected anesthetic agent is begun. The plastic tubing or the catheter is advanced to the twelfth thoracic space for patients in early labor, since the lower 2 thoracic nerves carry the afferents of uterine pain to the posterior columns of the spinal cord. Often the 2 test doses will relieve completely the pain of uterine contractions. In early labor no other nerve block is needed. (The maintenance dose with the catheter at the twelfth interspace is 5 to 7 cc. of any of the solutions commonly employed for extradural anesthesia.) The solution should be injected slowly so that it diffuses only around the eleventh and the twelfth thoracic nerves and the first lumbar nerve.

When the fetus begins to distend the vagina,

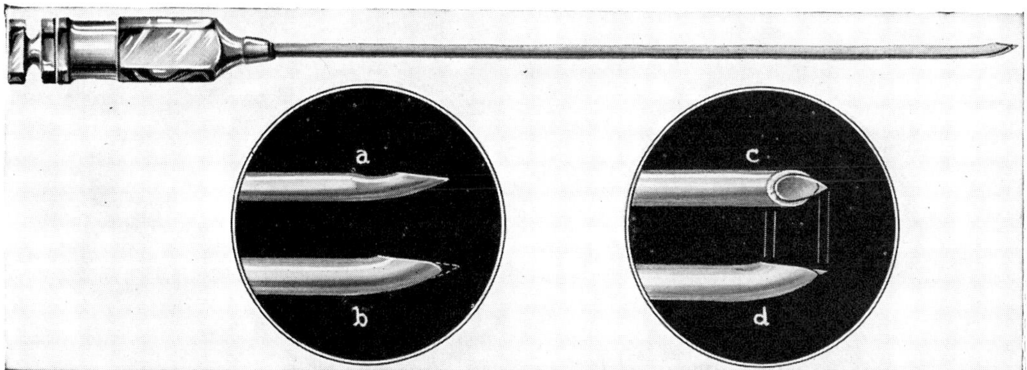

Fig. 62. Flowers-Hingson modification of Tuohy's spinal needle. (a) Stilet detail; (b) needle showing blunted bevel; (c and d) additional detail views. This needle is used for lumbar peridural anesthesia, when the blunted bevel is helpful in determining the location of the ligamentum flavum. (Pitkin's Conduction Anesthesia)

there is pain transmitted by the pelvic afferents to the sacral plexus. At this time, the sacral plexus as well as the eleventh and the twelfth thoracic nerves must be blocked. This may be done in two ways. One may utilize the sitting position and increase the maintenance dose during the last hour of labor so that the patient receives from 8 to 12 cc. of the local anesthetic every 15 to 20 minutes until the perineum is anesthetized. (Or following the lead of Cleland [*see* following section] a second catheter can be inserted into the caudal canal and the birth canal anesthetized with a single relatively small dose of anesthetic solution.)

The catheter is sent caudad for patients in late labor or for multiparous women who are expected to have rapid labor. The nerves of the sacral plexus are anesthetized with the lumbar and the lower thoracic nerves. But for delivery and forceps operations, the sacral nerves must receive an intense block, since at this time considerable pressure is placed upon them. Delivery must be anticipated by 30 to 45 minutes, during which time the patient should be placed in the sitting position and receive 2 or 3 therapeutic doses of 10 to 15 cc. of one of the local anesthetics, each dose being separated by a 10-minute interval. When full dilatation is reached, patients should be encouraged to exert abdominal and diaphragmatic force with each uterine contraction to aid descent of the fetus.

For cesarean section the catheter is sent cephalad to the level of the twelfth thoracic or the first lumbar interspace. The dose requirement is the same for patients in labor. The anesthetic level should include the tenth thoracic dermatome, to relieve pain in the region of the bladder. The level may be extended to the sixth thoracic to eliminate peritoneal traction pain in complicated cases with numerous adhesions. The operation should not begin sooner than 20 minutes after the first test dose, in order that the nerves may be anesthetized completely. Best results are gained if at least 3 therapeutic doses are given during this interval.

Whether peridural anesthesia is used for labor or cesarean section, one always must realize that the exact dose and the time interval depend upon the somatic level of each patient. The level of anesthesia should not rise above the tenth thoracic nerve in order not to inhibit the motor nerves of the uterus. Likewise, the level of anesthesia should not fall below the twelfth thoracic nerve, if one desires complete relief of obstetric pain.

The somatic level of anesthesia and the blood pressure must be observed carefully. (The operator should bear in mind also that a high spinal anesthetic may result inadvertently, even in the face of a negative test dose, and be prepared to give intratracheal oxygen if respiration fails.

Cleland's Combination Block

John G. P. Cleland (1949), recognizing the advantages of economy of drug administration in extradural anesthesia for obstetrics, devised the combination block, in which 2 plastic tubes or catheters are inserted into the extradural space, 1 caudad and 1 peridurad. In caudal anesthesia for obstetrics, it is necessary to inject a volume of solution sufficient to fill the extradural space

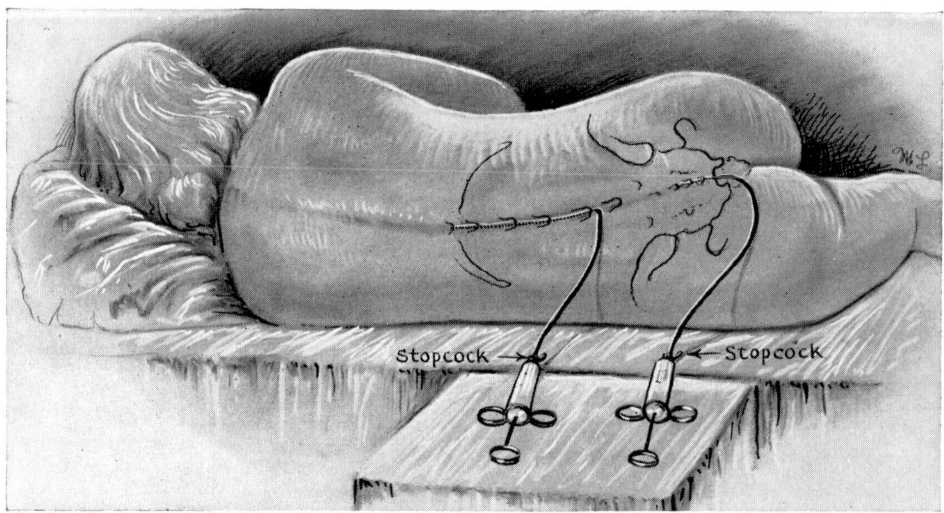

FIG. 63. Cleland's combined peridural and caudal block for relief of pain during labor and delivery. (Pitkin's Conduction Anesthesia)

from the sacral hiatus to the region of the eleventh and the twelfth thoracic nerves, but there is little or no need to block the intervening lumbar nerves. Lumbar peridural anesthesia for obstetrics fails sometimes to give adequate block of the birth canal. These disadvantages can be overcome by installing 2 plastic tubes or catheters in the extradural space, 1 in the sacral canal and 1 in the extradural space near the eleventh and the twelfth thoracic nerves, as Cleland has described. A small dose of solution (10 cc. of 1% Xylocaine) through the sacral plastic tube will anesthetize the birth canal any time that relief is required, and a smaller dose (2 cc. of 1% Xylocaine at 2- to 3-hour intervals), injected through the peridural catheter or the plastic tube, will relieve the pain of uterine contraction. The arrangement of the plastic tubes is indicated in Figure 51.

This is a moderately spectacular form of conduction anesthesia—called "the double whammy" by 1 obstetrician at least—which appears to be complex: in reality, it is quite sound, logical and desirable from the standpoint of low drug dosage; technically, it is not difficult for the expert extradural blocker.

Saddle-Block and Isobaric Spinal Anesthesia

During the past decade these methods have been used widely in large and in small hospitals throughout the United States. On the basis of sales of individual spinal ampules by the pharmaceutical companies, there is evidence that more than 400,000 deliveries per year are managed in this way. If the dosage of the anesthetic drugs is kept within the suggested range and the proper safeguards surround the parturient and her baby and the proper obstetric and anesthesiologic technics are employed, these methods are most satisfactory. However, it should be emphasized that from our file reports of complications and mortalities from the major American hospitals, more than 50 deaths have resulted recently from injudicious and overwhelming spinal anesthesia dosage. On the other hand, in the 7 largest maternity hospitals of Cleveland, the authors'

1. Disinfection and surgical asepsis.
2. Local anesthesia of the skin.
3. Introduction of wing needle 2 to 3 cm.

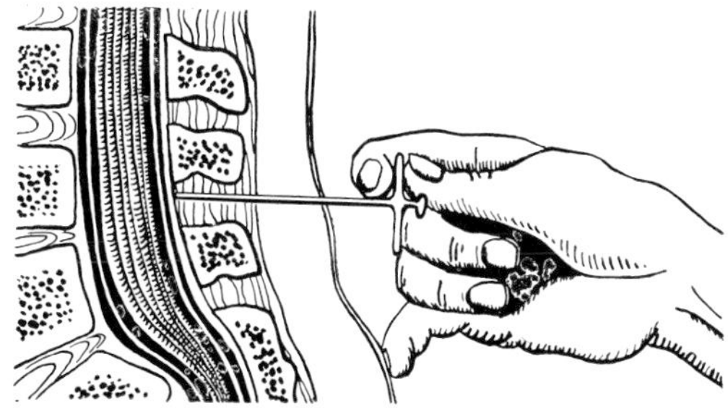

4. Withdraw the stilet and attach to the needle the automatic Iklé syringe, previously charged with physiologic saline solution.

5. Activate the syringe by moving the piston 1/4 turn; push the assembled syringe and needle forward.

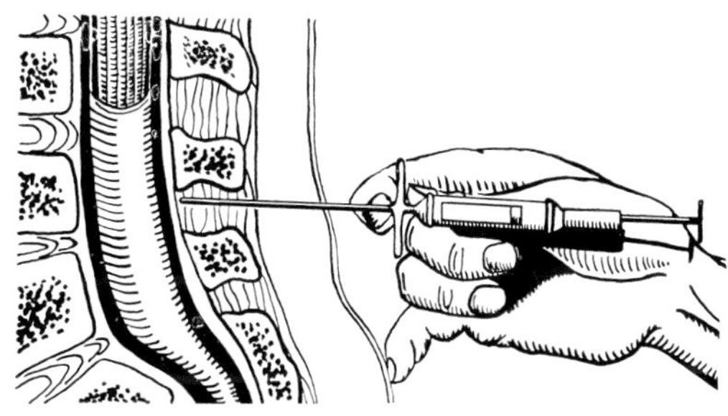

6. The syringe empties automatically when the point of the needle penetrates the peridural space.

7. Apply the 3 security tests: (1) aspiration; (2) easy injection of 5 to 7 cc. of air; (3) injection of test dose of 10 cc. of 1.5 per cent Xylocaine. Wait 5 minutes while examining the patient for signs of subarachnoid injection.

8. Proceed with the injection of the predetermined full dosage of the anesthetic solution.

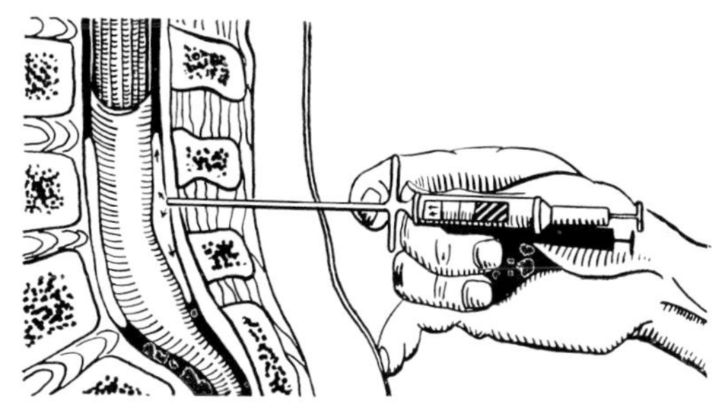

For obstetrics, a Touhy-type needle often is utilized. A fine polyethylene catheter is introduced through it into the peridural space, and the needle is withdrawn, leaving the catheter in place. The anesthesia is maintained by periodic reinjection through the catheter.

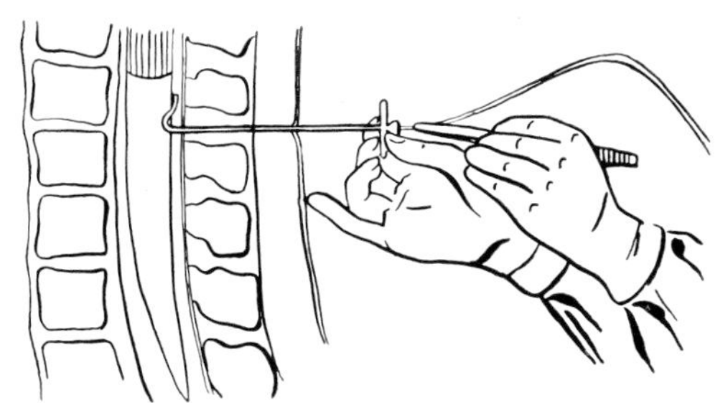

FIG. 62. The Iklé technic of administering lumbar peridural anesthesia, developed by Dr. F. A. Iklé. The steps are shown and explained above.

survey revealed 78,000 obstetric spinal anesthetics for delivery with only 1 maternal death from any cause in the period 1940 to 1955.

Frequently, the dosage of anesthesia in obstetrics is less than is seen in patients of comparable size and weight in surgery. This is particularly true in spinal and in saddle block anesthesia, where the dose may be reduced from one half to one third the usual amount. See below the safe maximum single-dose schedule for spinal or saddle block anesthesia that can be depended upon for vaginal delivery.

Safe Maximum Single-Dose Schedule

For vaginal delivery:

1. Procaine hydrochloride: 30 to 50 mg., with or without dextrose
2. Piperocaine hydrochloride: 22 to 30 mg., with or without dextrose
3. Tetracaine hydrochloride: 2 to 5 mg., with dextrose 5 per cent
4. Dibucaine hydrochloride: 2.5 to 3.75 mg., with dextrose 5 per cent
5. Lidocaine hydrochloride: 25 to 40 mg., with or without dextrose

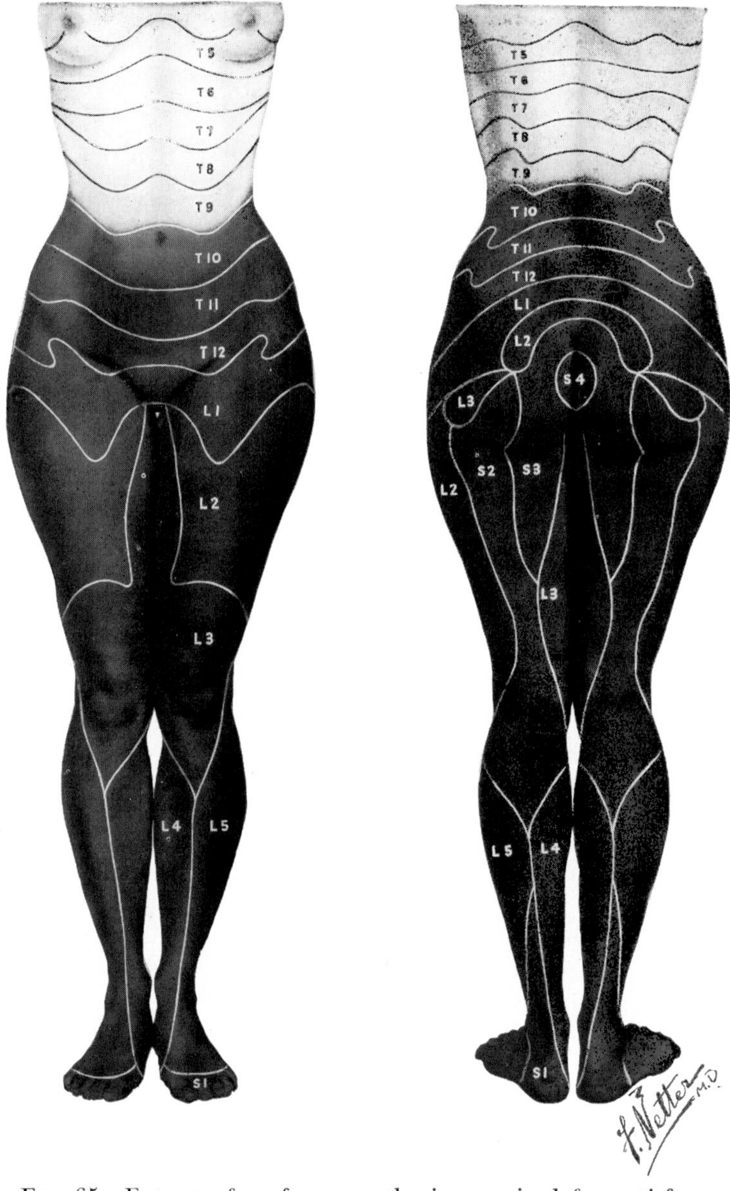

Fig. 65. Extent of surface anesthesia required for satisfactory relief of obstetric pain. (Copyright—Ciba Pharmaceutical Products, Inc.)

For cesarean section:

1. With continuous spinal anesthesia, doses listed for vaginal delivery should not be repeated more frequently than at 30-minute intervals.

2. With single-injection spinal anesthesia, tetracaine might be used in doses up to 10 mg., and dibucaine up to 5 mg., but procaine, piperocaine and lidocaine alone are frequently too short acting to permit the operation to be completed with safety.

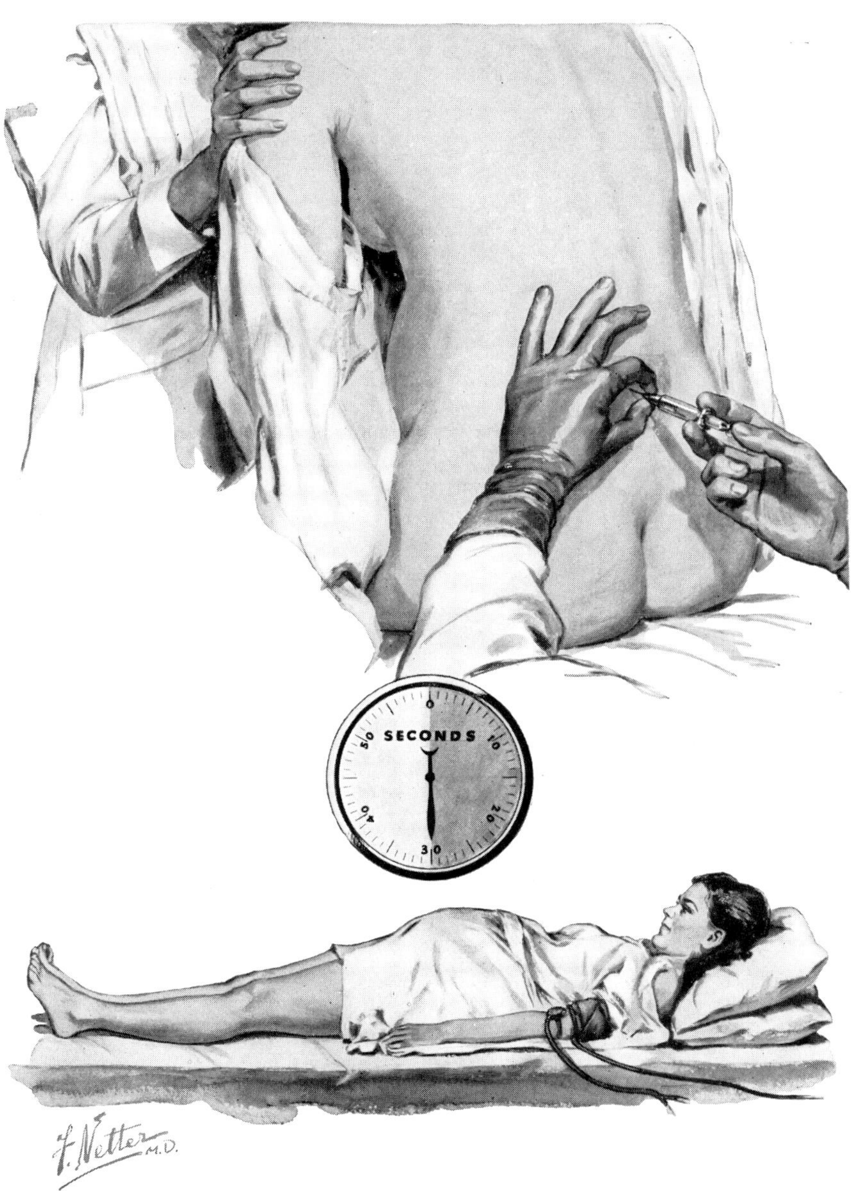

FIG. 66. Injection made to the count of one-and-two-and-three will be complete in from 2 to 3 seconds. Patient remains sitting *exactly* 30 seconds. Patient then is placed *immediately* in a recumbent position with 2 pillows under the head. (Copyright—Ciba Pharmaceutical Products, Inc.)

Isobaric Spinal Anesthesia

If there is perineal bulging, the use of this method with a short-acting agent such as procaine or piperocaine is preferred to the saddle block technic because with the latter there is danger of injury to the baby's head when the mother assumes the sitting position. In such instances, the injection is made with the mother in the lateral reclining position in maximum flexion for injection.

Hyperbaric (Saddle Block) Anesthesia

Advantages:

1. It will localize spinal anesthetic

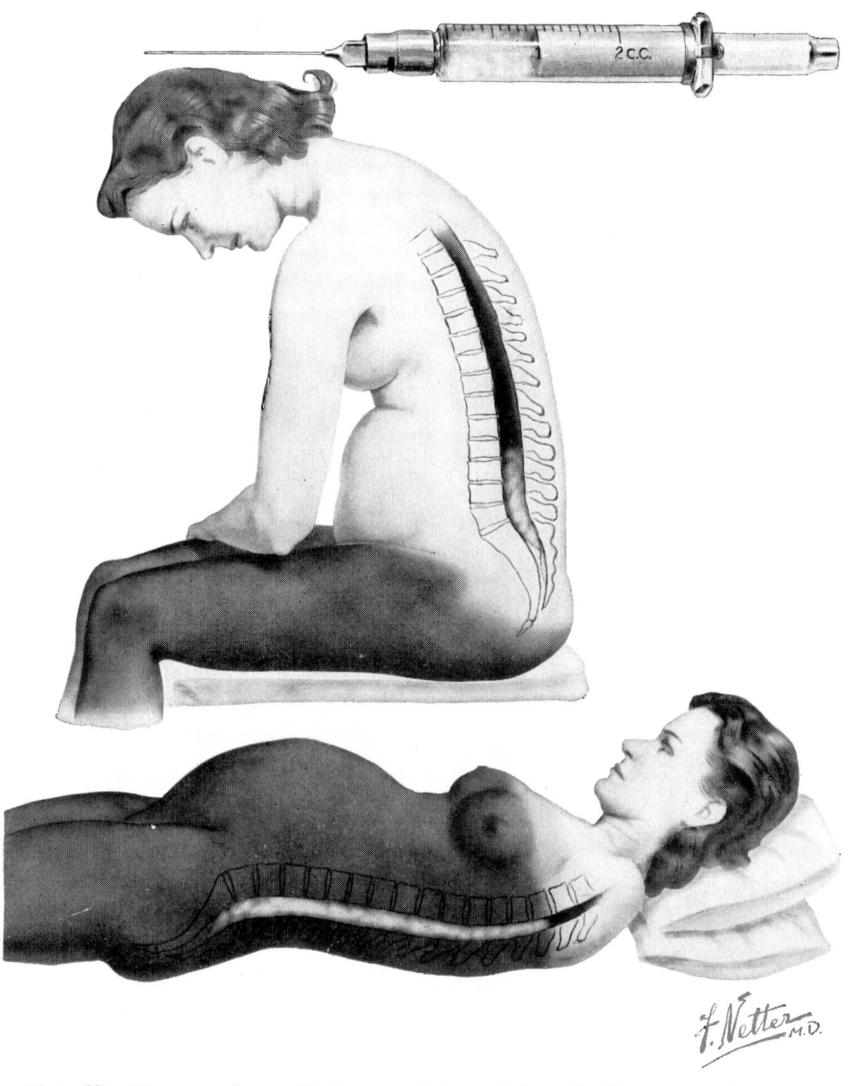

Fig. 67. Nupercaine will be precipitated by alkali present in soap or alkaline tap water. All needles and syringes should be rinsed in acidified water prior to sterilization. Pain will not be completely abolished if the patient sits up too long or the injection is made too slowly. Motor nerve involvement may interrupt labor if patient lies down too soon or the injection is made during uterine contraction. (Copyright—Ciba Pharmaceutical Products, Inc.)

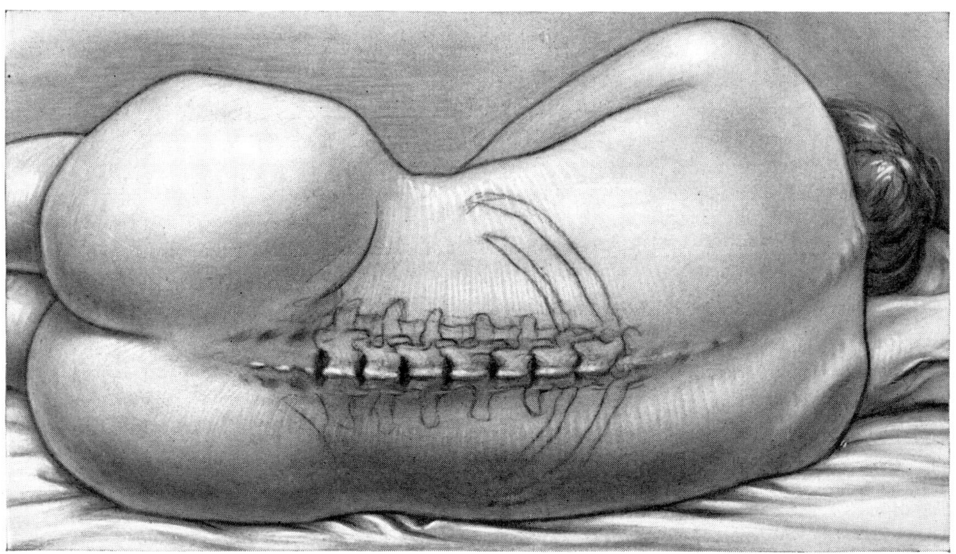

FIG. 68. Patient on side, spine flexed to open interspinous spaces, which are marked with thumbnail pressure on the skin. (Pitkin's Conduction Anesthesia)

agent to provide painless delivery and repair without greatly reducing power of abdominal or uterine musculature.

2. Sensory nerves from fundus and birth canal are affected, and surface anesthesia reaches almost to umbilicus, but there is only major motor involvement of cervix, perineum and, to a lesser extent, legs.

Technic:

1. After pains of early labor have been controlled by analgesics or sedatives, saddle block is instituted only after cervix is 60 per cent effaced and dilated 8 to 10 cm. Patient sits upright with back flexed, legs over side of bed, supported by attendant.

2. 1 cc. of anesthetic drug is drawn into syringe, and lumbar puncture is performed at fourth interspace (level of iliac crest).

A. If difficulty is encountered, use third interspace.

B. Use sharp, short bevel, 20- to 22-gauge spinal needle.

C. Leakage of spinal fluid following tap is minimized if bevel faces laterally.

D. 24- and 26-gauge needles have been used with and without sleeves; this 2-needle technic decreases incidence of postspinal headache.

3. Attach syringe to spinal needle. Aspirate only 0.1 cc. of spinal fluid to ensure free flow. Between uterine contractions, inject anesthetic to the count of "1-and-2-and-3" (injection completed in 2 to 3 seconds).

4. Patient remains sitting exactly 30 seconds following injection. A longer or a shorter period in this position will result in improper height of anesthesia. During the past 5 years in the University Hospitals of Cleveland we have performed these hyperbaric spinal anesthetics with the patient in the lateral flexed position with excellent results.

5. With the aid of the physician and the attendant, the patient is immediately made recumbent in the dorsal supine position, and then pillows are placed under her head.

6. Injection of patient in lateral position is more comfortable in advanced labor. Patient then is placed in a 5° Trendelenburg position.

Precautions:

1. Long bevel needle permits aspiration of spinal fluid but causes extradural injection of anesthetic, resulting in failure to obtain analgesia. Always use a short bevel needle.

2. Dibucaine is precipitated by alkali in soap or alkaline tap water; therefore, needles and syringes should be rinsed in distilled water prior to autoclaving.

3. Anesthetic may go too high, involving motor nerves and interrupting labor, if:

A. Injection is too forceful.

B. Injection is too rapid.

C. Injection is performed during uterine contraction.

D. Patient lies down too soon or is not moved carefully (straining may cause a shift in level of anesthetic)

4. Anesthetic solution will settle unduly, and pain will not be completely abolished if:

A. Patient sits up too long.

B. Injection is too slow.

Complications:

1. **Hypotension.** Treatment is required in only about 5 per cent of cases. Blood pressure should be taken frequently. If severe hypotension occurs, treat it promptly, since death of fetus may result.

Treatment. Raise patient's legs to vertical. This drains blood pooled in leg veins into systemic circulation. If this is ineffectual, inject intravenously 15 mg. of ephedrine or Wyamine Sulfate or some comparable vasopressor. Give parenteral fluid and oxygen inhalation if blood pressure falls below 90 mm. of mercury.

2. **Postspinal Headache.** Since this usually is a result of leakage of spinal fluid, incidence will decrease as technic improves and as smaller gauge needles are used.

Treatment. Apply tight abdominal binder and administer intravenous fluids. Rapid relief is obtained with caudal or extradural injection of 30 to 50 cc. of sterile physiologic saline, which raises sagging subarachnoid pressure by compression within the essentially closed space of the vertebral canal and by counterpressure preventing continued leakage of spinal fluid.

INTRAVENOUS ANESTHESIA

Thiopental Sodium (Sodium Pentothal) or Surital Sodium for Delivery

A recent study shows that a period of 11 minutes was required for equilibrium to be established between anesthetic concentrations of thiopental sodium in maternal and fetal-cord blood, and 5 to 6 minutes was required before an appreciable amount crossed the placenta to the fetal blood. This latent period makes possible the delivery of unnarcotized babies to mothers who require anesthesia for this period of time or less. This method of anesthesia is more prompt than nitrous oxide, ethylene or ether, but it must be conducted by an anesthetist and an obstetrician working as a team. *It is not a technic for the occasional or the inexperienced anesthetist.*

Contraindications

1. Mid-forceps or major obstetric manipulations
2. Patients without premedication with atropine or scopolamine
3. Patients delivering premature babies estimated to weigh 2,500 Gm. or less
4. Primiparas delivering babies through breech mechanism
5. Twin gestation or other multiple births
6. Patients with asthma
7. Patients with clinical cyanosis from

cardiac or respiratory disease, asthma or suspected gastric retention

8. Patients in labor with hypotension

Indications

1. Rapid spontaneous deliveries
2. Some cases of toxemia, where convulsions are likely
3. Patients with central nervous system disease, such as epilepsy and mania

Technic of Administration

1. Place patient on delivery table and insert into a good arm vein an 18-gauge needle attached to tubing and syringe.
2. Apply transparent face mask for oxygen inhalations.
3. Give test dose of 2 cc. of a 2.5 per cent solution of thiopental to observe for exaggerated effect, especially on respiration, during catheterization, cleansing of perineum and application of sterile drapes.
4. Reassure patient constantly that anesthesia will provide instantaneous relief at the moment required. Patient is required to bear down, with the promise that this pleasant anesthesia is readily available when she makes sufficient progress.
5. Coincident with "crowning" and on indication from the obstetrician, administer an induction dose of 6 cc.
6. After a full circulation time of 30 seconds, a second dose of 2 to 4 cc. is administered when it is verified that respirations are not obtunded. Usually a total of 12 cc. is adequate for spontaneous delivery in multiparas. An additional 6 to 10 cc. in 2-cc. doses 1 minute apart may be required for spontaneous delivery in primiparas.
7. For outlet forceps delivery:

A. Patient is anesthetized promptly as for operation of dilatation and curettage until the mid-second plane of surgical anesthesia is reached.

B. When patient's respirations are adequate and desired anesthetic depth is reached, obstetrician beings application of forceps and the episiotomy.

C. After baby is delivered, cord is clamped and cut promptly, and anesthesia is continued for third stage and repair.

D. Use of 50 per cent nitrous oxide-oxygen mixture will reduce amount of thiopental required.

E. Administration of 25 mg. of intravenous Demerol after test dose will provide higher degree of analgesia as a synergistic supplement, thereby reducing the requirement of the almost pure soporific effect of pentothal. The mere fact that this technic works so well in normal uncomplicated obstetrics indicates that its excellent and instantaneous control of the disturbed psyche is strong forte.

INHALATION ANESTHETICS FOR OBSTETRIC LABOR

Chloroform

This agent still is used widely as a method of pain relief in home obstetrics and is, perhaps, the general anesthetic agent of choice in tropical and equatorial countries. It may be administered by either the open or the closed technic. The high oxygen concentration that can be added to it in the closed system is a most important factor in protecting the maternal liver from toxic damage. We believe that regardless of the method chosen, the obstetrician who uses chloroform should have oxygen at hand so that he can administer it to his patient in the event of respiratory depression with its attending anoxia.

Analgesia "à la reine" in Labor

Chloroform was the type of anesthesia that was administered by Sir John Snow to Queen Victoria during her eighth confinement. Since chloroform in the liquid state will produce severe irritation and burns of both the skin and the conjunctiva, a drop of castor oil or mineral oil should be placed in each conjunctival sac before its administration is begun. Cold cream, petroleum jelly or lard should be rubbed generously round the patient's external air passages and round the mouth. First, the patient should be resassured that slow, regular inspiration of chloroform will relieve her pain. Also, she should be told that her co-operation is an important part of the success to be obtained with this agent. She should indicate to the anesthetist the exact second of the onset of each pain.

Method of Administration:

1. Any of the ordinary types of higher basket masks covered with a few thicknesses of gauze or porous cotton cloth should be placed a few inches above the patient's nose.

2. Two or three drops of chloroform should be placed on the cone of the mask and the patient instructed to breathe deeply in and out. The chloroform should be administered by the open drop method at the rate of 4 to 10 drops per minute during the height of the uterine contraction. At no time should the mask encircle the mouth and the nose tightly. As soon as the painful contraction has passed, the analgesic agent should be withheld until the patient indicates its return. With this technic the patient will not be placed in any of the deep stages of anesthesia. She can understand the command of the anesthetist and can co-operate with the obstetrician upon request.

Chloroform is the most potent and generally complete of the inhalation analgesic and anesthetic agents.

Chief factors concerning inspired atmosphere:

1. Concentration must be minimal.
2. Oxygen must be adequate.
3. Carbon dioxide must be removed with certainty.

Premedication:

Atropine, 1 mg., is advisable to counteract possible bradycardia or cardiac arrest caused by augmented vagal nerve impulses during induction. Initial ventricular fibrillation need not be considered, because its clinical occurrence is yet to be proved.

Induction and Maintenance:

1. Open drop, insufflation, semiclosed or closed method of administration may be used.

2. Holding mask 3 fingerbreadths from face when open administration is begun aids in minimizing dosage and maintaining oxygen-carbon dioxide balance.

3. If breath-holding occurs, mask should be removed instantly. Continued dropping of the agent, followed by as few as 2 subsequent respiratory exchanges of nearly vital capacity, has produced cardiac arrest. Prompt and vigorous inflation with oxygen may reverse the effects of such maladministration.

Cessation of Administration:

1. Begun as soon as closure of operative field is started.

2. Analgesia is prolonged, and a patient who is conscious and responsive to questions will not object to or give evidence of knowledge of placement of sutures at end of operation.

Muscular Relaxation:

1. As estimated by usual signs of depression, relaxation is approximately as great in second to third plane of surgical anesthesia with this agent as in third to fourth place with any of the other general anesthetic agents.

2. If great depth of anesthesia is not forced, satisfactory relaxation will prevail for the surgeon, and stable levels of blood pressure will be maintained for any surgical procedure done in a reasonable length of time.

As Supplement to Ethylene, Nitrous Oxide or Basal Agents:

Chloroform added to these agents in such low concentrations as to be scarcely detectable to the anesthetist by its odor (0.05-0.2%), produces adequate anesthesia for procedures for which muscular relaxation is not required.

Chief Uses:

1. When nonflammable inhalation agent is needed
2. When nonirritating inhalation agent is needed

Because of severe toxic effects on circulation and liver, it is seldom used now in this country.

Precautions:

1. For oxygen deficiency caused by reduced minute exchange with open drop method, enrich atmosphere under mask by flow of 1 to 2 L. of oxygen per minute.
2. This is advisable also when possibility of potential pathologic condition exists, such as hepatic, renal or coronary damage.
3. These pathologic conditions are aggravated by carbon dioxide accumulation; therefore, rigorous attention to its removal is necessary at all times.
4. Control of oxygen and carbon dioxide still is more important when chloroform is administered with an anesthetic machine.
5. Since chloroform vapor is relatively pleasant, sweet and nonirritating to inhale, untoward cardiovascular accidents have occurred from rapid and unwitting overdosage.
6. If spilled on face, it may cause burns of eyes and mucous membranes of nose and mouth.

Chloroform Anesthesia for Delivery

Usually, the administration of chloroform anesthesia is begun toward the terminal portion of the first stage of labor at the time the cervix is almost completely dilated. But when the presenting part is distending the perineum, more than analgesia is necessary to relieve pain. The chloroform mask for the open drop technic is placed lightly over the nose and the mouth. Then the chloroform is administered at the rate of 4 to 10 drops during the first minute as a trial for pharmacologic effect. Its rate of administration can be increased or decreased as indicated. The patient will be placed in one of the planes of anesthesia somewhat swiftly. It will be noticed that she goes through the following stages:

1. The stage of analgesia, during which the "edge" will be removed from the painful contraction.
2. The stage of excitement, when the patient may struggle, talk incoherently, scream, cry or laugh. It is not unusual for the patient to attempt forcefully to grab the arms of the anesthetist or to try to knock the mask from her face. She should be restrained firmly but gently by the assistants who, in the hospital, would be nurses, and, in the home, members of her family. Even in this stage she should be reassured by the anesthetist and told to breathe deeply in and out. Occasionally in this stage vomiting occurs. The anesthetist should be ready at all times to remove food particles or fluid from the mouth, the throat and the nose. When vomiting occurs, the mask should be removed and the patient's head turned to the side. As soon as the patient has re-established regular respirations, the anesthetic may be continued.
3. The patient then passes into the first plane of the third or surgical stage of anesthesia. Her respirations, during this period, are quite noisy and deep. The pupils begin to dilate. Increased salivation and increased secretion from the lacrimal glands causing "tearing" are not unusual. This is the stage most fre-

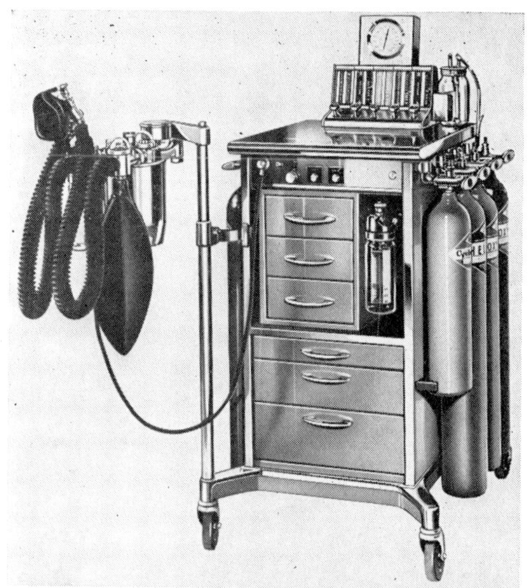

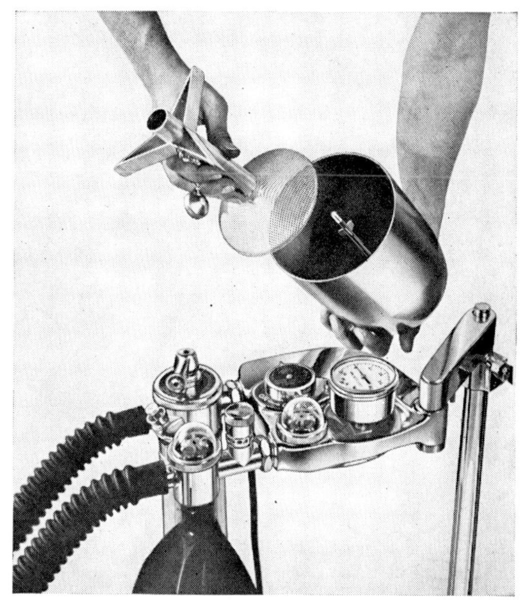

Fig. 69. Heidbrink new cabinet kinetometer G-25 machine with enlarged view of soda lime circuit and vaporizer. (Ohio Chemical & Surgical Equipment Co., Madison, Wis.)

quently used for uncomplicated obstetric delivery. The average patient with chloroform anesthesia can be placed in this stage within 2 to 5 minutes from the onset of the induction. The uterine contractions are not yet abolished. This is the stage most frequently employed for spontaneous delivery. Episiotomy in indicated cases can be performed without pain to the patient. After the head of the baby is born, the anesthetist should be instructed to remove the chloroform mask and permit the patient to breathe air freely. In the ideal situation, the patient at this stage would be administered 100 per cent oxygen. If several minutes are required to resuscitate the baby, the patient often will recover consciousness from the anesthesia. However, in hospital practice, many anesthetists and obstetricians prefer to keep the patient completely anesthetized until the completion of the third stage and the repair work has been performed. For the repair of the episiotomy or for any intra-uterine manipulations for removal of the placenta, complete relaxation of the patient is required, so that she has to be put into the second plane of the third stage of surgical anesthesia. In this stage the respirations are regular and more shallow. The pupils are beginning to dilate, the pulse is slow and regular. The patient should be given enough air or oxygen to maintain a pink color of the skin.

Anesthesia for Operative Delivery

Patients who require delivery by decomposition of the breech and the performance of internal podalic version must be perfectly relaxed to the point that uterine contractions are no longer present. This state is reached in the second plane of the third stage. There is no form of surgical anesthesia that provides the relaxation of the patient as rapidly and as efficiently as chloroform. Because of its accelerated rate of action and its property of obtaining complete muscular relaxation in a brief period of time, for such emergencies as prolapse of the cord, or when quick termination of the labor is necessary to save the child, it is a satisfactory form of anesthesia.

Technic for the Closed System

With the Heidbrink, the McKesson and the Foregger gas machines, chloroform may be administered with high concentration of oxygen with or without the carbon dioxide eliminator. Light anesthesia may be maintained with 1.35 volumes per cent; deep anesthesia, with 1.65 volumes per cent. As indicated in the drug discussion in Chapter 1, 2 volumes per cent may produce cardiac and respiratory arrest. However, in the induction stage, until the alveolar tissues and the circulating blood have absorbed an anesthesia level, 4 volumes per cent may be necessary. In unusually robust individuals, and in women undergoing agonizing pain near the termination of labor, as high as 10 to 18 volumes per cent is required for the induction. This induction stage lasts only for 1 to 5 minutes. The anesthetist should be more skilled in interpreting physical signs of pharmacologic action with this method than with any other form of inhalation anesthesia. Usually, cardiac irregularities that occur during the stages of induction indicating myocardial irritability will disappear and will be replaced by a regular bradycardia once the first plane of the surgical stage of anesthesia has been passed. Lundy has condemned the use of Adrenalin for any of the cardiac "emergencies" during this form of anesthesia.

Once the induction stage is over, the

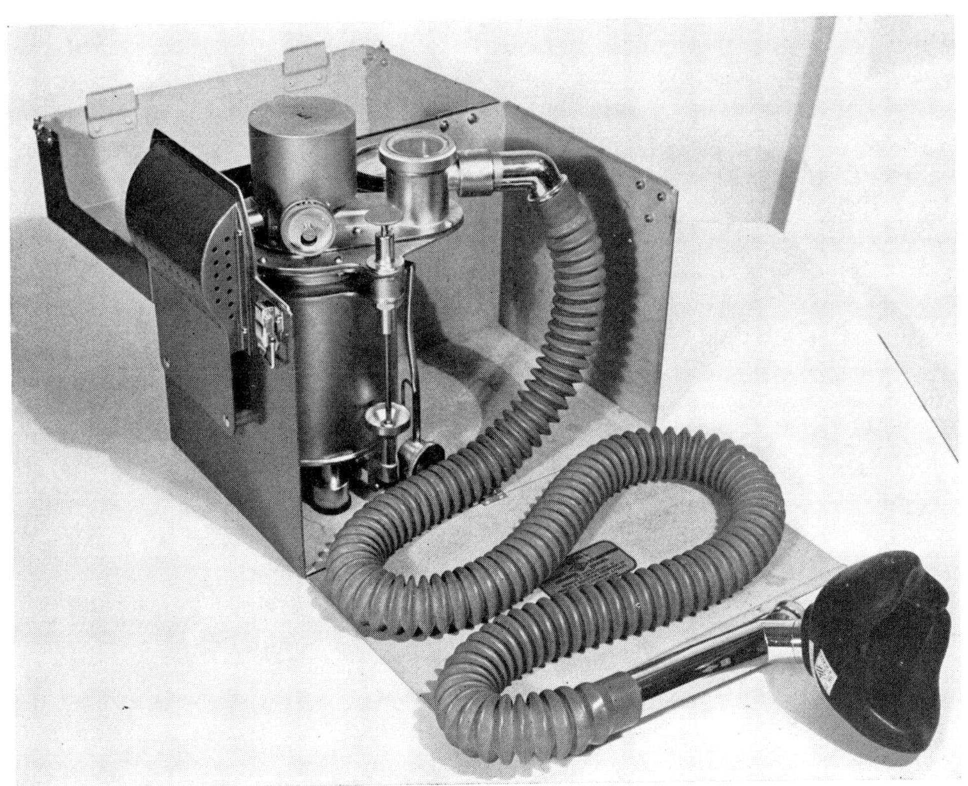

FIG. 70. Emotril inhaler.

amount of chloroform administered to the patient should be reduced markedly to below 2 volumes per cent. The rebreathing bag should be emptied and refilled with 100 per cent oxygen.

Chloroform still is used extensively today in private homes and in tropical countries, but its administration in modern hospitals is so infrequent that very few anesthetists are familiar with its action.

It has been said that chloroform is not dangerous in pregnancy, and that pregnant women are particularly resistant to its toxic effects. According to the experiments of Whipple, direct evidence was produced to the contrary. In his experimental work in drugs he found that young animals during the first 4 weeks of life did not succumb to 2 hours' administration of chloroform anesthesia. Beyond this time it was shown that the usual marked liver necrosis occurred. According to Graham, the fact that pups were resistant to chloroform poisoning was due to protection by glycogen in the liver.

It is admitted that many thousands of confinements have been conducted with the use of chloroform inhalation, but, in view of the fact that the margin of safety with chloroform is not comparable with ether, and since the factor of mortality outweighs the factor of morbidity in choosing the anesthetic agent, chloroform has been discarded gradually in favor of ether. Today it remains an inhalation anesthetic that should be used in obstetric practice only when other forms of analgesia and anesthesia are not available, or when they are made inefficient or undesirable because of climate or exposure to open flames or electricity.

Trichloroethylene in Labor

Trichloroethylene (Trilene) during the last half of the first stage of labor and for delivery.

The Emotril Inhaler has been developed by the Nuffield Anesthesia Department of Oxford University to provide a constant and controllable concentration of Trilene for analgesia. Trilene is a liquid with a pungent but not unpleasant smell in light concentrations. It is nonexplosive. It is a potent analgesic and a light anesthetic agent. Trilene will provide fair analgesia if the inhaled mixture of air contains 0.375 per cent. It will provide light anesthesia suitable for spontaneous delivery and easy outlet forcep extraction of the infant if the concentration is delivered at 0.5 per cent. The Emotril Inhaler can be standardized according to room temperature by matching the simple color chart with the color graduations on the temperature scale; to provide for 0.375 per cent concentration, set at the "weak" designation, and for 0.5 per cent concentration, set at "normal" concentration. There is a special expiratory valve that prevents the rebreathing of exhaled mixtures.

A special mask is provided for self-administration of the agent. The patient is instructed to apply the mask and to inhale regularly and normally during uterine contractions. With the increasing intensity of uterine contraction discomfort, the patient is encouraged to keep the mask, set appropriately as mentioned, over her face for longer periods of time. As she feels more relaxed, she can remove the mask. As she approaches delivery, she is encouraged under the surveillance of the anesthetist to keep constantly over her face the mask set at "normal" to provide an 0.5 per cent concentration. Under this form of management a great many patients co-operate intelligently and bear down upon instruction. They are seldom out of contact with the environment, and they will answer questions and carry through the instructions of the anesthetist. However, it should be emphasized that deepening of the anesthetic beyond the first plane of the surgical stage is characterized frequently by a bradycardia or an irregular heart action and by the onset of curiously rapid, shallow respiration. Upon the onset of these symptoms, the anesthetic mask is removed, and 100 per cent oxygen is inhaled. A small percentage of the babies show the usual obtunding of the respiratory mechanism if they are born to mothers who had Trilene analgesia and anesthesia for longer than 20 minutes. Trilene should not be used with soda lime in a rebreathing closed circuit machine, since eighth nerve damage often results from inhaling metabolites of the mixture. The use of trichloroethylene in labor for any period absolutely contraindicates subsequent closed or semiclosed soda lime absorption technics for delivery.

USE OF CONTINUOUS CONDUCTION ANALGESIA FOR LABOR

Continuous Caudal

This technic, properly performed at the appropriate time during progressive labor, approaches the ideal. In the multipara, the cervix should be dilated 3 cm. or more, the presenting part in the pelvis and the uterine contractions occurring at 3 minutes apart or less and lasting for 40 seconds or more. In the primipara, the cervix should be dilated 5 cm. or more, the presenting part well fixed in the pelvis and uterine contractions occurring 3 minutes apart or less and lasting for 40 seconds or more before the analgesia is begun. The method demands hospital facilities and a degree of skill in administration that always will limit its availability to only a small percentage of cases. There is no doubt as to its efficacy, and on the Hardy-Javert dolorimeter scale it provides complete analgesia for labor and intense anesthesia for delivery. There is equally no doubt as to the increased forceps rate that follows its use and the dangers of such hazards of hypotension, infection and inadvertent spinal injection.

ANESTHESIAS FOR VAGINAL DELIVERY

The Volatile Anesthetics

Chloroform

Even though this method is rejected by most of the large American hospitals, we recognize from past experience that when administered drop by drop, and, more cautiously, drip by drip, to normal healthy parturients delivering healthy full-term babies, it is a very prompt and efficient agent for relief of pain. Since it is an irritant to conjunctivae, proper protection must be effected by the instillation of a drop of castor oil in each and by sufficient covering with a rubber shield. It must be given with high concentrations of oxygen or fresh air, which are ensured by supporting the mask always at least 1 fingerbreadth from the face. The finger of the anesthetist is kept constantly upon the maternal pulse, and the anesthetic induction is started. Within 2 to 4 minutes if the chloroform is administered at the rate of 10 to 15 drops per minute, the patient has passed into the first plane of surgical anesthesia. Upon the slightest indication of bradycardia, the mask is withdrawn and the patient is permitted to inhale 100 per cent oxygen or air.

In complicated obstetric emergencies at home and in hospitals that require prompt and relaxing anesthesia, in such cases as a prolapse of a pulsating cord that cannot be replaced easily and surely, it is an efficient agent of choice.

Ether

Because of its wide margin of safety, ether anesthesia still has a place in ob-

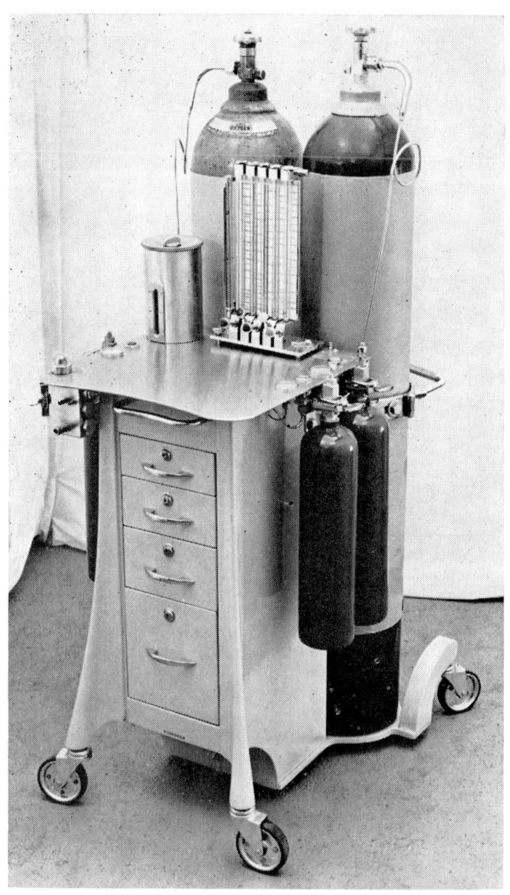

Fig. 71. Foregger cabinet model for large and small cylinders, rotameter-type flowmeters and copper kettle ether vaporizer. This machine permits the use of low cost K cylinders of commercial oxygen and G cylinders of nitrous oxide, in addition to the standard hospital size D tanks. A copper kettle ether vaporizer, described in Dr. Lucien E. Morris' paper, "A new vaporizer for liquid anesthetic agents," has its own oxygen-feed system to control the amount of ether vapor in addition to the conventional flowmeters for the remaining gases.

stetrics. It can be used either alone in the open drop method, or in the closed circuit machine, where it can augment a weaker agent, such as nitrous oxide. In these circumstances, at least 20 per cent oxygen should be provided during induction and at least 50 per cent of oxygen during maintenance. Usually, it requires from 6 to 15 minutes to procure adequate relaxation for forceps delivery with open drop ether or with ether and nitrous oxide technic. It is important that the patient should have had previously atropine $\frac{1}{150}$ gr. (0.4 mg.) as a preanesthetic preparation. Insufflation of ether anesthesia has been used by us promptly to relax a tetanic uterus that produces signs of anoxia in the child. Rectal anesthesia, according to the technic of McCormick, is a valuable alternative method.

Divinyl Ether (Vinethene)

Because of its more acceptable aroma, this anesthetic agent is inhaled more readily by the patients in the second stage of labor. Administered on a mask a little more sparingly than ether, it provides moderate relaxation for operative delivery with, perhaps, less pulmonary postdelivery complications than ether. Most advocates of this agent urge that it be used for contemplated short deliveries and obstetric manipulations that are expected to be less than 15 minutes in duration.

Trichloroethylene (Trilene)

This agent has been used in Great Britain for several hundred thousand deliveries. It is not used with soda lime. We have had experience in the use of this agent in more than 200 deliveries in the Johns Hopkins Hospital. Its technic of administration through the Emotril Inhaler has been described already. We do not feel that the Cyprane and the McGill Inhalers, which permit an unregulated amount of Trilene to enter the respiratory systems, offer the safety factors presented by the Emotril instrument. Many of our patients who have had previous general anesthetics with nitrous oxide and ether tell us that the induction with

Trilene is much more pleasant, and pain relief is more satisfactory. We have had no maternal complications in our series, and only 1 baby presented evidence of profound depression from this agent.

GAS ANESTHETICS

Nitrous Oxide

During labor, a good measure of analgesia can be maintained with 40 per cent nitrous oxide and 60 per cent oxygen. The patient approaching delivery will need more relief than that afforded by the lower concentrations of the gas. For the induction stage, with the Heidbrink, the McKesson and the Foregger machines with the semiclosed circuit method, a mixture of 80 to 85 per cent nitrous oxide and 15 to 20 per cent oxygen should be administered for from 3 to 5 minutes. The most satisfactory volumes of oxygen and nitrous oxide to obtain this percentage are: 5 L. of nitrous oxide per minute and 1 L. of oxygen per minute with the semiclosed technic. After 3 to 5 minutes the excess nitrogen has been expired from the patient's lungs, and the parturient begins to pass from the second to the third stage of anesthesia. Then the concentration of nitrous oxide is reduced to a running maximum of 80 per cent, and the concentration of oxygen is raised to a running minimum of 20 per cent. This can be maintained by the use of a flow of 2 L. of nitrous oxide and 500 cc. of oxygen per minute. This concentration is very satisfactory for spontaneous deliveries and obstetric operations that require 15 minutes or less. It becomes hazardous through a gradual build-up of nitrous oxide percentage due to the patient's consumption of oxygen. As soon as the baby's head is born, the nitrous oxide is shut off temporarily, and the rebreathing bag is flushed with 100 per cent oxygen until the cord is clamped.

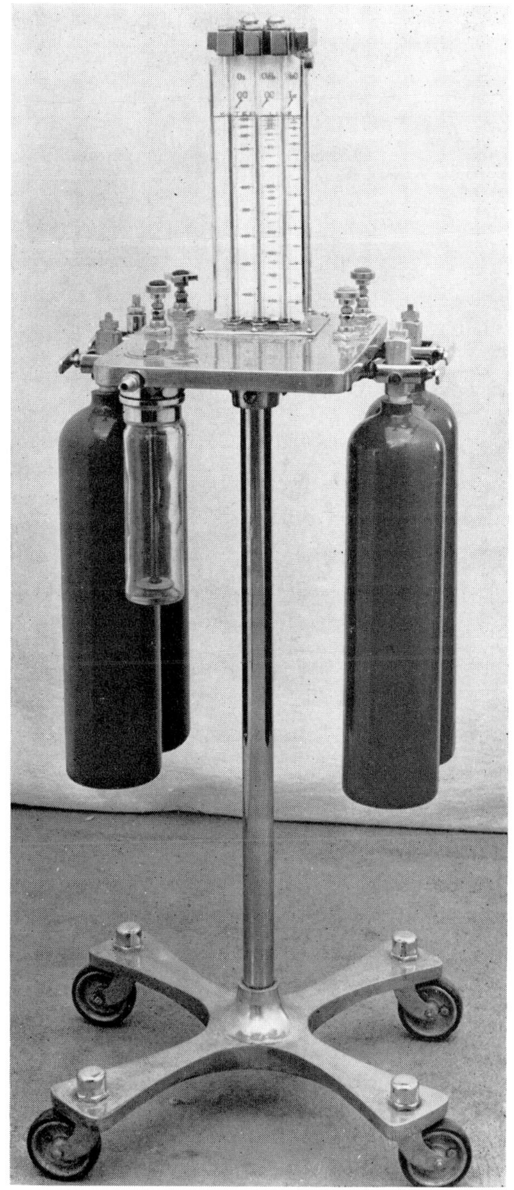

Fig. 72. Foregger 3-OF base and upright with built-in ether vaporizer, a small, light and readily transportable unit built with aluminum base and plate and equipped with ball-bearing wheels for mobility. An ideal unit for office use or outpatients, or for the small OB department where storage facilities, chart table, etc., are not required.

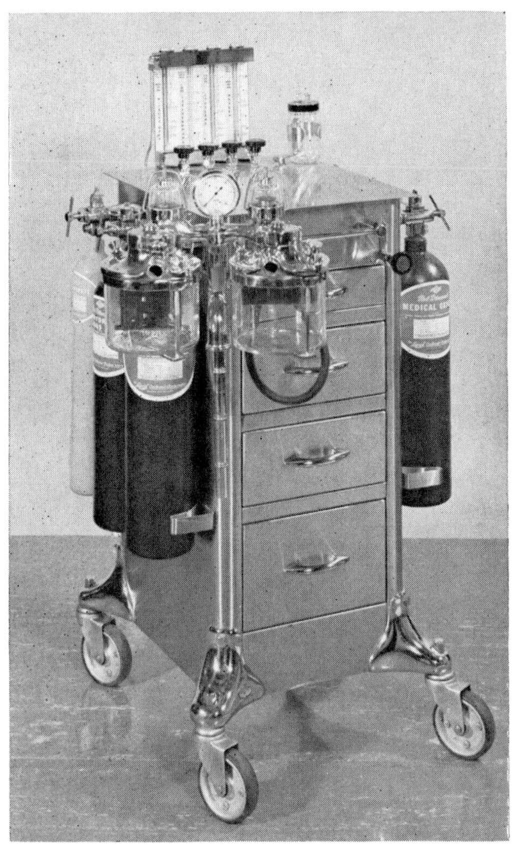

FIG. 73. The rotameter, cabinet model. (Chicago Anesthetic Equipment Company)

Should further relaxation of the patient be required at any time, ether is added slowly to the induction mixture with an enrichment of the oxygen concentration as anesthesia deepens.

ETHYLENE

Because of its explosiveness, ethylene never should be administered intermittently; therefore, it is not to be used as a method of analgesia early in labor. It is more satisfactory for continuous planned anesthesia, and, when it is used with the closed method with a well-grounded unit of administration, the explosion hazard is practically eliminated. For induction we have found that a mixture containing 85 per cent ethylene and 15 per cent oxygen will produce satisfactory obstetric anesthesia in 3 to 5 minutes. Then the concentration of ethylene is reduced to from 80 to 75 per cent, and the concentration of oxygen is raised 20 or 25 per cent.

CYCLOPROPANE

This is the most potent of the anesthetic gases. It may be administered with a higher concentration of oxygen than any of the other agents. From 3 to 5 per cent will produce analgesia in 5 to 10 minutes; from 6 to 8 per cent will produce unconsciousness in the same period of time; from 20 to 25 per cent will produce anesthesia in the average case. In some patients, respiratory failure with paralysis of the respiratory center begins at 35 per cent, and in most patients it is complete at 42 per cent. The gas has a sweet odor and is not irritating. It is an unsaturated hydrocarbon, and the explosion hazard attendant upon its use is great. Consequently, like ethylene, it should be administered by the closed method with the continuous flow technic. The uterine contractions are not decreased in light anesthesia, but they are abolished entirely in the third plane of surgical stages. The gas passes through the placenta to the fetus, whose oxygen content in arterial blood is decreased approximately 20 per cent because of the diminished respiratory excursions of the mother. Success with its use is proportional to the previous experience of the anesthetist. Because of the rapidity of its action, it is used best in terminal delivery.

With the technic described below, maternal cyclopropane blood level reaches 16 to 20 mg. per cent in 10 minutes. Simultaneous blood levels in fetal cord blood have been measured by us at 13 to 16 mg. per cent in the same period. In one second twin the blood level was 22 mg. per cent after 23 minutes of maternal anesthesia. This level corresponds with third-plane third-stage anesthesia.

It should be emphasized that cardiac irregularities under cyclopropane occur not infrequently. These irregularities may be merely a few extra systoles, auricular tachycardia, auricular flutter or fibrillation, and, if improperly managed, ventricular fibrillation. Thus, the mechanism of action of cyclopropane, because of the sensitization it causes in the myocardial mechanism, has been shown to be similar to that described for chloroform. One should remember that cyclopropane produces a vagal stimulating effect.

Closed Method of Administration

1. The patient should be given a few inhalations of 100 per cent oxygen before this concentration is diluted 50 per cent with cyclopropane. She should be asked to count audibly from 1 to 20.

2. When incoherent counting begins, the mixture may be reduced to 25 per cent cyclopropane and 75 per cent oxygen. The depth of anesthesia will increase markedly between pains. The quantity of cyclopropane should not be increased until after the birth of the baby, at which time the oxygen content is raised until the umbilical cord is severed. Manual assistance to respiration, by intermittent compression of the rebreathing bag, is required upon slightest evidence of hypoventilation. One must keep in mind the classic picture of cyclopropane postanesthesia shock from CO_2 shift from retention during unassisted respiration while asleep to altered low levels when awake.

If an episiotomy or a laceration has to be repaired or if some other obstetric maneuver is required, the concentration of cyclopropane may be raised to any percentage between 20 and 35 that is necessary to provide the adequate amount of relaxation desired. The incidence of the third stage and postpartum hemorrhage is increased when this agent is used to provide third plane third stage surgical anesthesia. Fetal deaths have been reported with this anesthetic agent both in obstetric delivery and for cesarean section. Pitocin and/or Ergotrate should be used as the oxytocics, since pituitrin with cyclopropane is more likely to initiate dangerous ventricular fibrillation.

The anticipated duration of the labor and the delivery and the severity of the pain are the important factors to consider when the choice and the concentration of analgesic and anesthetic gases have to be made. The use of the gases during internal podalic version is not so satisfactory as with ether or chloroform. Usually, in cesarean section ether is not added to the gaseous mixture until the child is delivered from the uterus, and just preceding the extraction of the child the oxygen intake is increased again. Following the extraction of the child and the clamping of the umbilical cord, the addition of ether gives a better relaxation and permits the anesthetist to have better control of the patient during the closure of the uterus and the abdominal wall. The use of cyclopropane in nonexplosive helium buffered and dampened mixtures is described in the section on the Reserve Midget, page 167.

In summing up the use of the inhalation anesthetics as analgesic agents during the first stage of labor, it might be said that although all of them may be used, there have been so many other methods that seem to be more satisfactory for this stage that they are being replaced rapidly. In the use of the inhalation anesthetics for actual anesthesia, one has to choose the anesthetic and the type of machine available in his surroundings. We perfer nitrous oxide-oxygen with or without ether to the various other drugs, and, again, the choice of the anesthetic agent among this group has to be selected according to the condition of the patient, the requirements for relaxation and the duration of the obstetric procedure to be carried out. It is essential that the soda lime absorber be used with all the gas anesthetic mixtures. An increase in the carbon dioxide content of the mixture certainly would produce a pharmacologic stimulation of the fetal respiratory center. This would initiate in some cases undesired inspirations by the fetus of infected amniotic fluid or meconium-stained fluid into the respiratory tract of the infant.

BARBITURATES

Utilizing the technic established by Hellman and Eastman, more than 5,000 deliveries have been conducted with Pentothal Sodium in the Johns Hopkins Hospital during the past decade. These investigators have determined with spectrum studies that a period of 11 minutes is required for establishment of equilibrium of the anesthetic concentrations in both maternal and fetal cord blood. Of greater significance is the fact that a period of 5 to 6 minutes is required before an appreciable amount of Pentothal Sodium crosses the placenta to the fetal blood. This latent period makes possible the delivery of unnarcotized babies to mothers who have a smooth anesthesia for this period of time or less.

Contraindications

1. Mid-forceps or major obstetric manipulations
2. Patients who have eaten a meal within 6 hours of induction
3. Patients who have a suspected gastric retention
4. Patients who have not been premedicated with atropine or scopolamine
5. Patients delivering premature babies estimated to be 2,500 Gm. or less in weight
6. Primiparas delivering babies through the breech mechanism
7. Twin gestation or other multiple births
8. Patients with asthma
9. Patients with clinical cyanosis from cardiac or respiratory disease

Indications

We believe this method of anesthesia to be indicated for:

1. Rapid spontaneous deliveries
2. Patients who have had massive hemorrhage with and without shock in placenta previa and premature separation. (These patients always should have 100 per cent oxygen by mask. They can be managed usually with one half of or less than the usual dose.)
3. Some cases of toxemia in which convulsions are likely
4. Patients with central nervous system disease, such as epilepsy and mania

Technic of Administration

1. Place the patient on delivery table and insert into good arm vein an 18-gauge needle attached to Pentothal Sodium tubing and syringe.
2. Apply transparent face mask for oxygen inhalations.
3. Give test dose of 2 cc. of 2.5 per cent solution of Pentothal Sodium to observe for exaggerated effect during catheterization, cleansing of perineum and application of sterile drapes.
4. Reassure patient constantly that anesthesia will provide instantaneous relief at the moment that she requires it. Patient is instructed to bear down, with the promise that this pleasant anesthesia is readily available when she makes sufficient progress.

5. Conicident with "crowning," upon indication from the obstetrician an induction dose of 6 cc. is administered.

6. After a full circulation time of 30 seconds, a second 4 cc. is administered when it is verified that respirations are not obtunded. Usually, this total dose of 12 cc. is adequate for spontaneous delivery in multiparas. An additional 6 to 10 cc. is required in 2-cc. doses 1 minute apart for primiparas during spontaneous delivery.

7. When outlet forcep delivery is anticipated, the patient is put to sleep promptly as for the operation of dilatation and curettage until the mid-first, or second, plane of surgical anesthesia is reached. Upon indication from the anesthetist that the patient's respirations are adequate and that the desired anesthetic depth is reached, the obstetrician begins the application of forceps and the episiotomy. After the baby is delivered the cord is clamped and cut promptly, and the anesthesia is continued for the third stage and repair, as in surgery. The use of 50 per cent nitrous oxide-oxygen mixture will reduce the amount of Pentothal Sodium required.

This method of anesthesia is more prompt than nitrous oxide, ethylene or ether, but it must be conducted by an anesthetist and an obstetrician who will work as a team. It is not a technic to be used by the occasional anesthetist or by the inexperienced.

CONTINUOUS CAUDAL AND EXTRADURAL ANESTHESIA FOR DELIVERY

The use of these methods in the terminal part of labor was described earlier. When it is anticipated that the patient is approaching delivery, a careful recheck of the intensity and the somatic level of anesthesia is made by pin prick and by observing the motor power of the patient's lower extremities. If the patient has not had a supplementary injection within 20 minutes, and if the level of nerve block is not above the umbilicus, she is given another 20 cc. of 1.5 per cent Metycaine, or 0.15 per cent Pontocaine, or 1.0 per cent Xylocaine, or 2.0 per cent procaine, and prepared in the usual manner for delivery. With the patient herself holding the mask, 100 per cent oxygen inhalations are administered. She is more comfortable with her head on 1 or 2 pillows. The patient can cooperate and bear down when desired and instructed to do so. Spontaneous deliveries can be accomplished in most multiparas and in about one third of the primiparas. Instructions of mechanisms of labor and the active part required by the parturient are just as important here as for the physiologic childbirth group.

However, the incidence of necessary outlet forceps is increased. Generally, third stage blood loss is reduced because of the better contraction of the uterus. Usually, 0.2 mg. of Ergotrate is injected after the delivery of the placenta and is the only oxytocic required. It is important to guard the patient from hypotension below 100 mm. systolic. Small intravenous doses of 5 mg. of desoxyephedrine or 15 mg. of ephedrine will raise the pressure promptly from hypotensive levels. The use of intravenous fluids with 5.0 per cent glucose is especially beneficial in extremely hot weather as a supportive measure.

DIRECT INFILTRATION AND PUDENDAL ANESTHESIA

After a wide experience we agree with J. P. Greenhill that a great degree of safety accompanies local anesthesia in obstetrics not achieved with other methods. The advantages of direct infiltration anesthesia are:

1. There is practically no mortality due to this method.

2. There are no pulmonary complications directly attributable to the procedure. This is of special importance in the delivery of women who have pulmonary conditions, such as tuberculosis, bronchitis, asthma and influenza.

3. There are no local or general complications. There are only 3 possible sources of trouble:

The first is that a needle may break during an injection, especially if an old or a rusty one is used, but this is extremely rare. To prevent this, only good needles should be used. Furthermore, since a needle always breaks near the hub, one never should insert the needle its full length.

The second possible source of trouble is injection of the solution directly into a vein. This might cause disturbing symptoms, which, fortunately, last only a short time. To avoid this, before injecting the solution into an area one always should pull up on the plunger of the syringe to see if any blood is drawn into the barrel of the syringe. If blood is seen, a new area must be selected for the injection. Furthermore, the needle should be kept in constant slow motion while the solution is being injected.

The third possible complication is an idiosyncrasy for procaine, but, fortunately, this complication is rare.

4. The technic is simple, and it may be used at home as well as in hospital.

5. There are no ill effects on such vital organs as the liver, the lungs, the heart, the circulatory apparatus and the central nervous system.

6. No special knowledge is required. The physician carries out the procedure and, therefore, is not dependent on another individual.

7. No special after-care is required.

8. There is a striking reduction of bleeding in the field of operation, so that the amount of blood lost is almost negligible.

9. There is no interference with the action of the uterus, of the abdominal wall or of respiration.

10. Gastro-intestinal symptoms after operation are uncommon.

11. The patient may take liquid and carbohydrates by mouth before, during and immediately after the operation, when this is necessary.

12. Asphyxia of the child, such as may occur after the use of any general anesthetic, is absent.

13. There is seldom need to hurry through an operation.

14. The tissues must be handled gently, and this is advantageous to the patient.

15. There is less wound infection, because trauma is diminished and the patient's general resistance has not been lowered.

16. Local anesthesia is much cheaper than any general anesthetic. Infiltration anesthesia should not be employed if sulfonamides are to be used locally, because procaine inhibits the action of these drugs.

For these procedures we recommend procaine in 1 to 2 per cent solution, Metycaine in 1.5 per cent solution, or Xylocaine (lidocaine) in 1 to 2 per cent solution. The last mentioned drug, introduced only recently, is by far the most rapid and intense in action. The anesthesia may be begun at the time delivery is imminent. If a more profound anesthesia is desired, additional wheals may be made at the upper portion of each labium, and a line of infiltration may be directed downward to join the previously infiltrated areas. As a rule, 30 cc. of solution should suffice. In using local anesthetic agents, a more prolonged action may be obtained if epinephrine is added so that the final dilution of this substance is between 1:100,000 and 1:200,000.

In the event of operative delivery, more profound anesthesia may be obtained if the pudendal nerves are blocked. With the patient in lithotomy position, draped and prepared for delivery, bilateral wheals in the skin are made with a hypodermic needle midway between the anus and the tuberosity of the ischium. The index finger of the left hand is inserted into the vagina or the rectum, and the left ischial spine is palpated. A No. 20 spinal needle 10 cm. long is passed horizontally through the wheal on the left side to a point just below and beyond the spine (Plate 20). Injury of the rectum is prevented by the left index finger in the rectum. About 15 cc. of solution is injected; this anesthetizes the internal pudendal nerve. The needle is withdrawn to a point just beneath the skin, the direction then is changed laterally, and the needle is inserted directly toward the tuberosity of the ischium until the bone is reached, where 5 cc. of solution is injected.

The needle is withdrawn again to just beneath the skin, and the labia on the right side is infiltrated. With the right index finger in the rectum, the procedure is repeated on the right side. Relaxation of the perineal muscles and anesthetization of the skin of the perineum follow in a few minutes. Uterine contractions are not interfered with, so that the co-operation of the patient in the way of voluntary expulsive efforts may be utilized during the course of operation. In difficult forceps operations, it is advisable sometimes to block the ilio-inguinal nerve which supplies a few fibers to the anterior portion of the vulva and the clitoris. This is done easily, for the nerve runs directly beneath the fascia along Poupart's ligament.

PARACERVICAL BLOCK ANESTHESIA IN OBSTETRICS

All sensory nerve fibers reach the uterus by way of the so-called utero-vaginal plexuses. These are paired structures that lie in the extraperitoneal connective tissue at the base of the broad ligament just above the uterovaginal junction. The uterine innervation is blocked easily by infiltration of local anesthesia into the paracervical (parametrial) area.

Injections are made into the lateral fornix of the vagina on each side at approximately the three and the nine o'clock positions. They can be made at any time during the first stages of labor. The procedure is facilitated by the use of a guide that consists of a long spinal needle of a larger bore than the needle through which the anesthetic agent is injected. The guide first is carried up to the junction of the cervix and the vagina with 2 fingers of 1 hand, and with the proximal end up. The needle on the syringe then is threaded through the guide, and the injection is made. The needles are selected for length so that the injection needle projects approximately 1½ cm. beyond the guide. This increases the safety of the procedure by limiting the depth of the injection. The usual technic for sterile vaginal examination is used. Sterile gloves are worn. The field is draped with sterile towels. A quantity of aqueous Zephiran 1-1000 is instilled into the vagina prior to injection.

Xylocaine 1 per cent with epinephrine is the agent producing the best results. The optimum amount of anesthetic agent to be used is 20 cc. on each side.

In general, paracervical anesthesia has the advantages of all local anesthetics. Apparently it is nearly completely safe for mother and baby. The technic is easy, and it can be done on almost any patient. There are no postdelivery reactions, and no pulmonary or general complications are to be expected. There is little or no interference with the normal process of labor and delivery, and no interference with the establishment of respirations in the infant. At the same time, the degree of pain relief obtained is complete or nearly complete in more than 90 per cent of cases.

There are several objections to the method. The block can be done only during the first stage of labor. Additional anesthesia is required for delivery. Intravaginal manipulations during labor always involve the hazard of introducing infection. While the procedure is simple, it is somewhat time consuming.

ANESTHESIA FOR CESAREAN SECTION, HYSTEROTOMY AND RUPTURED ECTOPIC GESTATION

At least 2 per cent of American parturients require anesthesia for one of these operations each year. These women have a previous cesarean section scar, a severe toxemia, some type of metabolic disease or some degree of shock associated with exsanguination of an intrapartum hemorrhage. Also, in many of these situations the fetus has been endangered by hemorrhage, toxemia or anoxia. The maternal mortality associated with cesarean section in the United States is approximately 1 per cent. In 1949, a report was presented to the Congress of Obstetrics in Great Britain of 7,760 cesarean sections from the 13 largest and best-staffed maternities in the British Isles, from which 77 maternal mortalities resulted. An analysis of factors that contributed to these mortalities were associated closely with the management of anesthesia:

1. Hemorrhage and shock
2. Inadequate oxygenation and inadequate fluid replacement
3. Reactions, prolonged inductions and aspiration of vomit
4. Infection
5. Continuation or accentuation of the disease by the depressing effects of the anesthesia

On the basis of our experience in the management of more than 3,000 cesarean sections, the following vital safeguards should be considered prerequisites for every case:

1. Crossmatch and have available in the operating suite Rh compatible blood
2. Experienced and competent anesthetists
3. An indwelling 18-gauge or larger needle or catheter in a proved vein with fluids running at the start of every operation
4. Implementation of every anesthetic, whether general, intravenous or conduction, with high oxygen atmospheres
5. Oxytocic drugs in the syringe and readily available for administration upon delivery of the placenta
6. Proper choice of the anesthetic to fit the individual case

We believe that the safety of the method selected depends more upon the judgment and the skill of the anesthetist than upon the drug or the technic. In view of the fact that agents should be selected that have the minimum of depression upon the baby, the following methods have yielded the best results in our hands:

1. Continuous and single spinal or extradural with low dosage as required and continuous caudal analgesia have been used in our departments for 4,000 cesarean sections with only a single maternal mortality (unrelated to anesthesia) within 8 days of operation.

2. Local anesthesia supplemented after the birth of the baby by intravenous Pentothal Sodium as required.

3. Cyclopropane anesthesia with and without curare supplement for those patients operated upon in profound shock from overt or concealed hemorrhage in premature separation of the placenta or from ruptured ectopic pregnancy or from placenta previa.

Technics

Continuous Spinal Anesthesia

Currently we are using the Tuohy 17-gauge spinal needle and the plastic catheter of divinyl and polyethylene types. With the distal end of the catheter inserted into the subarachnoid space to the level of the second lumbar spine from the third interspace.

1. 30 mg. of Metycaine or 50 mg. of procaine is administered in a 1 to 2 per cent concentration.
2. Coincidentally, in the normotensive or the hypotensive patient, 10 mg. of desoxyephedrine is injected into the intravenous tubing of the drip.
3. 100 per cent oxygen inhalation is begun.
4. In 5 minutes, if the intensity is insufficient or the level of anesthesia has not reached the eighth thoracic segment, a second dose of 15 mg. of Metycaine or 25 mg. of procaine is administered.
5. This is adequate for an operating period of 30 to 40 minutes, when another serial dose of the same proportions is administered each 30 minutes and as required by the patient throughout the operation.

Because of a vasomotor instability, an occasional patient will develop shocklike hypotension in being placed on her back on the operating table. Such a patient should have her blood pressure raised by a full intravenous infusion of 5 per cent glucose and saline and a vasopressor drug to a range greater than 100 mm. of mercury systolic blood pressure before the start of the operation.

Local Anesthesia and Pentothal Sodium

A fortifying local anesthetic technic, recently developed and recommended, is the "arrowhead" block by Frankis Evans, of London. This block takes advantage of the fact that in the anterior axillary line between the lower border of the twelfth rib and the upper border of the iliac crest course the somatic branches of the tenth, the eleventh and the twelfth thoracic and the first lumbar nerves.

1. A skin wheal should be made equidistant between these lateral flank bony landmarks.
2. A 22-gauge 2-in. needle should be injected through each wheal perpendicularly through the fascia and the muscles of the externis and the internis and the transversalis abdominae to the preperitoneal fat.
3. Several cubic milliliters of 1 per cent anesthetic solution (Xylocaine preferred) should be injected in all planes as the needle is inserted and as it is withdrawn.
4. Through the same skin wheal further injections are made as the needle shaft delineates an arrowhead in a superior oblique and inferior oblique direction.
5. A total of 20 cc. of anesthetic solution thus deposited in each flank will provide for a nearly perfect abdominal wall block.
6. Fortifying ilio-inguinal blocks on both sides now are performed by raising a skin wheal 1 in. medial and 1 in. lateral to the anterior superior iliac spine. Through these wheals perpendicular insertions of a 2-in. 22-gauge short beveled block needle will reveal the definite release of the resistance of the fascia abdominis oblique. At this point, in a

small circle of fanlike injections, an additional 5 cc. of anesthetic solution is deposited.

7. An ideal waiting time before surgery is from 15 to 20 minutes to permit thorough anesthetic effect, during which time the patient breathes high oxygen concentrations.

8. Incision then is performed, and the operation is completed down through the peritoneum.

9. Obviously, intraperitoneal and intra-uterine manipulation after incision for the extraction of the baby will produce the need for supplementary Pentothal Sodium or considerable discomfort will ensue. Of course, in the most complicated cases it is necessary to complete the operation with local anesthesia alone. For this type of poor-risk case, we have developed the following alternate supplement: At the moment of incision of the peritoneum 0.5 Gm. (25-50 cc.) of a 1 to 2 per cent solution of sterile Xylocaine is poured over the uterus, the bladder and other viscera as a topical intraperitoneal anesthetic. We have tested all phases of this procedure from the standpoint of toxicity or local irritant effect and have verified its safety. Within 2 minutes the discomfort of the patient is dissipated entirely, and operation can proceed with minimal or no discomfort.

10. The thiopental supplement consists of the injection of approximately 10 to 30 cc. of 2.5 per cent Pentothal Sodium in divided doses. It should be remembered that 5 to 8 to 12 minutes must elapse before thiopental blood levels in the mother are matched by the transplacental blood levels in the baby. Obviously, in the standard operations the baby is delivered in less time; thus, most babies are delivered without major narcosis.

11. However, there are cases associated with fetal emergencies that will not permit preparation with local block supplement. In these cases the operator must proceed with prompt dispatch, since there can be no doubt of resultant fetal narcosis in those babies whose mothers received Pentothal Sodium 20 minutes or more before the delivery. Every facility for infant resuscitation must be at hand to protect such babies from anoxia and depression.

CHLORPROMAZINE (THORAZINE) IN OBSTETRICS

During Labor and Delivery

1. It exerts a quieting effect, reducing apprehension, anxiety and psychomotor excitement; it induces a phlegmatic acceptance of pain.

2. It aids in the relief of pain by the potentiation of analgesics, sedatives and anesthetics, allowing a substantial reduction in the amounts of these agents.

3. It controls vomiting during labor and delivery, considerably lessening a potential anesthetic hazard.

Analgesia, Sedation and Hypnosis

Since chlorpromazine potentiates analgesics and sedatives, these agents can be reduced approximately one half. Patients given chlorpromazine in doses of 25 to 50 mg. in combination with reduced amounts of analgesics or sedatives in the first stage of labor usually become calm and quiet. Many will doze off between contractions, but they can be aroused promptly. Amnesia has occurred in a few patients. Also, chlorpromazine controls the psychomotor hyperactivity encountered occasionally with the use of barbiturates and scopolamine.

Furthermore, apprehension and anxiety seem to be dispelled. The patients appear to take detached attitudes toward their course and environment. Generally, they assume a quiet, phlegmatic acceptance of pain.

In addition, it also lessens the requirement for inhalation anesthetics. Satisfactory depth of anesthesia can be reached with smaller amounts of ether, nitrous oxide or cyclopropane. In a few instances, those who were given the drug delivered spontaneously with no additional anesthesia. Although the effect of chlorpromazine on local anesthetics is not defined clearly at this time, it appears that regional anesthesia may be prolonged by chlorpromazine.

Nausea and Vomiting

The incidence of nausea and vomiting in all 3 stages of labor is reduced significantly by chlorpromazine. From a study of 214 patients, Benaron, Karp *et al.* reported that the total incidence of nausea and vomiting in 114 receiving this drug was approximately half that in the control group of 100 patients who did not receive chlorpromazine.

Duration of Labor

Although variations have been observed, the duration of labor in patients receiving chlorpromazine and in those in control groups (without chlorpromazine) was found to be similar. In some patients, labor seemed to be accelerated; in others, there was no change. Occasionally, there appeared to be a reduction in the strength of uterine contractions and of active abdominal pressure, which prolonged labor. Whether or not these variations were due to chlorpromazine is undetermined.

Deliveries with chlorpromazine have been satisfactory. Hershenson and his associates observed, "The emergence phase is pleasant and uneventful."

Condition of Babies

Hershenson and his associates state that the condition of the babies at birth was satisfactory, with good reflex irritability and muscle tone. The authors agree.

Special Consideration in Obstetrics

It is imperative that the possible hypotensive effect of chlorpromazine be considered always during labor. In order to prevent any sudden drop in blood pressure, the patient always should be kept recumbent.

In obstetrics, the average drop in blood pressure, when it occurred, was 10 mm. Hg in systolic and diastolic readings. In a very few instances, greater hypotension occurred in toxemic hypertensive patients and in a few others immediately following the induction of spinal anesthesia.

For this reason *spinal anesthesia is not recommended* for use with this drug at this time. Although it has been used satisfactorily in a few deliveries with low spinal block, more studies are needed for a critical evaluation of the use of chlorpromazine with spinal block in obstetrics.

Chlorpromazine should be used with caution in patients with hypertensive toxemia of pregnancy, cardiovascular disease or other conditions where a drop in blood pressure is undesirable. In these cases, the blood pressure should be checked at frequent intervals throughout the period of labor, delivery and recovery.

Ordinarily, in the event that a serious drop in blood pressure does occur, it can be controlled by placing the patient in a tilted position with head lowered and legs raised. If it is desirable to administer a vasopressor drug, *nor-epinephrine appears to be the most suitable. Epinephrine should not be used,* because chlorpromazine may reverse its action.

In obstetric patients, the effect of chlorpromazine on body temperature has not been significant. The temperature was reduced about ½° to 1° F. in most patients.

Jaundice has been observed in a small number of patients receiving chlorpromazine for a week or more. However, since the use of chlorpromazine in deliveries is for such a short period of time, the likelihood that jaundice will occur in these patients is negligible. In the obstetrical service of one of the authors in the Kings County Hospital, Brooklyn, 2 patients under treatment for pernicious vomiting of pregnancy with chlorpromazine developed signs and symptoms of myocardial damage which reappeared each time the drug was continued. This drug still must be considered as in the evaluation stages.

Contraindications

Chlorpromazine is contraindicated in obstetric patients with eclampsia or severe hypertension, and in conjunction with spinal anesthesia. (See above.)

Administration and Dosage

In the *obstetric patient,* it is suggested that chlorpromazine be started when the cervix is dilated 3 to 5 cm., or when strong labor is established.

The recommended dosage of chlorpromazine is 12.5 to 25 mg. (½-1 cc.) given *slowly* by *deep intramuscular* injection. At the same time, half the usual dosage of an analgesic or sedative agent and, if desired, 0.4 mg. of scopolamine should be given by injection. (Chlorpromazine should be given separately, not mixed with other agents in the syringe.) The combination dosage may be repeated in 3 to 5 hours if labor is prolonged or if more sedation is desired. The repetition of dosage should be guided by observations in blood pressure and respiration.

Intravenous administration of chlorpromazine is not recommended in obstetrics at this time.

OXYGEN IN OBSTETRICS

A normal adult weighing about 140 pounds during rest metabolizes between 300 and 400 cc. of oxygen per minute. This means that in a patient breathing 20 times per minute, 20 cc. of pure oxygen must pass the respiratory surface membrane into the blood stream. In disease, during fever and during obstetric labor, this minimum oxygen requirement may be increased two- or threefold. Hyperthyroidism, scopolamine-activated metabolism and uncontrolled emotional distress of painful labor further increase the parturient's demand for oxygen. Therefore, oxygen therapy should be regarded as fundamental, both during obstetric labor and as an adjuvant to safe anesthesia for obstetric delivery. It never should be regarded as last-resort therapy for patients manifesting the symptoms of hypoxia. In many of the vascular diseases associated with pregnancy, as in anemia, it is a necessary safeguard for the mother. Likewise, in these conditions oxygen therapy with enriched atmospheres is just as important to the fetus in utero, which must depend upon the deficient maternal transport system for its transplacental "staff of life."

The value of saturating the mother with 100 per cent oxygen in fetal emergencies induced by tetanic contractions of the uterus, maternal hypotensive crises, abruptio placenta, placenta previa and partial obstruction through an umbilical cord compressed between the presenting part of the baby and the rigid parts of the birth canal can be appreciated only when one observes the improvement in the fetal heart beat within a few seconds following this essential therapy. Furthermore, when one realizes that fetal anoxia and disturbances of extra-uterine respiration are mainly responsible for perinatal injuries and death, the availability of this lifesaving gas becomes the cardinal requirement in all areas of the modern maternity hospital. In the 1952 Chicago study conducted by Bundesen and his associates,

10,021 deaths in the newborn were analyzed. Abnormal pulmonary ventilation was listed as the leading cause of mortality. Courville, in a recent review of etiologic relationship of anoxemia to brain disease, states the concept that oxygen deprivation may be an early factor in the development of certain clinical syndromes, including cerebral palsy. Eastman, Corner and Anderson, of Johns Hopkins University, and the authors share this concept. Eastman joins the authors in the belief that oxygen inhalations of near 100 per cent mixtures prior to the birth of the baby would preserve more baby life and brain cortex than any other procedure, regardless of the type of anesthesia.

Intra-uterine Anoxia

This complication to the fetus is the most frequently misdiagnosed in obstetrics. Primary oxygen want is responsible for most intra-uterine fetal deaths. Our present knowledge leads us to believe that most substances are transferred across the placenta in amounts greatly exceeding fetal requirements. Singularly, oxygen is transferred in amounts barely sufficient for fetal survival at term. In fact, during the terminal 2 weeks of pregnancy, the fetus exists in a constant state of hypoxia with only approximately 50 per cent arterial saturation of oxygen. With this precarious margin of safety, the special mechanisms described previously are necessary to keep the fetus alive. In fact, this may account for the fetal polycythemia.

In general, anoxia may produce temporary or permanent damage to the fetal tissues within the central nervous system. Temporary anoxia depression of the respiratory center is a factor in the production of neonatal asphyxia. Fetal asphyxia is recognized best by a steady but gradual slowing of the fetal heart rate. This sign is of greater diagnostic value than are those of excessive fetal movements or the presence of meconium.

Torpin, of Georgia, has raised and answered an important question:

> During labor what is to be done for the fetus? Few textbooks have given the subject much consideration. Moreover, the fetus is subject to exhaustion quite parallel to that of the mother and often to some factors not affecting her. Both need plenty of fluid. Dextrose is the most easily assimilated food and is most valuable and often neglected. Oxygen administered to the mother is of prime use for the fetus, and when there is evidence of actual or impending fetal exhaustion, oxygen should be administered constantly. The conditions which reduce the oxygenation of the maternal blood stream are convulsions or come of eclampsia, pneumonia and other infections, anemia, cardiac decompensation, morphine and other drug depression. Besides these there are conditions in which the oxygen of the maternal blood stream may be adequate ordinarily, but the fetus has reduced ability to obtain or use it, such as premature separation of the placenta, placenta previa, cord entanglements, prelapse of the cord, some cases of velamentous insertion of the cord, and hypertonicity of the uterus, which sometimes may be so extreme as to be tetanic. In all these conditions oxygen administered to the mother may be life-saving for the fetus, tiding it over until delivery. Nothing is more dramatic than the improvement in the depressed fetal heart rate by administration of oxygen to the mother. By administering it to all eclamptic patients in convulsions or coma, the fetal salvage rate may be greatly augmented.

Waters, of Wisconsin, has reported that all the drugs that relieve pain have the added characteristics of interfering with the normal functions of respiration and circulation—with the transport of oxygen from the environmental atmosphere to the tissues. The factors of duration of exposure, of innate resistance of the cells and of disease states, as well as the degree of lowered tension of oxygen, will determine the reversibility of effect. One must be prepared to recognize hypoxia, its cause and the proper means of treating it lest it advance to anoxia with permanent loss of function of some or all of the cells of the body.

An adequate oxygen supply to the fetus in utero is dependent upon the following physiologic factors:

1. Adequate oxygen level of the maternal blood. This is dependent upon both the relatively normal hemoglobin level of the maternal blood and the adequate oxygen percentage of the inhaled gases administered to the mother during labor. Although nitrous oxide is of inestimable value in preventing labor pain, it may be administered with a low concentration of oxygen so continuously that the mother experiences hypoxia for a prolonged period. In many instances, when the mother—and, therefore, the fetus—undergoes relatively severe oxygen want, it is due to the failure to interrupt administration of anesthetic mixtures with inhalations of high concentrations of oxygen, preferably with 100 per cent oxygen.

When excessive doses of analgesic drugs have produced relaxation of the lingual and the pharyngeal musculature, respiratory obstruction may be produced with accumulation of mucus and, at times, gastric contents from emesis. In addition, drugs that slow the respiratory rate result in a lowered volume of ventilation with resultant arterial anoxia.

2. Sufficient relaxation of the uterine musculature is necessary to permit adequate quantities of arterial blood to fill the placental lacunae. In tumultuous labors with uterine contractions of 2 minutes or less in frequency, there often is a mechanical interference with the placental circulation. Long-sustained contraction of the uterus due to the use of oxytocics may interfere with placental circulation to such an extent as to produce fetal anoxia. Also, in those cases in which the tone of the uterine musculature rises to a flattened tetanic plateau, as indicated by tocographic studies, the arteriovenous interchanges of blood through the placenta may be diminished.

3. The placental attachment must be sufficient to permit adequate interchange of oxygen. This condition is not present in some cases of premature separation of the placenta and in placenta previa with hemorrhage.

4. Mechanical obstructive complications of the umbilical cord, as exemplified by prolapse, tight loops round the neck or the arms or voluntary occlusive constriction by the baby's fists round the cord. We have seen the last-mentioned complication in 2 instances of babies born by cesarean section. Both babies were born with fists tightly clamped round the umbilical cord in such a manner that they had to be pried loose.

5. The relatively normal blood pressure of the mother must be maintained in order to deliver sufficient oxygenated blood to the placenta. We have found that fetal bradycardia develops invariably within 5 minutes after the maternal blood pressure has fallen below 80 mm. of mercury, systolic pressure. This may be combated with one or all of the following measures: (A) elevation of the mother's legs to right angles for a period of 2 or 3 minutes in such a manner as to administer an autotransfusion with specific increase to maternal circulating blood; (B) administration of 100 per cent oxygen; and (C) administration of a vasopressive drug such as ephedrine, Methedrine, Neosynephrine or Wyamine.

Irving, of Harvard, has noticed a beneficent effect from 50 mm. of ephedrine administered to the mother by intramuscular injection 10 minutes before the expected birth of the baby. He recommends the use of this procedure in all cases in which general anesthesia is superimposed upon deep sedation. (We have used ephedrine with benefit when caudal analgesia was associated with hypotension.) He has found that often this dosage of ephedrine, so administered, not only raises the blood pressure of the mother but also it seems to stimulate the central nervous system, with the effect on the baby of initiating early respiration and spontaneous and vigorous crying of the infant. We have verified this observation in numerous cases. Further, we have observed that patients deeply sedated often become alert and very keen mentally immediately after the ephedrine takes effect. We have noticed also that the babies appear to be somewhat stimulated.

Thus, in the treatment of the intrauterine anoxia, we should proceed as follows:

1. Administer 100 per cent oxygen as long as necessary and particularly during the actual birth and the moments before the umbilical cord is cut
2. Maintain normal blood pressure by means of autotransfusion or vasopressor drugs
3. Control uterine contractions in such a manner that drugs that produce uterine tetany are not administered.

Greenhill has said that "drug depression, independent of anoxia, is of limited duration." We must emphasize that central depression related to anoxia is capable of producing changes of permanent duration. In an extensive review of obstetric factors underlying cerebral palsy, as observed at the Johns Hopkins Hospital, Anderson states that 41.3 per cent of premature infants and 21.5 per cent of full-term infants died from the type of intracranial hemorrhage observed in experimental animals asphyxiated in laboratory studies.

Eastman has re-emphasized in his address, "Mount Everest in Utero," that fetal bradycardia is the most reliable sign of fetal distress. It is our belief that this complication represents the *sine qua non* indication for reducing immediately the administration of anesthesia to the mother and the use of 100 per cent oxygen therapy.

Dunlap and Brown reported that physiologic uterine contractions were accompanied by increased oxygenation of the blood stream. Therefore, immediate clamping of the umbilical cord at birth is to be condemned, since this practice may deprive the newborn of one

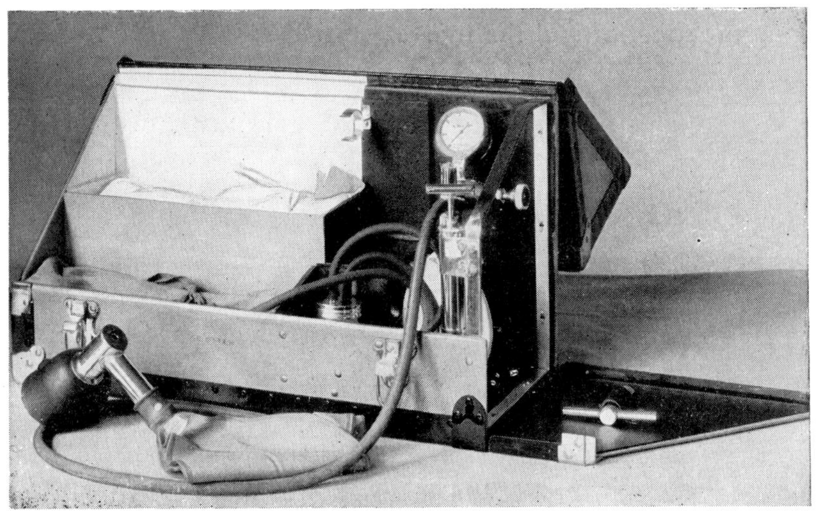

Fig. 74. P.A.D. resuscitation apparatus, ambulance model. (Flagg, Paluel J.: The Art of Anaesthesia, ed. 7, Philadelphia, Lippincott)

fourth its total blood volume and the oxygen it carries. Engel reported in 1885 that mortality in premature infants in whom the cord was tied immediately was twice as great as in those in whom the cord was tied later. Although the fetus can live for a considerable period after blood oxygen has been exhausted, as Windle has pointed out, the questions that confront us are: What will be the ultimate result? And will such serious deprivation be reflected later in mental deficiency of some degree? In Windle's studies, guinea pigs that survived 20 minutes' asphyxiation at birth were inferior to litter-mate controls, as shown by subsequent maze testing.

Various protective mechanisms function in the fetus to ensure an adequate supply of oxygen:

1. Fetal blood contains more hemoglobin and more red cells per unit volume than does the blood of the mother.
2. Fetal red blood cells are larger and take up oxygen with greater avidity in the lower ranges of oxygen tension.
3. The oxygen-carrying capacity of fetal blood at normal full-term birth is 21.5 volumes per 100 cc., whereas that of the mother's blood is 15.5.
4. Crossing the superior and the inferior vena cava streams permits access of oxygenated blood from the inferior vena cava to the brain and the heart by way of the foramen ovale.
5. In the presence of acute anoxia, the fetus apparently is aided temporarily by anaerobic glycolysis, through which it can obtain oxygen by utilizing its own blood sugar.

As shown by the early investigations of Barcroft, in 1932 and 1936, and the studies of Kramer and Luft on dogs, the spleen contracts during severe hypoxia, providing an additional temporary safeguard for the portal circulation. Therefore, it is estimated that a reserve of at least 40 cc. of oxygen in combination with hemoglobin is present constantly in the human fetus at term, under normal conditions, and provides a measure of safety during the birth process. In answer to Windle's question, "Is this reservoir of oxygen adequate to meet great emergencies?," our experience leads us to believe that it is not. Therefore, we urge administration of 100 per cent oxygen as a routine protective procedure—not as a last resort to counteract fetal distress that may indicate exhaustion of the natural safeguards and perhaps an irreversible respiratory failure. We believe that in some cases a disregard of the safety measure of administration of 100 per cent oxygen is capable of producing irreversible changes that may cause the infant to become a permanent cerebral palsy invalid. However, once respiration in the newborn has been established, usually room air is sufficient for adequate oxygenation of the term infants, and 40 per cent oxygen is sufficient for maintenance of viable prematures. We emphasize the dangers of higher concentrations of oxygen for prolonged fetal inhalations in the initiation of retrolental fibroplasia.

CURARE

Synthetic Substitutes (Flaxedil, Succinylcholine) As Adjuncts in the Conduct of Labor

It is recognized generally now that the grandiose complex pachymolecule of curare, which competes with acetylcholine at the myoneural junction, is capable of producing muscle relaxation comparable with the depolarization of the somatic axons achieved by spinal anesthesia within a period of 1 to 3 minutes. The leptocurare substitutes Flaxedil and succinylcholine are capable of achieving a similar type of muscular relaxation through depolarization of the muscle fibers themselves within 40 to 60 seconds. However, there does appear to be a latent period of total or partial blockade by the placenta that spares the fetus from curarization and its implied respiratory paralysis. Certainly it has been our experience clinically to utilize these drugs with general anesthesia in cesarean section and 5 to 10 minutes later to deliver infants who breathed and cried with physiologic vigor. We agree with Potter and Whitacre that the judicious use of these agents reduces the total amount of general anesthesia required for cesarean section, thus the infant is spared excessive depression of the central nervous system.

Another indication for curare in obstetrics is for use in delivery of large babies by breech mechanism. Curarization seems to block out perineal musculature before total respiratory paralysis, thus providing the maximum relaxation of the perineum.

In a series of 20 patients we used a very conservative dosage of curare (3-9 mg.) in conscious patients without sedation. These patients indicated some relief of pain, which we interpreted to be on the basis of muscular spasm relaxation.

The dosage for cesarean section should be kept in the range of 6 to 12 mg. of *d*-tubocurarine as an initial dose. Even though we do not intubate our obstetric patients routinely under curarization, we emphasize the necessity of having this equipment immediately at hand in the event of an inadequate airway.

During the 4 years of the Johns Hopkins-Sinai Hospitals study, we found it necessary to intubate only 2 patients in 15,000 deliveries. Neither of these patients had any curare.

The Use of Succinylcholine in Obstetrics

Thus far sufficient evidence has not been presented in either the literature or our personal series to provide the assurance that succinylcholine will not immediately cross the placenta and paralyze the fetus. However, in view of its instantaneous peak action within 30 to 60 secconds, and its rapid metabolism within the circulating blood plasma, we know that this agent would be most effective in providing relaxation of masseter laryngospasm induced by drug or vomitus. In such emergencies, for intubation we recommend the use of 60 to 80 mg. succinylcholine with 100 per cent oxygen-controlled ventilations before intubation (or intratracheal aspiration of foreign bodies), which usually can be performed within 1 to 3 minutes after injection.

WESTERN RESERVE PORTABLE MINIATURE ANESTHESIA MACHINE, RESUSCITATOR AND OXYGEN INHALATOR IN OBSTETRICS

In 1954, one of us (Hingson), recognizing the importance of available and easily accessible oxygen in anesthesia and in states of hypoxia in either mothers or babies, developed a midget machine capable of administering 100 per cent oxygen for inhalation, for intermittent positive pressure resuscitation or for providing instantaneous anesthetic inductions. A laboratory tested nonexplosive mixture of 40 per cent cyclopropane, 30 per cent helium and 30 per cent oxygen in a 6-L. total quantity is packaged in 2 thumb-size cylinders. This mixture can be released in toto into the rebreathing bag of the machine by a double turn of the wrist round the 2 side-arm containers of the instrument. This entire device weighs less than 2 pounds and can be carried easily in the coat pocket or in the physician's satchel.

The total amount of cyclopropane available and properly dampered with helium in a specially pin-indexed cylinder is 2,200 cc. of free volume gas, or the amount required to keep an adult anesthetized in a closed system for a period of 10 to 20 minutes. This premeasured quantity provides anesthesia promptly to the depth of Plane 2 of Stage 3 surgical anesthesia with a blood-stream concentration of 18 to 24 mg. per 100 cc. of circulating blood within 8 to 20 breaths. Anesthesia remains at this peak plateau for 3 to 5 minutes and then slowly recedes as the tissues take up the anesthetic from the blood stream. The patient regains consciousness within 1 or 2 minutes if the mask is removed from the face, or within 12 minutes if the mask is kept tightly in position.

The soda lime or the baralyme canister, freshly filled with 100 cc. of the pellets, is capable of maintaining the carbon dioxide content below 3 volumes per cent for 20 minutes. A cylinder of oxygen-helium is required each 5 to 6 minutes that the mask is left on the face.

The chart depicted in Figure 79 defining the explosive and flammable range of oxygen-cyclopropane mixtures illustrates the principle of initiating the anesthetic outside the flammable range at the designated point (A) and maintaining the mixture safely outside the range of both flame and spark ignition for the duration of each pair of cylinders at designated point (B). In order to determine this range, the authors have developed an anesthesia gas laboratory with apparatus capable of providing exhaled samples from the rebreathing bag each desired sequence of parturient breaths. The patient depicted in the chart had a gas sample each 10 breaths with the study carried on for 6 minutes. In several hundred patients studied it was determined that the cyclopropane crossed the respiratory alveolar surfaces into the blood stream just slightly more rapidly than oxygen, thus assuring the anesthetist of a diminishing cyclopropane proportion in the rebreathing bag. The oxygen percentages remained higher than the normal 20 of room air for the 5- to 6-minute life of the cylinder. Helium, which is an inert gas, remains in the lung and in the rebreathing bag, prop-

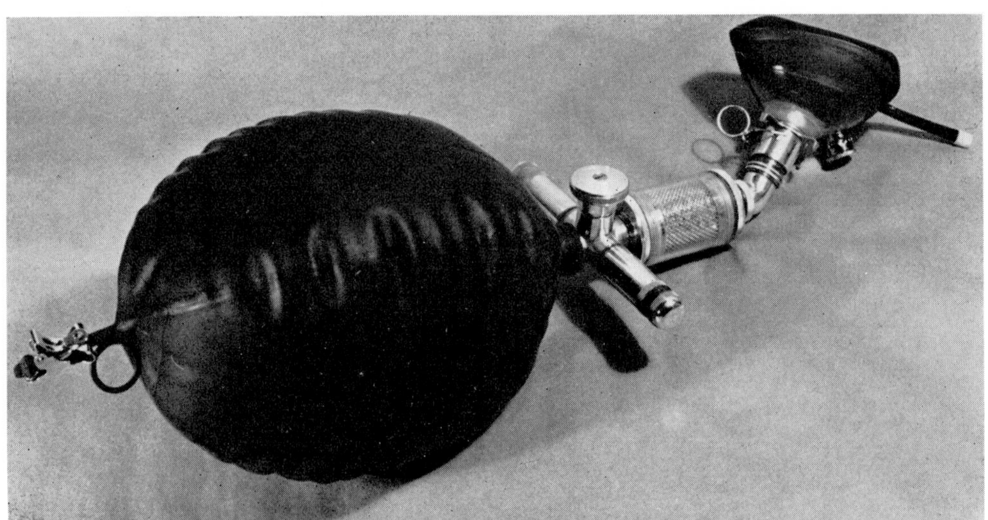

FIG. 75. The Western Reserve Portable Miniature Anesthesia Machine with inflated 6-L. bag containing contents of 2 side-arm cylinders. Note the pressure-limiting valve (20 mm. Hg) on plastic dome of mask and metering valve on central axial body.

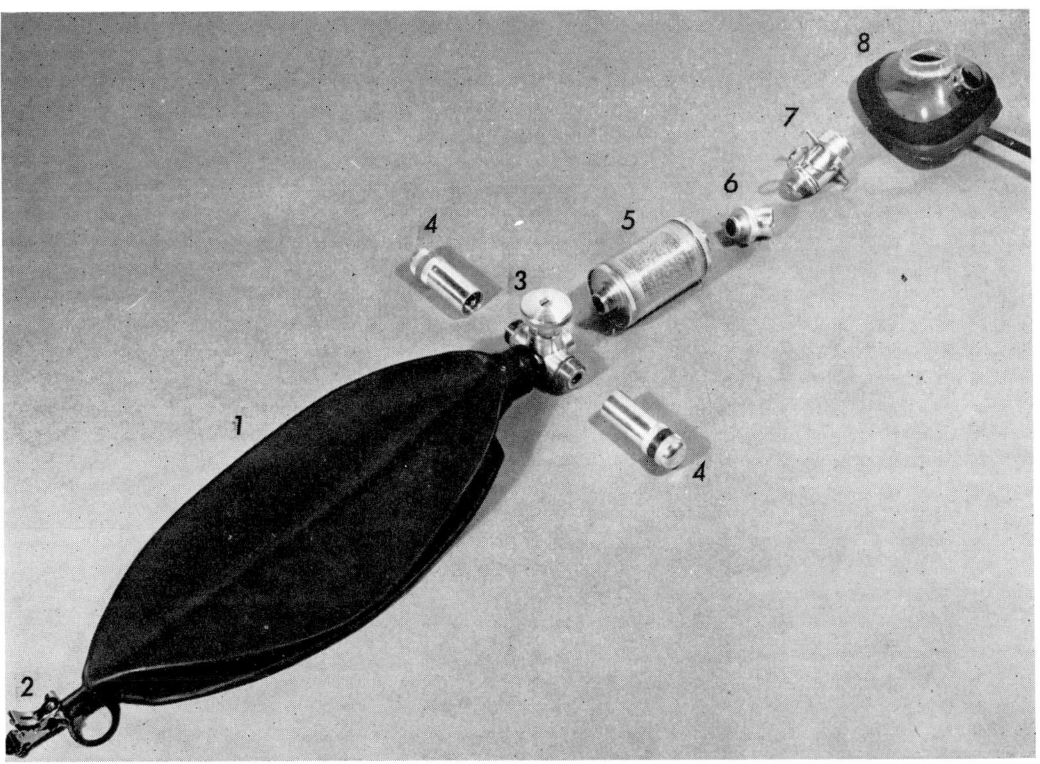

Fig. 76. The Western Reserve Portable Miniature Anesthesia Machine subassembled. (1) 6-L. conductive rubber bag with (2) snap clamp on distal end and (3) attached central axial member on other end, opposed laterally (4) by 2 aluminum side-arm containers and proximally (5) by plastic canister, (6) angle piece, (7) slide-valve assembly and (8) mask.

erly mixing with the inert nitrogen to provide the dampening effect. Thus, the concentrations of both helium and nitrogen rise to provide greater safety from explosions as the oxygen and the cyclopropane cross over into the blood stream of the patient. The mixture is not unpleasant to breathe, and it is adequate to provide instantaneous anesthesia for a wide variety of obstetric problems and emergencies:

1. Precipitous labor. (Since surgical anesthesia with this machine and mixture is provided within 6 to 12 inhalations, we have found this method to be 2 to 6 minutes faster than that achieved with all previously developed equipment in which there is at least 1 to 2 L. of dead space containing air as a diluent in the rebreathing tubes and canister chambers.)

2. Relaxation for version and extraction. On several occasions, the authors have been able to provide this anesthesia in 10 to 12 breaths for this type of delivery of the second of twins whose heart rate indicated through the auscultated bradycardia a dangerous hypoxia.

3. Manual removal of a retained placenta in a previously unanesthetized mother. One of us (Hellman) has utilized this method in a series of 86 such cases in the Kings County Hospital with no major anesthetic complications.

4. As an adjuvant to inadequate or anesthetic failure with the conduction

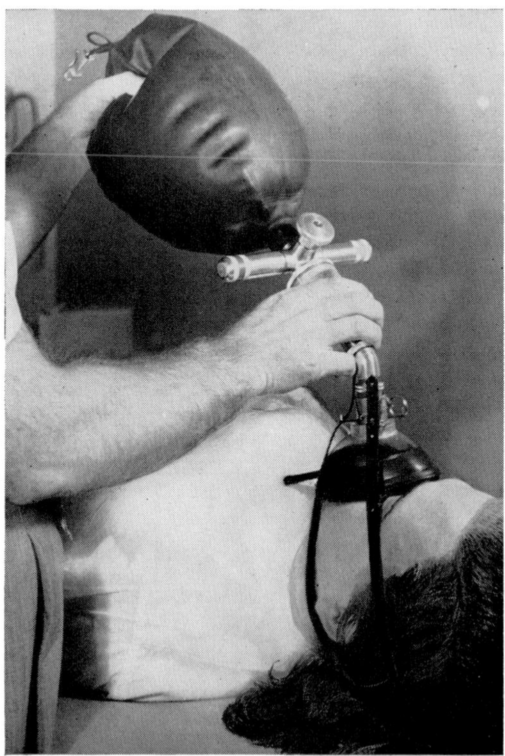

FIG. 77. The Western Reserve Portable Miniature Anesthesia Machine in use as resuscitator.

anesthetics of pudendal block, caudal and saddle block spinal for forcep delivery. In many of these cases the anesthesia of the block type was satisfactory until the crucial moment of forceps traction or extension of the head or the delivery of a shoulder dystocia. Extreme pain stimuli to the mother at this point indicated postponement of the obstetric maneuver until general anesthesia could be induced. The universal experience with anesthetic equipment and agents used frequently is that at least 3 to 12 minutes is required for satisfactory anesthesia. Such double anesthetics under the stimulus of pain and maternal fear and excitement are associated frequently with vomiting, breath-holding, laryngospasm, hypoxia from tongue obstruction and a thrashing excitement phase of induction. The obstetric emergency indicates frequently the immediate delivery of the infant who gives evidence of hypoxia. With the Reserve Portable we effect routinely the desired degree of anesthesia within 6 to 10 breaths. In a series of more than 80 such cases we have avoided the usual complications mentioned above that are seen with the slow inductions.

5. Occasionally we have an excited or a thrashing patient with scopolamine amnesia or an emotionally un-co-operative patient who will not maintain the flexed lateral position for spinal or caudal anesthesia. In such cases the incidence of conduction block anesthesia failure is high or induction is impossible, or the likelihood of needle breakage is great. In a dozen such cases we have had the patient relaxed and immobile after 4 to 10 respirations with the anesthetic mixture administered by the Reserve Portable.

It should be pointed out that the machine and snap-lock valve mask can be removed at any time, and a refilled bag of 6 L. of pure oxygen can be reapplied as an inhalator or a resuscitator should a respiratory emergency require it.

6. As a supplement to the management of patients delivering under physiologic relaxation technics. Many of these patients carry themselves very well until the actual moment of birth and then become uncontrollable for the delivery of a difficult shoulder or at the moment of episiotomy or as the head crosses the perineum. It is our policy to explain the speed of action of the Reserve Portable to such patients and to use it for 2 to 4 breaths upon their own or the obstetrician's request for these situations. Analgesia of a profound degree can be achieved after a 15-second circulation time following 1 full breath, and unconsciousness is achieved easily in 3 to 4 breaths. Then the mask is removed; the

snap-lock valve conserves the mixture for a second or a third use as required by the obstetrician. It is our opinion that with 1 breath of this mixture a degree of analgesia can be achieved that is superior to that seen with 20 to 40 breaths of 80-20 nitrous oxide or of trichlorethylene or ether and as good as that seen with 10 breaths of chloroform.

7. As a method of anesthesia for repair of unexpected lacerations of normal multipara who deliver precipitously but require anesthesia for sutures of 2 to 5 minutes of operation.

8. As a method of anesthesia for postpartum inspection of the cervix or intrauterine exploration for secundines after delivery.

Since May, 1954, in our combined clinics we have used this instrument for more than 400 obstetric procedures without major complication.

Prolonged anesthesia can be provided with the same mixture as described in Section 5 of the instructions listed below, or induction may be provided rapidly by the Reserve Portable, and then nitrous oxide-oxygen mixtures of 80 to 20 or 66 to 33 per cent may be maintained through the removal of the Midget apparatus and the use of the closed or semiclosed circle absorber technics with the Heidbrink, the Foregger or the McKesson standard machines.

Since this technic for the Reserve Portable is not available in any present anesthesia text, it is included below under the 6 designated sections:

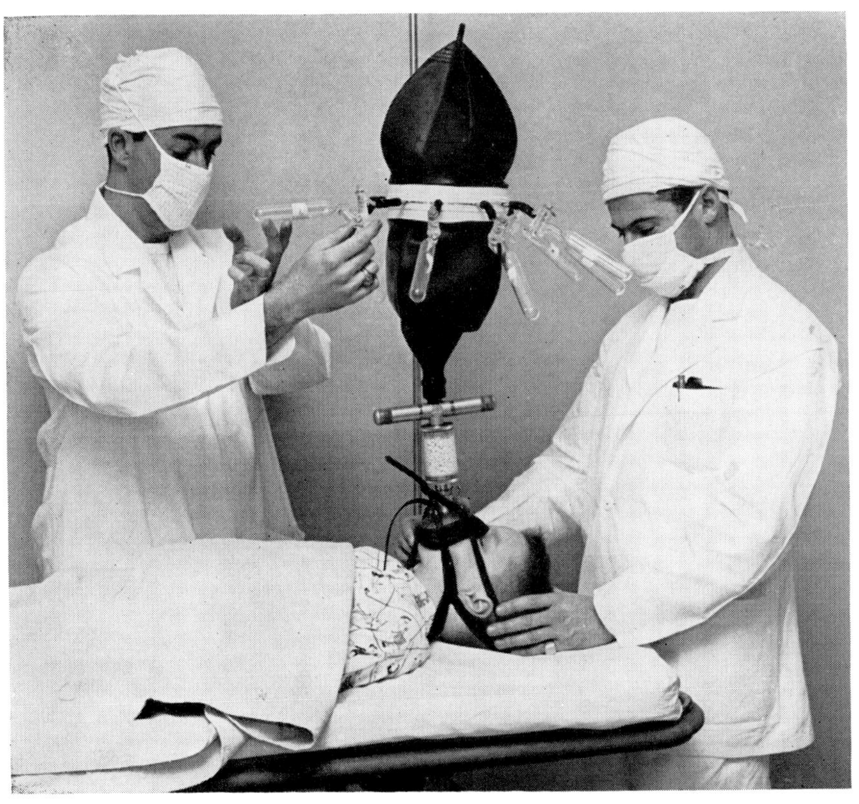

Fig. 78. Gas sampling apparatus for testing anesthetic mixtures, designed by one of the authors (Hingson) for serial cyclopropane determinations.

1. For Use As a Resuscitator
(See exploded view, Fig. 76)

A. First close the snap clamp on the terminal port of the rebreathing bag. For use with central reservoir oxygen supply see Instruction 1C.

B. Insert green cylinders (oxygen) in both side-arm containers, with the tapered neck of the cylinder facing the perforating pin in the central axial body. Each cylinder contains 3,400 cc. of pure oxygen, which is released instantaneously into the rebreathing bag by clockwise rotation of the side-arm container on to the threads until the gas cylinder is pierced by the perforating pin. Two cylinders will inflate fully a 6-liter bag. Provided there is no leak round the face mask, this is adequate oxygen for approximately 12 to 15 minutes of resuscitation.

C. As an alternative, oxygen may be supplied from tank or wall reservoir through a flowmeter set at 300 to 600 cc. per minute by opening the snap clamp and attaching the flowmeter to the terminal port of the rebreathing bag by means of a glass connector and rubber tubing.

D. The plastic canisters filled with 100 cc. of fresh Baralyme or soda lime is adequate to keep carbon dioxide levels

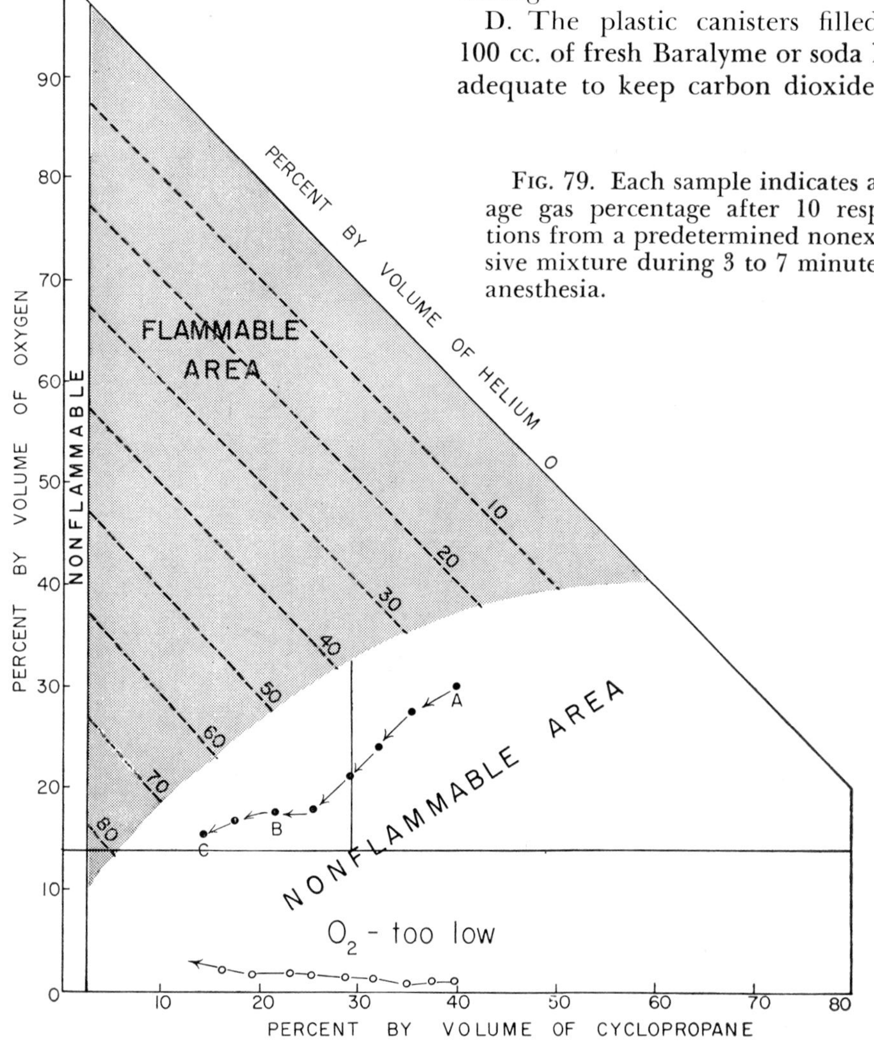

Fig. 79. Each sample indicates average gas percentage after 10 respirations from a predetermined nonexplosive mixture during 3 to 7 minutes of anesthesia.

below 2 per cent by volume for 15 to 20 minutes.

E. Be sure that the patient's airway is clear of foreign bodies, regurgitated fluid, blood or mucus. Place headstrap under patient's head. Moisten surface of mask cuff which comes in contact with the skin, place snugly on patient's face.

F. Open the ports immediately to the rebreathing bag by holding the central axial body and exerting slight downward pressure against the mask until the sliding member covers the red band above the plastic dome.

G. Then hook the snap lock into position to hold the ports open. As a visual check, if the red band is exposed, it means that the snap lock is not hooked properly and that the breathing ports in the face mask are closed.

H. **Secure mask** on patient's face with headstrap.

I. **Lift tongue** from posterior pharynx by protruding lower jaw with one hand. Squeeze bag rhythmically with other hand slowly for 1 second, releasing quickly to allow 1 second for exhaling and pausing 1 second before repeating the cycle (12-20 complete cycles per minute). This should provide effective means of artificial respiration, giving visual evidence of good chest expansion and deflation during each respiratory cycle. If a patient's airway is not maintained satisfactorily by this maneuver, release the snap lock to close the ports, remove the mask, insert to proper position soft rubber oral pharyngeal airway of proper size, reapply mask and resume the resuscitation procedure, starting with Instruction 1F.

J. As absorption of oxygen deflates the rebreathing bag, additional supplies of oxygen can be provided as required by replacing empty cylinders and reinflating the bag as described previously.

K. The soda lime canister should be replenished after approximately each 20 minutes of use in prolonged cases of resuscitation.

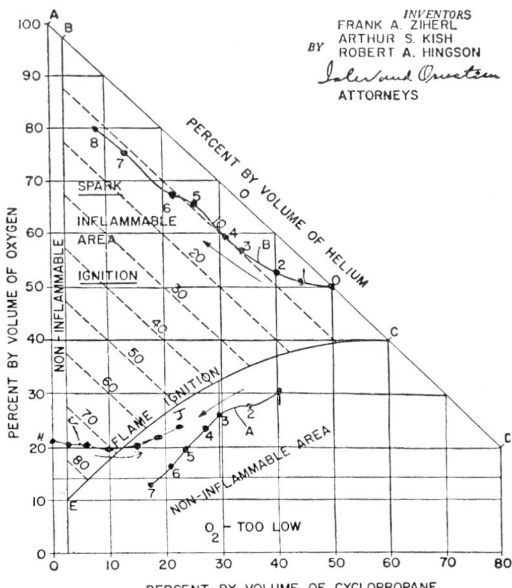

FIG. 80. The superior line graph B represents the standard method of inducing cyclopropane and oxygen anesthesia with a 50-50 mixture that obviously is high in the explosion range and becomes more dangerous from the point of view of spark ignition after each succeeding minute as the cyclopropane is reduced and the oxygen is increased to 80 per cent.

Line graph A shows the completely nonexplosive and nonflammable curve achieved with the Western Reserve Portable Miniature Anesthesia Machine with nonflammable mixtures of cyclopropane, helium and oxygen.

Line graph C between points H and J shows the theoretical mixture that may be achieved with a constant flow of oxygen at 20 per cent, helium at 60 per cent and cyclopropane at 20 per cent. Such a mixture passes through the flammable range during the induction and becomes nonflammable after several minutes.

2. FOR USE AS AN INHALATOR

A. Firemen, rescue squads and aviators may use the machine as an inhalator by self-administration of 100 per cent oxygen through the mechanism described above.

B. Cardiac patients, asthmatics and smoke-asphyxiated victims may inhale oxygen under direct supervision of experienced personnel, or they may be trained to administer therapeutic inhalation of oxygen and helium upon a doctor's prescription and instructions at home or at high altitudes.

3. Uses in Anesthesia—Basic Rules

A. It is recommended that no physician or dentist who is untrained in the management of the airway of the unconscious patient should use this machine.

B. It is recommended also that only properly trained personnel who understand thoroughly the pharmacology, the preparation of the patient, the technic of administration of cyclopropane and the treatment of complications resulting from its uses should use this machine in anesthesia.

C. This machine should not be used in anesthesia in areas without available suction, mechanical or pharyngeal airways and instruments for visual intubation.

D. The cylinders provided contain cyclopropane and oxygen and helium in nonexplosive proportions, with a special safety perforating mechanism within the central axial body of the machine that makes impossible the use of 2 cyclopropane cylinders at the same time. However, it is possible to use pure oxygen or oxygen and helium for resuscitation by repetitive filling from the green side-arm container.

E. When using cyclopropane, a filled oxygen-helium cylinder must be released into rebreathing bag after each 6 minutes of use to meet patient basic oxygen requirements.

4. Induction of Anesthesia

A. The green cylinder with the brown band (oxygen and helium) should be placed in the side arm with the green band and the contents emptied into the rebreathing bag, the procedure described under Instruction 1B being used.

B. Only after the bag is half filled at least by this maneuver should the orange cylinder with the brown stripe (cyclopropane and helium) be released from the orange band (opposite) side arm into the bag, thus filling the 6½-liter bag with a mixture containing 2,400 cc. of cyclopropane, 1,700 cc. of oxygen and 1,700 cc. of helium.

C. This mixture will produce a loss of consciousness in the adult or the child within 6 to 10 breaths. Surgical anesthesia at about Plane II or III is provided in from 20 to 30 breaths.

D. With a snug fit, this mixture is safe for inhalation for a period of 4 minutes. In more than 10 per cent of our laboratory testing of patients of all sizes, the mixture was revealed to be nonexplosive.

5. Prolonged Maintenance of Anesthesia

A. The anesthesia may be prolonged beyond this period by adding additional cylinders of oxygen and helium to the mixture each 4 to 5 minutes by repeating Instruction 4A.

B. One cylinder of cyclopropane and helium and 3 cylinders of oxygen and helium are sufficient for anesthesia from 10 to 20 minutes.

C. Should additional cyclopropane be required, it may be added to the mixture by following Instruction 4B.

Note: The alternate technic of using oxygen or oxygen and helium mixtures without simultaneous addition of cyclopropane and helium brings the mixture back into the flammable range for a few breaths after each cylinder evacuation.

6. Optional Metering Procedure

A. The operator may use the specially designed metering valve mechanism that

TABLE 11. RESERVE MIDGET PORTABLE ANESTHESIA MACHINE

APPLICATIONS MARCH 1, 1954 TO SEPTEMBER 30, 1955 Cleveland: University, City,* Huron Road and St. Luke's Hospitals Montreal: Queen Elizabeth Hospital† Chicago: University of Illinois Research Hospital‡ New York: Kings County Hospital§ London: St. Bartholomew	NUMBER PATIENTS	CARDIAC IRREGULARITY OR BRADYCARDIA BELOW 60	APNEA REQUIRING CONTROLLED VENTILATION	OTHER COMPLICATIONS: LARYNGOSPASM; EMERGENCE DELIRIUM, CONVULSIONS, ETC.
ANESTHESIA				
Dentistry:				
Adult dental extractions	155	3	3	6
Pediatric dental extractions	490	8	3	6
Obstetrics:				
Precipitate delivery	350	4	3	2
Supplement for failed or inadequate conduction blocks	50			
Maternal or fetal emergencies, versions, extractions, etc.	80	2		1
Anesthesia required for un-co-operative patients receiving spinal anesthesia	8			
Rapid induction for maintenance with another anesthetic	5			
Surgery:				
Induction for tonsillectomy in children	1,450	8	4	8
Pediatric, orthopedic and general surgery	300	1		2
Adult short surgical operations	80	2		
Anesthesia for eye operations	110			
Induction of anesthesia for adult surgery	144		2	1
Anesthesia for intubation	80			
Removal of burn dressings and surgical packs and sutures	54			
Electroshock anesthesia	40			
Anesthesia for experimental testing depth and volume uptake, cyclopropane (medical students, residents and nurses)	78			
	3,474	28	15	26
THERAPY				
Postanesthesia hyperventilation	120			
Acute cerebral hemorrhage and cerebral thrombosis	2			
Oxygen and/or helium in asthma and cardiac disease	93			
Oxygen at high altitudes—mountains and aircraft	76			
Testing with fireman's mask under simulated rescue conditions and mobile evacuation maneuvers	156			
Total Uses	3,921			

*175 Pediatric and adult surgical cases
† 65 Intubations
‡150 Pediatric dental cases
§ 85 Obstetric cases

permits the administration of serially titrated doses of cyclopropane at will by opening and closing the valve as indicated. Thus, anesthesia can be prolonged.

B. The operator should be aware of the fact that at least 300 cc. of oxygen per minute should be available in the bag for the adult and at least 200 cc. per minute for the child.

C. Since the meter valve mechanism is an alternate technic, it will be used by anesthesiologists conversant with the minute-volume requirements of cyclopropane to achieve the necessary patient relaxation. It is not necessary to use this alternate technic at all for short operations.

D. The machine can be used most advantageously with balanced anesthesia in which there is proper premedication, supplemented with intravenous anesthesia and/or conduction nerve block anesthesia.

E. However, it is sufficient alone in a wide variety of other operations, such as: dental extractions; inductions for all pediatric anesthesias; the setting of simple fractures; myringotomies; the incision of abscesses; obstetric deliveries; a supplement to nerve block and spinal anesthesia; the control of hemorrhage and the removal of foreign bodies; the removal of surgical packs and sutures; the changing of burn dressings; and prolonged anesthetics with alternate technic.

INCOMPATIBILITIES IN ANESTHESIA WITH ERGOT OXYTOCICS

Clinical research at the School of Medicine, Western Reserve University, has demonstrated, in a study of 4,296 deliveries, a 1.5 per cent incidence of unexplained postpartum hypertension in the apparently normal mother, i.e., from 20 to 80 plus mm. of Hg elevation of systolic blood pressure. In the patient who either received a vasopressor during delivery or had hypertensive cardiovascular disease, a 6.3 per cent incidence of untoward postpartum hypertensive phenomenon was observed; in the patient with hypertensive cardiovascular disease who received a vasopressor, a 12 per cent incidence of unexpected untoward hypertensive sequelae was recorded in the subsequent postpartum period.

This report should serve as a warning against the use of unnecessary dosage of vasopressor drugs in combination with the Ergotrate and the Ergometrine oxytocics.

BIBLIOGRAPHY

Corcoran, John W., and Hingson, Robert A.: A new portable resuscitator and anesthetic gas machine, Dental Digest (in press).

Hingson, R. A.: New portable anesthetic gas machine and resuscitator—preliminary report, J.A.M.A. **156**:604–606, 1954.

Tricomi, V., and Hellman, L. M.: The uses of the Reserve Midget in Obstetrics, Am. J. Obst. & Gynec. (in press).

5 Psychological Principles of Pregnancy and Delivery

Formerly, it was considered that good obstetrics had been practiced if a living mother and child were obtained, and if the pains of labor were alleviated sufficiently so as to leave no lasting psychic trauma. More and more we are coming to look upon childbirth as one of life's most important experiences for women. As such, it furnishes an opportunity for emotional growth and stability far in excess of anything that a woman has experienced previously or is likely to experience in the future. Upon the obstetrician falls the burden of creating an environment in which this emotional experience can yield the best possible results. Particularly at the time of labor the anesthesiologist may play an important role.

Anxiety more than any other factor is a detriment to emotional growth. The anxieties of pregnant women are not particularly well understood, nor have they received adequate study. Klein and Potter, in a small but excellent book on the subject,* investigated a group of indigent women in a large city obstetric service. Perhaps the most significant point brought out was that fear of pain during parturition did not constitute the major source of anxiety for these patients. Death of the baby, possibility of malformation and increase in financial burdens all were of greater import. These anxieties were solved in as many ways as there were personalities involved. Frequently, great dependence was placed upon the physician or, in this particular case, the hospital. The fears and the anxieties of this stratum of society are different from those of private patients, and even in this latter group there is great variability in this matter.

Today's mothers are different from those of a generation or so ago. Then labor was expected to be, at the best, a dreary experience and frequently an extremely painful one. Tales of its difficulties form part of woman's folklore and were told and retold with amplification over the nation's bridge and luncheon tables. Surely, in retrospect, the age of amnesia when the best of the country's obstetricians allowed their patients to experience no memory following admission to the labor floor can be understood.

The years of adequate pain relief have brought a change in this type of thinking. No longer do the majority of mothers tell their daughters of the frightfulness of the process. In these young people, one encounters curiosity regarding pain relief but little or no fear that labor and delivery itself will be an impossibly painful process. There is an expectancy that the doctor chosen will play his part well and adequately. Also, at least in the mentally sound, there is an anticipation of partaking consciously in the event.

However, the fear of pain in childbirth has been a part of the intimate conversation of women since time immemorial. It is not dispelled easily by the attitudes developed in one short generation, but in all probability it still exists only a short distance beneath the con-

* Klein, H. R., Potter, H. W., and Dyk, R. B.: Anxiety in Pregnancy and Childbirth, New York, Hoeber, 1950.

scious surface of thought in many women. This fear is all too ready to emerge should a careless word or thoughtless act shatter a mother's confidence. It is no easy task to dispel or to keep submerged these age-old fears. The obstetrician must instill in his patient a confidence, not only that he is a friend and is anxious to spare her all unnecessary discomfort compatible with her welfare and the safety of her child, but also that he is quite capable of meeting each problem as it arises with confidence and skill. Qualities such as these cannot be taught, nor can their writing impart them to the physician who is so unlucky as not to have them. They form an attitude that, as Eastman so aptly says, "comes only as the result of long nights in the labor room and then only to those of understanding heart. It is the very substance of which good doctors are made, and it is at once the safest and the most welcome of obstetric anodynes."

Information about labor analgesia is given frequently during the first visit of the patient to her obstetrician, for the majority of private patients exhibit some curiosity in this regard in the first conversation. The obstetrician should discuss this matter carefully and intelligently with the patient. He should make no promises regarding any specific type of pain relief, nor should he guarantee the patient a completely painless delivery, for such, even today, exists rarely. Perhaps, it is well not to dwell too deeply upon this subject during the first visit, for the obstetrician should have some opportunity to become acquainted with his patient and her attitudes before offering her, or even considering, any specific type of pain relief. Sometime during the prenatal course it would be well for him to explain to her the various types of pain-relieving programs that exist. He should tell her that amnesia can be produced with little or no memory of the process, or that pain can be lessened with certain analgesic drugs and blocked completely by certain methods of conduction anesthesia.

Pain can be brought to a frightful nearness through the telescope of fear. Fear can be greatly accentuated and magnified through the microscope of pain. These two processes are pathologic psychic gemini which, when present in an uncontrolled form, may periscope into the sensorium an irreversible emotional trauma. The control of pain is achieved by 2 methods: (1) the anatomic approach, i.e., by blocking pain impulses at their source, as in local, spinal and regional anesthesia and in caudal analgesia; (2) the encephalic approach, i.e., by obliterating pain at its site of interpretation in the central nervous system through various forms of general, intravenous and rectal anesthesia. Some measure of control is afforded by obtunding the memory of pain through the use of drugs that produce amnesia or forgetfulness. Sometimes the control of fear is the more difficult of the two and can be managed by the establishment of the patient's confidence in her physican and by the maintenance of comfort in her surroundings. The patient in whom fear is controlled completely is the ideal one for the use of the anatomic approach. The one in whom fear is uncontrolled can be relieved usually more satisfactorily by one of the forms of general anesthesia or amnesia.

In the past decade Grantly Dick Read, of England, has written extensively on the psychological factors of labor. He has stated:

> The great intensifier of stimulus interpretation is fear. This emotion, like pain, is protective and produces through the sympathetic nervous system a state of tension within the body. Thus, we have the three great evils, pain, fear and tension. It is this syndrome which is responsible for the pain of labor. My contention is that the pain of labor is the result of an assault upon a primitive function which was intended to be painless. The attack is made by

> forces against which no protective apparatus has been developed, because the forces have not been understood and, which is probably more important, the method by which the attack is made has not been recognized. If there is any truth in this theory, it should be possible to demonstrate in practice how and where this vicious circle may be broken through. Modern science has laid the smoke screen of anesthesia in order to hide its own lack of perception. It appears, however, that a more rational method of approach to this problem would be to discover the vulnerable point at which to make a counterattack, not only to resist this dangerous invader which we call fear, but also to set up an efficient protective mechanism so that the primitive function of painless childbirth may be recognized by civilized women for all time as both natural and sound. . . .
>
> The perfect painless labor will be obtained not by the administration of drugs and agents to destroy consciousness. By careful and patient investigation of the phenomena of labor, observations will be made from different aspects. Chemical, neurological, psychological, mechanical, electrical and even metaphysical facets to this physiological gem will flash some new methods to those who care to look and in time these varied observations will be correlated and sifted until the truth of natural painless labor is obvious to all.*

The reading of the above statements carefully shows Read to possess the zeal of a metaphysical apostle. There can be no doubt that he anticipated the complete relief of pain through the obliteration of fear and tension. He did not mean that these psychological approaches should require the additional benefit of pain-relieving drugs. However, as time has passed, it has been realized by his disciples that childbirth should not be conducted without anesthetic aids, nor can it be made completely devoid of pain. A rational regimen of natural childbirth realizes that most patients experience pain to a greater or a lesser degree, and analgesic and anesthetic drugs should be administered when indicated. Regardless of Read's apostolic crusade, which, in itself, was in many aspects unscientific, obstetricians are greatly indebted to him.

* Read, Grantly Dick: Childbirth Without Fear, New York, Harper, 1953.

There has arisen a whole new school of thought that has emphasized the emotional and psychological aspects of the process of childbirth. As Goodrich and Thoms* point out:

> Natural childbirth is a broad concept and represents an attempt on the part of those who care for pregnant and parturient women to understand the physiology of pregnancy and labor, especially in its emotional aspects, so that these important functions may be viewed with less apprehension and better understanding by patients and that greater skill in caring for them may be developed by the physician.

Natural childbirth entails prenatal education designed to eliminate fear. As such, it encourages conversations between the patient and her physician regarding many of the physiologic processes that are taking place within her body. It encourages the physician to deal frankly with the process of labor and even to have his patient conducted on a tour during late pregnancy through the labor rooms and delivery suite. If these facilities are modern and designed competently, they will have many attributes that contribute to the patient's mental well-being. These rooms will be air-conditioned, soundproofed and decorated in a tasteful manner, which should be reminiscent of the woman's boudoir rather than the bare walls of the old-fashioned facilities. In view of the fact that there are 4 million births a year in the United States, it is amazing that it has taken so long to realize the necessity for more adequate labor rooms.

MUSIC DURING OBSTETRIC LABOR

The labor rooms should be equipped to satisfy not only the physical comforts but also the mental demands of the woman. Adequate reading material is a help, but more useful than this—at

* Goodrich, F. W., Jr., and Thoms, H.: Clinical study of natural childbirth; preliminary report from teaching ward service, Am. J. Obst. & Gynec. **56**:875, 1948.

least in our experience—has been music. Music has been used as an instrument of healing for as long as history has been recorded. It has been recognized as an intimate part of all primitive life. Four songs have been used by the Seminole Indians—for lumbago, for a sick baby, for childbirth and for death. The Chippewa, the Cherokee and the Winnebago Indians all have developed special types of music for the treatment of specific diseases. The medicine man in equatorial Africa used music in his therapy as often as he did potions of herbs.

In civilization also, the value of music in the alleviation of symptoms of disease is well recognized. In 1 Samuel 16: 23, it is recorded:

> And it came to pass, when the *evil* spirit from God was upon Saul, that David took an harp, and played with his hand: so Saul was refreshed, and was well, and the evil spirit departed from him.

There are similar accounts of such alleviation of melancholy in Hindu, Chinese, Hebrew, Arabian and other religious writings. In 1744, John Armstrong wrote in *The Art of Preserving Health* the following little poem:

> Music exalts each joy, allays each grief,
> Expels diseases, softens every pain,
> Subdues the rage of poison, and the plague;
> And hence the wives of ancient days ador'd
> One power of psychic, melody and song.

More than 2 decades ago, Dr. Joseph B. DeLee, the Chicago authority on obstetrics, was among the first in this country to use music as a therapeutic aid with local anesthesia. For the last 5 years, the University of Chicago Surgical Unit has employed earphone transmitters of music to patients being induced with gas anesthesia. They have observed that patient-fright thus is minimized, inductions are shorter, and higher concentrations of oxygen can be given with nitrous oxide anesthesia.

The Jewish Hospital in Brooklyn has used music as an adjunct to gas anesthesia for the past number of years. They have experimented by trial and error to find the type of music most suited to this method of combined management. The following selections are presented in order of their effectiveness:

Clair de Lune, by Debussy
Moonlight Sonata, by Beethoven
Dream Pantomime, by Humperdinck
Evening Star, by Wagner
Forest Murmurs, by Wagner
Poème, by Chausson

During the period of the anesthesia study program in the Department of Obstetrics at Johns Hopkins and Sinai Hospitals, of Baltimore, not only was music supplied to each labor room by "Muzak" but these rooms were redecorated and air-conditioned. The comparatively harsh finish of old-style hospital rooms gave way to cool, pastel tints following established rules of color therapy. There was a "peach" room and a "blue" room, another was tinted a soothing gray, and still another had a pinkish glow. Light fixtures were varied and modern, avoiding the grim standardization so widely accepted as inevitable. These rooms devoted to the mother's comfort were hung with Venetian blinds and draperies of hand-blocked Chinese linen, and attractive mirrors were added to the wall. All rooms were furnished differently, some with oil paintings and others with water colors. The paintings were selected to suggest peace and quiet, with no suggestion of human conflict.

An attempt was made to evaluate the effects of this type of therapy upon the patients within 24 hours of delivery. They were interviewed by a trained nonmedical observer and were asked to state in the order of their preference the benefit from the various facilities. First choice was:

1. Staff	76
2. Medicine	17
3. Music	7
4. Air-conditioning	0
5. Interior *décor*	0
	100

The second choice was:

1. Music	39
2. Medicine	28
3. Staff	23
4. Air-conditioning	0
5. Interior *décor*	0
6. Combination of all	6
7. No second preference	4
	100

In combining these choices it can be seen that 46 women found music of value in either first or second choice, 99 preferred the staff presence as first or second choice, and 45 preferred medicine in first or second choice.

In order to promulgate natural childbirth programs, many obstetricians refer their prenatal patients to group teaching clinics. If these teaching clinics are well run, they are of great benefit, as they give the mothers much information regarding the physiologic childbirth processes of reproduction and practical information regarding care of themselves and their children. The classes also include exercises. Probably these are of no direct value, but they do act as adjuncts to group therapy and, as such, are particularly enjoyed by many women.

The anesthesiologist usually comes into this picture quite late, that is, during labor, or even at the actual delivery. If the groundwork has been laid well during the prenatal period, his path is an easy one, and if he possesses the qualities of the good physician already described, then he can aid the obstetrician in making this process a comfortable one for all concerned. He should realize, perhaps even more than the obstetrician, that there are many methods of obstetric pain relief, each of which has its good points and its drawbacks. Also, he ought to realize that there is great variation in a patient's response to this situation, and even variation in her response from one birth to the next. Obstetricians, and even institutions, are apt to be enthusiasts for one method of pain relief or another. They are given to publishing figures showing that this or that method far excels all others. The anesthesiologist ought to realize that the obtaining of such data is fraught with difficulties and that it is apt to be biased by particular environmental situations or physician or patient enthusiasms. He should attempt to have available whatever sound statistical data he can bring to bear on the subject, but when his advice is sought, he ought to apply that method of pain relief that best fits the particular case and factors involved.

In an effort to obtain some data on the patient's own psychological evaluation of the various methods of pain relief, we conducted a control obstetric study at Johns Hopkins and Sinai Hos-

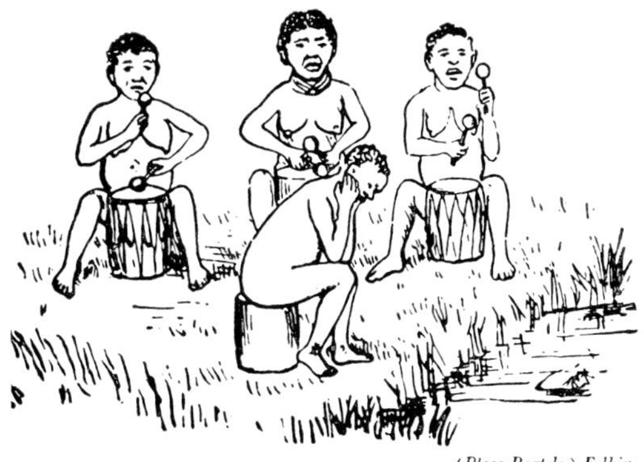

(Ploss-Bartels.) Felkin.

FIG. 81. Niam-Niam woman delivering on a crude birth stool on the bank of a river. Musical accompaniment. (Ploss & Bartels: Das Weib in der Natur- und Völkerkunde, Leipzig, Th. Grieben's Verlag)

pitals, in Baltimore, from November, 1948, to March, 1951. This study comprised approximately 9,500 mothers who received anesthesia for labor, as shown in Figure 82. In addition, certain groups of mothers were selected to test various methods and combinations of methods of anesthesia and analgesia. Our findings appeared in Table 13, page 185.

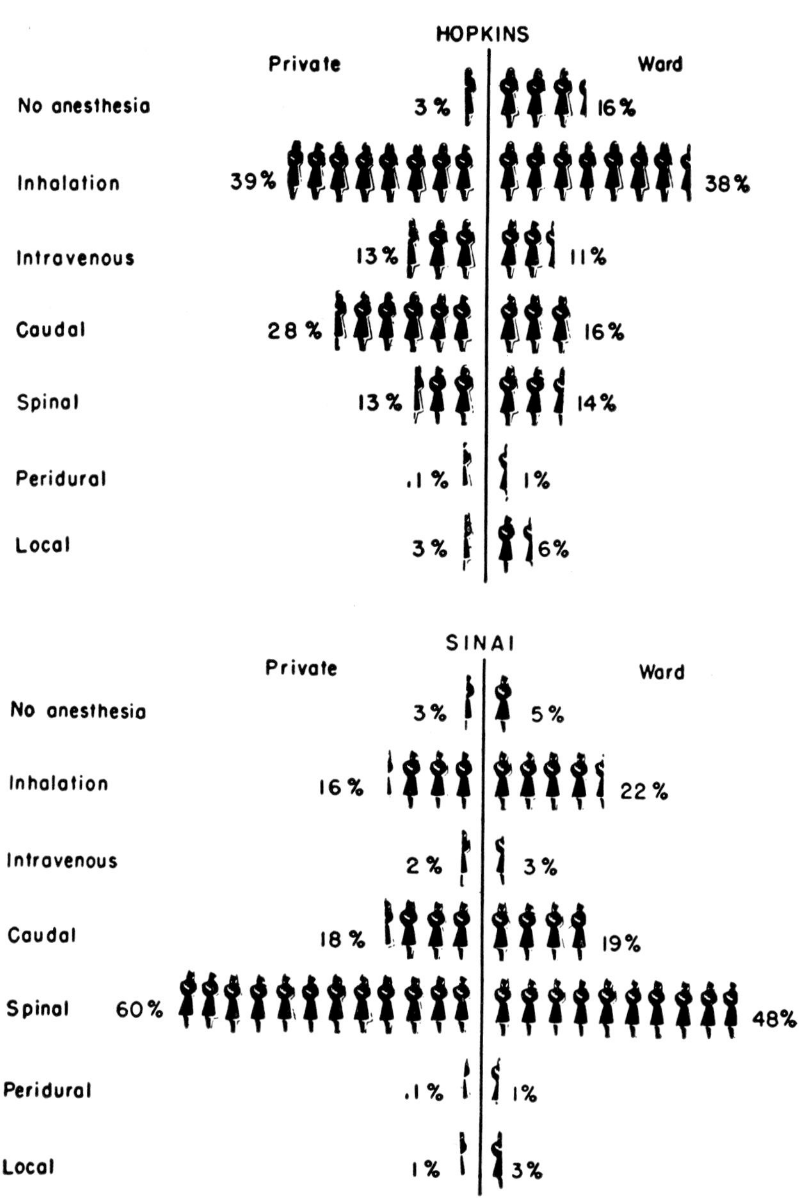

FIG. 82. Distribution of mothers in the Baltimore Obstetric Anesthesia Study.

EIGHT THOUSAND PARTURIENTS EVALUATE DRUGS, TECHNICS AND DOCTORS DURING LABOR AND DELIVERY

A Qualitative and Quantitative Assay of Obstetric Amnesia, Analgesia, Anesthesia and Psychological Lobotomy During Childbirth*

During the past decade progress in the understanding and the utilization of the principles of obstetric analgesia and anesthesia during childbirth has exceeded the accomplishments of the previous century introduced so dramatically and effectively by the lifework of Sir James Y. Simpson. More than 800 scientific articles and a half dozen texts in many languages have presented the evaluations of physicians of multiple methods used at present in the control of obstetric pain. The following is the first evaluation of obstetric amnesia, analgesia and anesthesia and psychorelaxation methods by a statistically significant group of parturients who themselves experienced the effects of these drugs or the lack of them during childbirth.

The study was a small part of a total evaluation of all methods used presently in the control of obstetric pain conducted in Johns Hopkins and Sinai Hospitals, in Baltimore, during 1948 to 1951 as a planned project supported by the staffs of the two hospitals in co-operation with the United States Public Health Service and nine pharmaceutical companies.†

The IBM punch cards were used throughout the study in the tabulating of 80 columns of medical, obstetric, anesthesiologic and pharmacologic data which were recorded frequently and regularly during labor and delivery and in postdelivery follow-up of all the patients by a specially trained team of special anesthesia assistant obstetric nurses who were available 24 hours daily for the 3 years of the study. The data were first recorded on the patients' charts, and on the same day they were transcribed to individual code sheets, a numerical system identical with the IBM cards being used. The final recording was made on the IBM cards with one for each mother and one for each baby by clerks in the department of obstetric statistics of the Johns Hopkins Hospital. The organization of the data into tables and charts was performed by the Section on Statistics in the Division of Public health Methods in the United States Public Health Service under the direction of Dr. S. D. Collins.

There were 9,347 mothers in this study. In order that certain heterogeneous variables could be removed, those mothers who delivered multiple births, infants who died in utero before labor and analgesia, infants with congenital abnormalities incompatible with life and those delivered by cesarean section were excluded. This left 7,704 mothers with live single fetuses in utero at the onset of analgesia, as can be seen by summary Tables 12, 13 and 14. There was a widespread distribution among all categories of primiparas and multiparas, white and nonwhite, private and ward patients. Also, as can be seen in Figure 82 and Tables 13 and 14, statistically significant groups were managed with each of the various methods of obstetric analgesia and anesthesia.

At the onset of the study, it was determined that parturients in the Hopkins Hospital would be managed with 1 of the 5 following group plans considered to embody the standard presently used methods of analgesia and anesthesia:

* From Am. J. Obst. & Gynec. 68:262-278, 1954.

† Made possible by grants to the obstetric anesthesia research program of the Johns Hopkins University and Hospital from Abbott Laboratories, Astra Pharmaceutical Products, Inc., Ciba Pharmaceutical Products, Inc., Eli Lilly and Company, Merck & Co., Inc., Parke, Davis & Company, Sharpe & Dohme, Inc., E. R. Squibb & Sons, Winthrop-Stearns, Inc., and Becton, Dickinson and Company.

TABLE 12. SUMMARY. TOTAL NUMBERS ONLY (NO EXCLUSIONS)

	BOTH HOSPITALS	HOPKINS	SINAI
Total infants	9,472	5,856	3,616
Live births	9,337	5,757	3,580
Neonatal deaths	130	103	27
Congenital malformations	32	23	9
Stillbirths	135	99	36
Infants who died before onset of labor and analgesia	110	83	27
Congenital malformations	3	1	2
Multiple births	249	179	70
First births	124	89	35
Second and third births	125	90	35
Deaths among multiple births	8	6	2
Stillbirths among multiple births	11	10	1
Premature infants	993	721	272
Private patients	271	103	168
White	264	96	168
Nonwhite	7	7	—
Ward patients	722	618	104
White	257	153	104
Nonwhite	465	465	—
Cesarean sections	105	83	22
Twins*	126	98	28
Total mothers	9,347	5,766	3,581
Ward mothers	5,354	4,233	1,121
White	2,497	1,377	1,120
Nonwhite	2,857	2,856	1
Private	3,993	1,533	2,460
White	3,928	1,472	2,456
Nonwhite	65	61	4
Primiparas	2,918	1,701	1,217
White	2,062	848	1,214
Nonwhite	856	853	3
Multiparas	6,429	4,065	2,364
White	4,363	2,001	2,362
Nonwhite	2,066	2,064	2
Mothers with breech	315	195	120
Mothers with cesarean sections	407	315	92
Mothers with diabetes	29	23	6
Mothers with heart disease	202	144	58
Mothers with hemorrhagic conditions	379	293	86
Mothers with obesity	200	130	70
Mothers with toxemia	997	755	243
Mothers with tuberculosis	159	134	25
Maternal deaths	6	6	—

* Twins counted as premature only when both twins weighed less than 2,500 Gm.

TABLE 13. PERCENTAGE OF MOTHERS WITH SPECIFIED PSYCHOLOGICAL EVALUATIONS ACCORDING TO METHODS OF ADMINISTERING DRUGS (HOPKINS AND SINAI)

	Percentage			*Number**			
METHODS	SATISFACTORY	PARTIALLY SATISFACTORY	UNSATISFACTORY	MOTHERS' KNOWN EVAL.	SATISFACTORY	PARTIALLY SATISFACTORY	UNSATISFACTORY
All Mothers							
Total mothers	81.7	10.2	8.1	7,704	6,297	785	622
No anesthesia	73.2	11.4	15.4	643	471	73	99
No anes. or anal.	69.3	10.4	20.3	374	259	39	76
Intravenous	79.9	11.8	8.3	558	446	66	46
Inhalation	77.4	12.4	10.2	2,153	1,666	267	220
Caudal†	86.1	7.3	6.6	1,529	1,317	111	101
Spinal	87.2	8.5	4.3	2,388	2,083	202	103
Local	69.5	17.8	12.7	197	137	35	25
Combination of methods	75.0	13.1	11.9	236	177	31	28
Primiparas							
Total mothers	85.5	8.2	6.3	2,483	2,122	204	157
No anesthesia	76.3	13.5	10.2	59	45	8	6
No anes. or anal.	61.5	23.1	15.4	26	16	6	4
Intravenous	80.1	11.8	8.1	186	149	22	15
Inhalation	79.9	10.9	9.2	523	418	57	48
Caudal†	89.4	6.0	4.6	587	525	35	27
Spinal	89.3	6.6	4.1	974	870	64	40
Local	72.5	14.5	13.0	69	50	10	9
Combination of methods	76.5	9.4	14.1	85	65	8	12
Multiparas							
Total mothers	80.0	11.1	8.9	5,221	4,175	581	465
No anesthesia	73.0	11.1	15.9	584	426	65	93
No anes. or anal.	69.8	9.5	20.7	348	243	33	72
Intravenous	79.9	11.8	8.3	372	297	44	31
Inhalation	76.6	12.9	10.5	1,630	1,248	210	172
Caudal†	84.4	7.9	7.7	942	792	76	74
Spinal	85.8	9.8	4.4	1,414	1,213	138	63
Local	68.0	19.5	12.5	128	87	25	16
Combination of methods	74.2	15.2	10.6	151	112	23	16

* Twins, cesarean sections, infants who died before onset of labor and analgesia, and infants with congenital malformations incompatible with life are excluded.

† Caudal includes a few mothers delivered by special conduction and peridural anesthesia.

Group 1. Systemic sedation for labor and general inhalation anesthesia for delivery with agents nitrous oxide, ether, cyclopropane and trichlorethylene.

Group 2. Systemic sedation for labor and intravenous barbiturate anesthesia for delivery with agents Pentothal Sodium, Surital, Seconal and Nembutal.

Group 3. No drugs exceeding 50 mg. Demerol during labor or delivery, but psychoanalgesia established with suggestion, comfortable air-conditioned envi-

TABLE 14. PERCENTAGE OF MOTHERS WITH SPECIFIED PSYCHOLOGICAL EVALUATIONS FOR EACH METHOD OF ADMINISTERING DRUGS ACCORDING TO HOSPITAL ACCOMMODATIONS (HOPKINS AND SINAI)

METHODS	*Percentage* SATISFACTORY	PARTIALLY SATISFACTORY	UNSATISFACTORY	MOTHERS' KNOWN EVAL.	*Number** SATISFACTORY	PARTIALLY SATISFACTORY	UNSATISFACTORY
All Accommodations							
Total mothers	81.7	10.2	8.1	7,704	6,297	785	622
No anesthesia	73.2	11.4	15.4	643	471	73	99
No anes. or anal.	69.3	10.4	20.3	374	259	39	76
Intravenous	79.9	11.8	8.3	558	446	66	46
Inhalation	77.4	12.4	10.2	2,153	1,666	267	220
Caudal†	86.1	7.3	6.6	1,529	1,317	111	101
Spinal	87.2	8.5	4.3	2,388	2,083	202	103
Local	69.5	17.8	12.7	197	137	35	25
Combination of methods	75.0	13.1	11.9	236	177	31	28
Private							
Total mothers	89.7	6.6	3.7	3,497	3,137	232	128
No anesthesia	93.1	5.9	1.0	101‡	94	6	1
No anes. or anal.	91.7	8.3	—	24‡	22	2	—
Intravenous	85.8	8.2	6.0	183	157	15	11
Inhalation	88.9	8.0	3.1	804	715	64	25
Caudal	90.6	5.4	4.0	795	720	43	32
Spinal	90.3	6.3	3.4	1,468	1,326	93	49
Local	84.2	10.5	5.3	38	32	4	2
Combination of methods	86.1	6.5	7.4	108	93	7	8
Ward							
Total mothers	75.1	13.2	11.7	4,207	3,160	553	494
No anesthesia	69.5	12.4	18.1	542	377	67	98
No anes. or anal.	67.7	10.6	21.7	350	237	37	76
Intravenous	77.1	13.6	9.3	375	289	51	35
Inhalation	70.5	15.0	14.5	1,349	951	203	195
Caudal†	81.3	9.3	9.4	734	597	68	69
Spinal	82.3	11.8	5.9	920	757	109	54
Local	66.0	19.5	14.5	159	105	31	23
Combination of methods	65.6	18.8	15.6	128	84	24	20

* Twins, cesarean sections, infants who died before labor and analgesia and infants with congenital malformations incompatible with life are excluded.

† Caudal includes a few mothers delivered by special conduction and peridural anesthesia.

‡ These 101 mothers represent only the residue of a much larger number of private patients who required drugs and anesthetics after a few hours' trial of psychoanalgesia in early labor.

ronment, therapeutic music and interior decorating.

Group 4. Systemic sedation for labor with terminal conduction block of spinal, caudal or local for delivery.

Group 5. Continuous conduction block without systemic narcosis during labor and delivery.

In the Sinai Hospital the staff and the directors of the obstetric department felt that a study of a group of patients receiving no analgesia or anesthesia should not be done. Consequently, 3 methods of management were decided upon that coincided entirely with the 4 groups in the Hopkins Hospital which were conducted with analgesic and anesthetic drugs. The sedation for labor and inhalation with intravenous anesthesia for delivery were combined into a single group designated as Group C. These 3 methods recorded in Table 14 are:

Group A. Systemic sedation for labor and terminal block with spinal (saddle block) for delivery.

Group B. Continuous conduction caudal or peridural analgesia for labor and delivery without systemic narcosis.

Group C. Systemic sedation for labor and inhalation or intravenous anesthesia for delivery.

Labor Room Environment

Comfortable and pleasing environment, while not directly linked with evaluation of drugs and other treatments, has a definite influence upon emotional and psychological reactions. Therefore, the standard type labor rooms in these hospitals, hitherto strictly functional, have emerged as chambers of restful grace. The new "climate" for labor is established in air-conditioned, soundproof rooms, where the comparatively harsh finish of old-style hospital rooms has given way to cool pastel tints following established rules of color therapy. Peach, cascade blue, soothing gray and pinkish glow rooms are equipped with modern indirect lighting fixtures, Venetian blinds and appropriately chosen draperies. Attractive wall mirrors, oil and water-color paintings of landscapes blend with the wall finish. Therapeutic background music is transmitted by "Muzak" into each labor and delivery room on a 24-hour per day optional basis. Individual volume controls permitted patient the use of the music to the volume tone desired, or she could eliminate it. The same environment was offered private and service cases and all races without exception. The patients themselves almost unanimously have appraised music as one of the most valuable and pleasant remedies for the emotional tension so frequently attending prodromal and active labor and delivery.

Method of Determining Psychological Evaluation

Twenty-four hours after delivery the patient was visited for the first time by a secretary trained for interviews who explained the purpose of her visit as a means of assaying the efficiency of analgesics, anesthetics and methods. The patient was encouraged to designate her pain relief during labor and delivery as "excellent, good, satisfactory, partially satisfactory or unsatisfactory." The data then were entered on the patient's code sheet and correlated with the evaluations of the physician and the obstetric nurse anesthesia assistant who managed this particular patient. In less than 0.5 per cent the patient did not wish to communicate any evaluation concerning drugs or methods used. Obviously, because of the use of the amnesic agents, some parturients remembered nothing of labor or delivery. Such cases were coded as excellent unless the parturient disclosed significant unpleasant symptoms resulting from the amnesia. When the patient remembered only single or occasional disjointed events of labor or delivery, the analgesia was coded as good.

Experimental Group

Since it was our object to evaluate the efficiency and the safety of the various methods designated by the 5 groups in a controlled study, 1,489 parturients, or about 20 per cent of the total, were managed in the 5 groups by a chronologic delineation from their hospital history numbers. These patients had their method of management chosen for them by the last 2 digits of their history numbers in the manner that all patients with numbers ending in 0 and 1 were managed by the Group 1 method; those with endings of 2 and 3 by Group 2; those with endings 4 and 5 by Group 3; those with endings 6 and 7 by Group 4; those with endings 8 and 9 by Group 5. In this manner the human choice factor was eliminated. However, both the experimental group and the larger heterogeneous groups with complications or patients removed from the experimental group for any of the reasons listed in Table 15 were analyzed in evaluating the various drugs and technics. There was no significant difference in the evaluation of the mothers, regardless of whether the physician or the history number digits determined the method.

Therefore, the 1,489 patients without complications in either mother or baby group (which represented 20 per cent of the study and were managed by methods as determined by the terminal digits of their history numbers) are not studied in detail here but have been reported in the *New York State Journal of Medicine,* December 1, 1953.

Instead, the entire group of 7,704 mothers who had single babies alive in utero before the onset of analgesia from both hospitals are reported upon here.

Combined Total Group

The controlled obstetric study at Hopkins covered deliveries during the period of November, 1948, through March, 1951. The Sinai study covered the period of October, 1949, through March, 1951.

Sixty-nine per cent of the infants at Sinai were born to private patients, as against 26 per cent at Hopkins. There were 5 nonwhite infants delivered at Sinai, as against 2,917 (51 per cent of total mothers) at Hopkins. By combining the total mothers in Tables 13 and 14, we believe there is a more representative sample of American obstetrics than would be the case in analyzing the cases of only one of the hospitals alone.

In Hopkins, 5,856 infants were delivered to 5,766 mothers—in Sinai 3,616 infants were delivered to 3,581 mothers—as recorded in Summary Table 12.

The specific type of delivery was controlled on the basis of the last digit of the hospital history number among ward patients only, unless one of the reasons presented in Tables 15 and 16 required the withdrawing of the intended method and the substitution of an indicated method on the basis of therapy, expediency or complications inherent in the method.

The percentage of mothers retained in each of the 3 study groups at Sinai is higher than at Hopkins. This may be due to the large number of nonwhite mothers in the Hopkins' groups who frequently came to the hospital late in labor and more frequently in precipitate labor. In Table 15 it can be seen that 1,287, or 30 per cent of the five groups combined, were precipitous labors, as against 207, or 18 per cent, at Sinai, as recorded in Table 16. Seventy-two per cent of the 1,287 were nonwhite mothers.

TABLE 15. PERCENTAGE OF MOTHERS (WARD) WHO REMAINED IN OR WERE REMOVED FROM THE EXPERIMENTAL GROUPS AND THE REASON FOR REMOVAL (HOPKINS HOSPITAL)

	Percentage						*Number**					
REASON	TOTAL	GROUP 1	GROUP 2	GROUP 3	GROUP 4	GROUP 5	TOTAL	GROUP 1	GROUP 2	GROUP 3	GROUP 4	GROUP 5
Total ward patients	100	100	100	100	100	100	4,233	842	870	820	876	825
All substitutions	75.41	65.44	77.59	83.05	76.71	74.30	3,192	551	675	681	672	613
Precipitous labor	30.40	32.07	39.08	4.03	41.33	34.18	1,287	270	340	33	362	282
Fetal distress	0.24	0.12	0.23	0.49	0.23	0.12	10	1	2	4	2	1
Insufficient staff	0.90	0.95	0.80	0.12	1.14	1.46	38	8	7	1	10	12
Maternal complications	19.47	18.05	24.48	18.90	17.70	18.06	824	152	213	155	155	149
Inertia, intrinsic	1.30	1.19	1.26	0.61	1.83	1.58	55	10	11	5	16	13
Inertia, extrinsic	0.14	—	0.23	0.12	0.11	0.24	6	—	2	1	1	2
Prematurity	4.91	6.29	5.17	5.00	4.79	3.27	208	53	45	41	42	27
Research	1.37	1.54	1.38	1.95	1.03	0.97	58	13	12	16	9	8
Teaching	0.92	1.07	0.92	1.34	1.14	0.12	39	9	8	11	10	1
Error	1.65	2.02	1.95	0.98	2.17	1.09	70	17	17	8	19	9
Failed insertion	2.06	—	0.35	—	2.74	7.27	87	—	3	—	24	60
Drug failure	0.17	—	0.12	—	0.11	0.61	7	—	1	—	1	5
Vomited	0.05	0.12	0.12	—	—	—	2	1	1	—	—	—
Analgesia indicated	1.04	0.12	0.12	1.46	0.23	3.40	44	1	1	12	2	28
Failure, method	9.38	0.24	0.12	47.32	0.34	0.36	397	2	1	388	3	3
Patient refused method	0.87	0.83	0.57	0.49	1.14	1.33	37	7	5	4	10	11
Unknown reason†	0.54	0.83	0.69	0.24	0.68	0.24	23	7	6	2	6	2
Experimental group	24.59	34.56	22.41	16.95	23.29	25.70	1,041	291	195	139	204	212

Group:
1—Sedation–inhalation
2—Sedation–intravenous
3—Psychoanalgesia
4—Sedation–terminal block
5—Continuous conduction

* Excludes second twins (81).

† Includes 6 infants who died before labor and analgesia but no substitution reason was given.

Failure of Psychoanalgesia Among Ward Patients

It is significant that in spite of the ideal labor room environment already described, 47 per cent of the ward patients designated by the history number digit method were failures in the psychoanalgesia method in which our staff attempted to conduct labor without analgesia or anesthesia with drugs. These patients became so miserable or uncontrollable with suggestion and attempted psychological lobotomy analgesia that it was necessary to substitute drug therapy for their own safety and the peace of the remainder of the hospital. This compared unfavorably with the 0.24 per cent failure rate in Group 1; the 0.12 per cent failure rate in Group 2; the 0.34 per cent failure rate in Group 4; and the 0.36 per cent failure rate in Group 5. This fact is accentuated further by the psychological evaluations of the ward patients recorded in Table 14, which shows that only 69.5 per cent of 542 ward mothers remaining in the Group indicated 24 hours after delivery that they were satisfied with the management of their pain relief. When we combine the 165 dissatisfied ward mothers with the 388 ward mothers removed from the group as indicated in Table 15, a total of 558 of 820

TABLE 16. PERCENTAGE OF MOTHERS (WARD) WHO REMAINED IN OR WERE REMOVED FROM THE EXPERIMENTAL GROUPS AND THE REASONS FOR REMOVAL (SINAI HOSPITAL)

Reason	*Percentage*				*Number**			
	Total	Group A	Group B	Group C	Total	Group A	Group B	Group C
Total ward patients	100	100	100	100	1,121	451	337	333
All substitutions	60.04	48.12	69.73	66.37	673	217	235	221
Precipitous labor	18.47	19.73	23.14	12.01	207	89	78	40
Fetal distress	0.18	—	—	0.60	2	—	—	2
Insufficient staff	10.08	0.45	12.46	20.72	113	2	42	69
Maternal complications	12.22	9.54	14.54	13.52	137	43	49	45
Inertia, intrinsic	0.45	—	0.89	0.60	5	—	3	2
Inertia, extrinsic	0.27	—	0.59	0.30	3	—	2	1
Prematurity	6.96	8.87	2.67	8.71	78	40	9	29
Research	0.53	0.45	0.30	0.90	6	2	1	3
Teaching	4.55	5.54	2.08	5.71	51	25	7	19
Error	1.34	0.67	2.08	1.50	15	3	7	5
Failed insertion	2.14	1.33	5.34	—	24	6	18	—
Drug failure	0.89	0.44	2.08	0.30	10	2	7	1
Vomited	—	—	—	—	—	—	—	—
Analgesia indicated	0.62	0.44	1.18	0.30	7	2	4	1
Failure	—	—	—	—	—	—	—	—
Patient refused method	1.07	0.44	2.08	0.90	12	2	7	3
Unknown reason†	0.27	0.22	0.30	0.30	3	1	1	1
Experimental group	39.96	51.88	30.27	33.63	448	234	102	112

Group:
A—Sedation—terminal block
B—Continuous conduction
C—Sedation—inhalation or intravenous
* Excludes second twins (12).
† Includes 2 infants who died before labor but no substitution reason was given.

mothers, or 67 per cent of the total, were failures or managed unsatisfactorily by this method. This compares unfavorably with better than 85 per cent success in spinal and caudal anesthesia.

This analysis explains somewhat the 93.2 and the 91.7 per cent satisfactory results from the patient standpoint described in the psychological evaluation of a small group of 101 mothers who elected with their obstetrician the psychoanalgesia technic as recorded in the private patient section of Table 14. This table does not take into account the larger number of private patients who elected to "remain in this group method of management as long as possible" but during the course of labor required, and were given, other forms of management using analgesic drugs and anesthetics.

Likewise, except among private patients, local anesthesia (pudendal block) succeeded in less than 70 per cent of 197 patients (Tables 13 and 14).

Substantiation of Necessity of Pain Relief in Childbirth from Britain

This analysis is entirely in line with the evaluation given by 196 British women doctor-mothers. The British Council of the Medical Women's Federation asked 300 doctor-mothers: Is relief of pain in childbirth necessary? The overwhelming response, reported by the *British Medical Journal:* Yes. Of 196 who replied, 184 were in favor of drugs in the delivery room; only 8 were definitely against. The women who answered have a combined experience of 425 confinements. Of these, 66 per cent were in hospitals or nursing homes, where it is easier to relieve pain; only 28 per cent were at home. But from 21 to 36 per cent wanted more relief than they received.

There was no doubt in the mind of the author of the report, Dr. Kitty Kate Conrad, 39, mother of 2. Said she:

> Even when one has seen 300 or more confinements, as I have, the severity of labor pains comes as an intense surprise. They are more excruciating than anything you can possibly imagine. I am certainly in favor of spreading the use of pain-relieving drugs in childbirth as widely as possible.

Some of our patients in their recorded comments were in complete agreement with Dr. Conrad. Some of them even agreed with Mrs. Leah Manning, Labor Member of Parliament:

> If some doctors had a labor ward of men to look after, I think it highly probable that for the defense of their sanity they would give their patients something more than a towel and tell them to pull on it.

However, in defense of the no anesthesia or analgesia method, we found enthusiastic supporters among the 101 of 3,497 private patients and among some of the 114 of the 820 ward patients. The small minorities in both extremes of the question for and against pain relief in obstetrics with analgesic and anesthetic drugs demonstrated a proficiency in verbalization. In between the extremes were the masses of women with a decided, though moderate, leaning toward the use of analgesics and anesthetics in childbirth.

Significance of the Subject in the United States

The mere mention of the approximately 4 million births per year in the United States, with use of some form of pain-relieving drugs in more than 75

TABLE 17. LABOR. PERCENTAGE OF SPECIFIED DRUG GIVEN IN LABOR OR DELIVERY THAT IS EVALUATED UNSATISFACTORY BY MOTHERS* (HOPKINS AND SINAI)

Name of Drug Alone or Augmented	*Percentage* Both Hospitals	Hopkins	Sinai	*Number†* Both Hospitals	Hopkins	Sinai
Demerol	13.67	18.81	11.21	3,050	989	2,061
Metycaine	13.71	15.93	12.00	3,166	1,375	1,791
Seconal	13.97	18.43	10.38	2,734	1,221	1,513
Scopolamine	14.18	17.59	11.73	3,943	1,649	2,294
Nupercaine	16.06	21.25	13.57	741	240	501
Nembutal	17.54	19.82	14.77	2,012	1,105	907
Xylocaine	19.48	18.53	22.22	349	259	90
Pentothal Sodium	19.58	20.33	12.50	669	605	64
Pontocaine	19.78	22.66	17.46	455	203	252
Nitrous oxide, ether	21.06	24.46	12.59	1,439	1,026	413
Nitrous oxide (no ether)	27.44	30.53	14.90	1,290	1,035	255

* Excludes mothers of twins.
† Excludes mothers with unknown or no evaluation.

per cent of them, indicates the importance of the subject. With an average $15 consideration to hospital or physician for each obstetric anesthetic there is a total investment made by 3 million women of approximately $45,000,000 in America for this service.

Evaluation of the Efficiency of Drugs and Anesthetics

In this study were used all the current analgesic and anesthetic drugs, including methadone, Nisentil, heroin, paraldehyde, cyclopropane, Surital, chloroform and Cyclaine, in addition to those listed in Tables 16 and 17. However, when an agent was used less than 50 times, it was not included in this study. It should be pointed out that cyclopropane, administered 20 times during delivery in our hospitals, was definitely a superior agent, but, because of the lack of adequate explosion-proof environment, it was not used as a major agent. Trichlorethylene was administered 45 times with 6 mothers, or 15.4 per cent, reporting unsatisfactory results.

Figure 83 presents the graphic incidence of unsatisfactory evaluation by the mothers of the 11 major agents used in this study. In this study it is evident that nitrous oxide alone during anesthesia, whether or not superimposed upon preliminary sedation in labor, gave the highest incidence of unsatisfactory reports from the mothers. It should be emphasized here that the technics used always maintained the oxygen at 20 per

TABLE 18. DELIVERY. PERCENTAGE OF MOTHERS BY PSYCHOLOGICAL EVALUATION WHEN ONLY ONE SPECIFIED DRUG WAS ADMINISTERED DURING DELIVERY (HOPKINS AND SINAI)

Drugs During Delivery	Percentage		Mothers' Known Report*	Number	
	Satisfactory	Unsatisfactory		Satisfactory	Unsatisfactory
Inhalation					
Nitrous oxide, oxygen	73.97	26.03	803	594	209
Nitrous oxide, ether, oxygen	79.27	20.73	1,283	1,017	266
Trichlorethylene	84.60	15.40	45	39	6
Intravenous					
Pentothal sodium	81.60	18.40	413	337	76
Continuous Conduction (Caudal or Peridural)					
Metycaine	88.50	11.50	1,148	1,016	132
Pontocaine	83.06	16.94	124	103	21
Xylocaine	84.26	15.74	108	91	17
Terminal Block (Saddle Block or Spinal)					
Procaine	88.71	11.29	62	55	7
Metycaine	88.82	11.18	1,368	1,215	153
Pontocaine	85.21	14.79	169	144	25
Nupercaine	85.11	14.89	658	560	98
Xylocaine	91.43	8.57	35	32	3

* Cesarean sections, twins, and infants who died before labor are excluded.

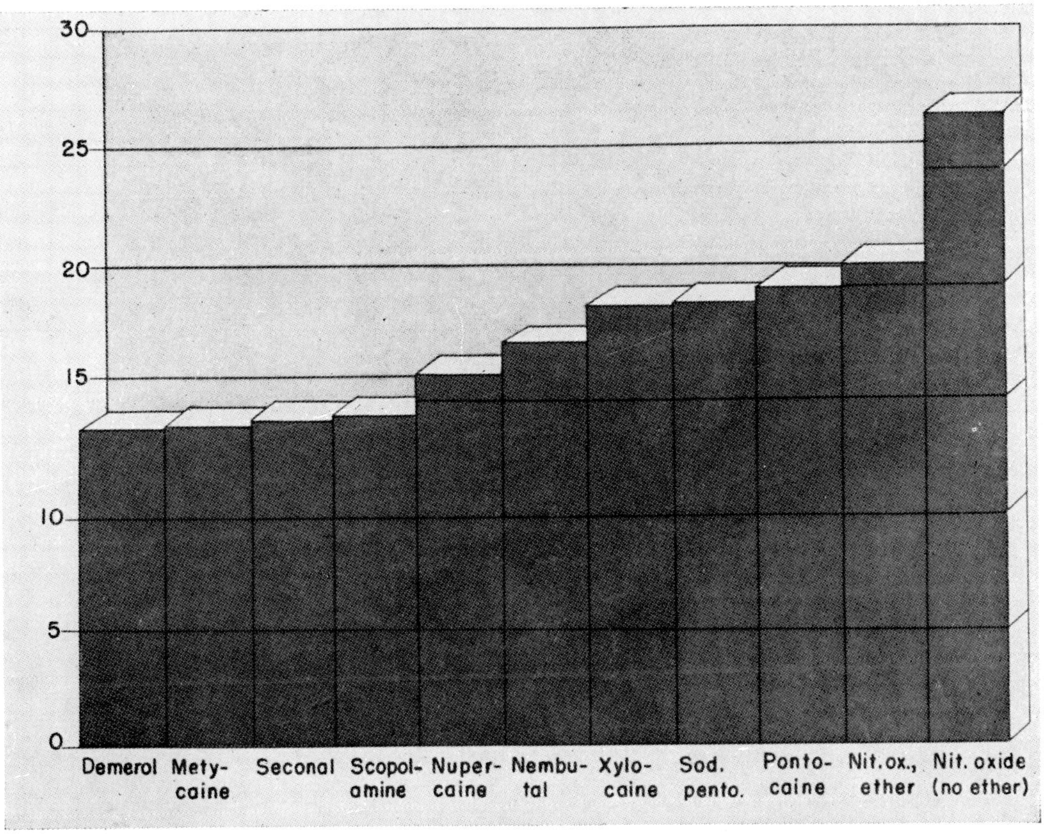

FIG. 83. Percentage of cases evaluated *unsatisfactory* by drug. (Baltimore Obstetric Anesthesia Study)

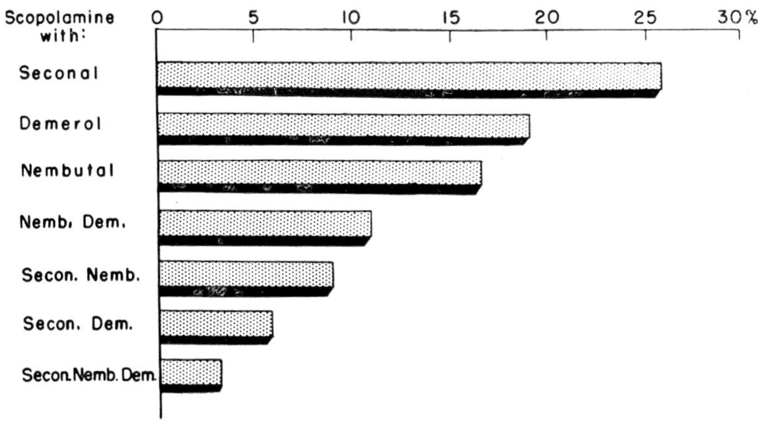

FIG. 84. Percentage of cases with *poor* evaluation by drug. (Baltimore Obstetric Anesthesia Study)

cent or above. These technics were used in complete accord with the pioneer studies of Eastman* which first showed that

If the concentration of oxygen is less than 15 to 20 per cent, anoxemia of the fetus results. Furthermore, prolonged use of this gas in higher concentrations may result in fatal maternal accidents as shown by Courville, Lowenberg and others.

The use of nitrous oxide–oxygen in a 90:10 mixture for 5 minutes reduces the oxygen saturation of the arterial blood of the fetus from 40 to 20 per cent and the oxygenation of the venous blood from 8 to approximately 2 per cent. Clinically, we became aware of the fact that the robust mother with normal hemoglobin in intense pain in the second stage of labor was unsubdued frequently to an adequate plane of anesthesia for delivery with mixtures of 80:20 nitrous oxide-oxygen even after 15-minute inductions. The patients themselves listed "oppressive dizziness," "frightful dreams" and "pain in subconsciousness" as major disadvantages of this agent.

* Eastman, Nicholson J.: Williams Obstetrics, ed. 11, New York, Appleton, 1956.

The addition of either analgesia or the substitution of ether anesthesia or the addition of Trilene analgesia to the mixture improves considerably the efficiency of nitrous oxide in patient acceptance in providing relaxation for difficult operative delivery. Yet the reactions of these mothers who reported 27 per cent unsatisfactory results with this agent should not be taken lightly, even though the procedure was safe. The words of Munroe Kerr and Chassar Moir* should be re-emphasized:

Of this may be said that it is no triumph of obstetric art to deliver a woman safely but to leave her mind so full of vivid and unhappy memories that she refuses to face childbed again.

Evaluation of Analgesic Drugs for Delivery

Scopolamine to produce amnesia was used widely in this study in average total doses of 1.5 mg. of scopolamine for each labor. Figure 83 and Table 18 present the efficiency of the various agents combined with scopolamine.

With Seconal alone there was a very high incidence, 26 per cent of those who

* Kerr, J. M. M., and Moir, J. C.: Operative Obstetrics, ed. 5, London, Baillière, Tindall & Cox, 1950.

TABLE 19. PERCENTAGE OF SPECIFIED DRUG GIVEN IN LABOR OR DELIVERY THAT IS EVALUATED UNSATISFACTORY BY MOTHERS* (HOPKINS AND SINAI)

Name of Drug Alone or Augmented	*Percentage*			*Number*†		
	Both Hospitals	Hopkins	Sinai	Both Hospitals	Hopkins	Sinai
Demerol	13.67	18.81	11.21	3,050	989	2,061
Metycaine	13.71	15.93	12.00	3,166	1,375	1,791
Seconal	13.97	18.43	10.38	2,734	1,221	1,513
Scopolamine	14.18	17.59	11.73	3,943	1,649	2,294
Nupercaine	16.06	21.25	13.57	741	240	501
Nembutal	17.54	19.82	14.77	2,012	1,105	907
Xylocaine	19.48	18.53	22.22	349	259	90
Pentothal sodium	19.58	20.33	12.50	669	605	64
Pontocaine	19.78	22.66	17.46	455	203	252
Nitrous oxide, ether	21.06	24.46	12.59	1,439	1,026	413
Nitrous oxide (no ether)	27.44	30.53	14.90	1,290	1,035	255

* Excludes mothers of twins.
† Excludes mothers with unknown or no evaluation.

became agitated with complete loss of frontal lobe control. This lack of good analgesia was reduced significantly by the substitution of Demerol or Nembutal, and reduced still further by the use of balanced analgesia with scopolamine for amnesia, Seconal or Nembutal for soporific effect, and Demerol for analgesia. The highest incidence of success was obtained with 100 mg. of Nembutal intravenously at the onset of active labor, 100 mg. of Seconal by mouth; 100 mg. of Demerol intramuscularly and 0.6 mg. of scopolamine intramuscularly with a repetition of 0.2 mg. of scopolamine each 2 hours. In this latter series the number with poor evaluation fell to 3 per cent. Of course, as the amount of analgesia and systemic narcosis increased, the more delayed became the breathing and crying time of the infants, as has been reported in other parts of this study.

The Parturient's Evaluation of Each Physician by Method of Pain Relief

As drugs and anesthetics vary in action in different patients, so do physicians in their personalities, patient acceptability and efficiency in the use of the various methods. Carl Gauss, who developed *Dämmerschlaf,* said in 1913: "Show me the average woman, and I will show you the average dose, but since there is no

TABLE 20. METHOD OF DELIVERY FOR MOTHERS BY PRIVATE PHYSICIAN (HOPKINS)

PHYSICIAN BY CODE NUMBER	TOTAL* MOTHERS	*Method of Delivery* NO DRUG	INHALATION	INTRAVENOUS	LOCAL	CAUDAL	SPINAL	PERIDURAL
Percentage								
Total	100	3.3	38.7	12.2	2.2	30.0	13.4	0.2
1	100	4.2	27.3	13.2	6.2	38.4	10.4	0.3
2	100	4.2	45.8	3.4	0.8	31.7	13.3	0.8
3	100	2.1	8.5	28.7	—	25.6	34.6	0.5
4	100	7.9	34.5	12.2	1.3	38.4	5.7	—
5	100	0.4	39.1	13.0	0.9	35.7	10.9	—
6	†							
7	†							
8	100	—	76.5	—	—	5.9	17.6	—
9	100	1.2	77.1	2.5	0.4	8.2	10.6	—
Number								
Total	1,418	47	549	173	31	425	190	3
1	385	16	105	51	24	148	40	1
2	120	5	55	4	1	38	16	1
3	188	4	16	54	—	48	65‡	1
4	229	18	79	28	3	88	13	—
5	230	1	90	30	2	82	25	—
6	1	—	1	—	—	—	—	—
7	3	—	1	—	—	—	2	—
8	17	—	13	—	—	1	3	—
9	245	3	189	6	1	20	26	—

* Excludes all cesarean sections.
† Less than 10 deliveries.
‡ One maternal death, thrombus and/or embolus.

TABLE 21. PSYCHOLOGICAL EVALUATION FOR EACH PHYSICIAN BY METHOD OF DELIVERY (HOPKINS)

METHOD OF DELIVERY	Percentage			Number	
	SATISFACTORY	UNSATISFACTORY	TOTAL* MOTHERS	SATISFACTORY	UNSATISFACTORY
Physician No. 1					
Total	85.6	14.4	360	308	52
No drugs	85.7	14.3	14	12	2
Inhalation	79.8	20.2	99	79	20
Intravenous	93.5	6.5	46	43	3
Local	95.0	5.0	20	19	1
Caudal	88.7	11.3	141	125	16
Spinal	76.9	23.1	39	30	9
Peridural	—	†	1	—	1
Physician No. 2					
Total	94.7	5.3	113	107	6
No drugs	†	—	5	5	—
Inhalation	94.3	5.7	53	50	3
Intravenous	†	†	4	3	1
Local	†	—	1	1	—
Caudal	94.3	5.7	35	33	2
Spinal	100.0	—	14	14	—
Peridural	†	—	1	1	—
Physician No. 3					
Total	91.1	8.9	168	153	15
No drugs	†	—	4	4	—
Inhalation	87.5	12.5	16	14	2
Intravenous	85.7	14.3	42	36	6
Local	95.7	4.3	46	44	2
Caudal	—	—	—		
Spinal	93.2	6.8	59	55	4
Peridural	—	†	1	—	1

* Excludes 28 cesarean sections for No. 1; 8 cesarean sections for No. 2; 20 cesarean sections for No. 3.

† Less than 10 deliveries.

average woman, there is no average dose." From the standpoint of safety and efficiency, we are convinced that the various drugs and methods are no more safe and efficient than the men who use them. There were 9 obstetricians on the private service in the Johns Hopkins Hospital. Each one of them was assigned a blind number on the IBM card so that the psychologist could interview and record the data from each private patient without knowing the name of the obstetrician. In this manner, another personal factor was eliminated. As can be seen by Table 19, there was wide variation in the individual physician's choice of agents and technics for his patients. One physician used inhalation agents in 77 per cent and intravenous agents in 2.5 per cent, while another physician used inhalation agents in 8.5 per cent, intravenous agents in 28.7 per cent and caudal in 25.6 per cent. The highest use of no drug during labor or delivery among all the obstetricians was 7.9 per cent, while all of them were encouraged to try the method occasionally.

Tables 20, 21 and 22 present the parturients' psychological grading of the methods of pain relief of each physician. The high rating of satisfactory results of better than 85 per cent in the averages

TABLE 22. PSYCHOLOGICAL EVALUATION FOR EACH PHYSICIAN BY METHOD OF DELIVERY (HOPKINS)

METHOD OF DELIVERY	*Percentage*			*Number*	
	SATISFACTORY	UNSATISFACTORY	TOTAL* MOTHERS	SATISFACTORY	UNSATISFACTORY
Physician No. 4					
Total	85.6	14.4	216	185	31
No drugs	94.1	5.9	17	16	1
Inhalation	82.4	17.6	74	61	13
Intravenous	75.0	25.0	24	18	6
Local	†	†	3	1	2
Caudal	90.8	9.2	87	79	8
Spinal	90.9	9.1	11	10	1
Peridural			—		
Physician No. 5					
Total	88.1	11.9	210	185	25
No drugs	†	—	1	1	—
Inhalation	82.7	17.3	81	67	14
Intravenous	88.5	11.5	26	23	3
Local	†	—	2	2	—
Caudal	93.8	6.2	80	75	5
Spinal	85.0	15.0	20	17	3
Peridural			—		
Physician No. 6					
Total	†	—	1	1	—
Inhalation	†	—	1	1	—
Physician No. 7					
Total	†	—	3	3	—
Inhalation	†	—	1	1	—
Spinal	†	—	2	2	—

* Excludes 11 cesarean sections for No. 4; 17 cesarean sections for No. 5.

† Less than 10 deliveries.

TABLE 23. PSYCHOLOGICAL EVALUATION FOR EACH PHYSICIAN BY METHOD OF DELIVERY (HOPKINS)

METHOD OF DELIVERY	Percentage			Number	
	SATIS-FACTORY	UNSATIS-FACTORY	TOTAL* MOTHERS	SATIS-FACTORY	UNSATIS-FACTORY
Physician No. 8					
Total	87.5	12.5	16	14	2
Inhalation	91.7	8.3	12	11	1
Caudal	—	†	1	—	1
Spinal	†	—	3	3	—
Physician No. 9					
Total	96.3	3.7	218	210	8
No drugs	†	—	2	2	—
Inhalation	95.9	4.1	169	162	7
Intravenous	†	—	6	6	—
Local	†	—	1	1	—
Caudal	94.4	5.6	18	17	1
Spinal	100.0	—	22	22	—
Peridural			—		

* Excludes 14 cesarean sections for No. 9.

† Less than 10 deliveries.

of all physicians, regardless of method used, points out the merit of the high type of competence in private practice in this hospital. Two physicians achieved the near-perfect score of better than 96 per cent satisfied patients in regard to their methods of pain relief. The lowest score of 75 per cent for a single technic was given the physician by 24 patients delivered by him under intravenous anesthesia. This same physician attained the highest rating with his 17 patients who used not a single milligram of narcotic or anesthetic drug during labor or delivery and whose method was recorded as satisfactory in 16 instances. More than 90 per cent of his patients delivered by caudal and spinal anesthesia were satisfied. This physician represents the type of personality who is at his best when his patients are awake and are a part of the thrilling events surrounding the delivery of the baby.

Summary and Conclusions

1. The parturients themselves should be given more opportunity to evaluate the efficiency of methods of analgesia during labor and delivery.

2. The majority of women in America, regardless of propaganda to the contrary, desire and require and deserve analgesia and anesthesia during labor and delivery. Certainly it is just as safe in most cases and safer in many to mother and baby to have the advantages of pain relief in childbirth in modern obstetrics.

3. Cognizant of the wishes of women who neither request nor require pharmacologic anesthesia or analgesia, obste-

tricians and anesthesiologists must understand psychoanalgesia also and carry it as far as is expedient without prejudice, yet always have close at hand the anesthesia so often required unexpectedly in obstetrics.

4. There is a hard core of parturients at present of 4 to 12 per cent in private practice and 12 to 25 per cent in ward practice as yet relieved or managed unsatisfactorily from their standpoint during labor and delivery. As new equipment and skills and technics are developed, this is the group requiring renewed efforts compatible with safety to make them comfortable.

5. It is evident from the reactions of the patients that more comfortable and pleasant environment, embodying air-conditioning in extremely hot weather, interior decorating, lighting and therapeutic music, is sometimes as important as doses of the narcotic.

6. The physician who administers the drugs and the anesthetics and manages parturition is just as important as the ratio of the recipe in the mind of the parturient.

»» 6 «« Control of Pain in Maternal and Fetal Complications

INTRODUCTION

The maternal complications chosen for discussion in this chapter are those which add materially to the hazards of pregnancy and delivery; they jeopardize both maternal life and fetal survival, and, in addition, present particular problems in anesthetic management.

These complications, as they occurred in the Baltimore study, are shown in the general summary tables 24 and 25. They are divided into 2 groups, according to whether the difficulty is medical or obstetric. Included along with the usual medical complications of heart disease, diabetes and tuberculosis is obesity. This includes women who weighed 200

TABLE 24. TOTAL LOSS AND INFANT MORTALITY ACCORDING TO MATURITY OF INFANTS AMONG MOTHERS WITH SPECIFIC COMPLICATIONS

Specific Complications	Total Fetal Loss	Premature* Total Loss	Premature* Stillbirths	Premature* Neonatal Deaths	Full Term Total Loss	Full Term Stillbirths	Full Term Neonatal Deaths
			Rate per 1,000 total births				
Heart disease	55.8	192.3	115.4	76.9	35.1	11.7	23.4
Diabetes	241.4	571.4	285.7	285.7	136.4	90.9	45.5
Tuberculosis	6.4	55.6	—	55.6	—	—	—
Obesity	46.4	315.8	263.2	52.6	17.1	—	17.1
Toxemia	51.3	204.8	120.5	84.3	19.8	13.6	6.2
Hemorrhagic conditions:	165.8	315.8	157.9	157.9	80.9	68.1	12.8
Placenta previa	133.3	200.0	—	200.0	85.7	85.7	—
Premature separation	321.7	500.0	340.0	160.0	184.7	138.5	46.2
Other antepartum hemorrhage	82.9	207.0	69.0	138.0	29.6	29.6	—
Breech	120.6	312.5	162.5	150.0	55.3	38.3	17.0
Cesarean section	92.5	250.0	72.9	177.1	42.7	16.4	26.3

Specific Complications	Total Infant Loss	Premature Total Births	Premature Stillbirths	Premature Neonatal Deaths	Full Term Total Births	Full Term Stillbirths	Full Term Neonatal Deaths
				Number†			
Heart disease	11	26	3	2	171	2	4
Diabetes	7	7	2	2	22	2	1
Tuberculosis	1	18	—	1	138	—	—
Obesity	9	19	5	1	175	—	3
Toxemia	50	166	20	14	808	11	5
Hemorrhagic conditions:	61	133	21	21	235	16	3
Placenta previa	8	25	—	5	35	3	—
Premature separation	37	50	17	8	65	9	3
Other antepartum hemorrhage	16	58	4	8	135	4	—
Breech	38	80	13	12	235	9	4
Cesarean section	37	96	7	17	304	5	8

* Mothers of twins are excluded.
† A premature infant weighs 1,000 to 2,499 Gm.

pounds or over at delivery. Although excessive weight is not commonly considered to be much of an obstetric complication, the figures here indicate that there is a materially increased fetal loss. This may have been due to an increase in the premature births, although it has been pointed out repeatedly in the past that these mothers were more prone to hypertension and to difficulties during labor. The obstacles to satisfactory anesthesia are well known. Not only do they include difficulties with inhalation anesthesia and the establishment of a good airway but, also, the anatomic approach is encumbered with formidable problems. Perhaps this is borne out in the general tables by the fact that obesity has the highest percentage of cases in which no anesthetic was given.

The purely obstetric complications include toxemia, hemorrhage, malposition, dystocia and cesarean section.

HEART DISEASE

In recent years heart disease has come to be the leading cause of maternal death in several obstetric centers of northeastern United States and in London. Rheumatic heart disease makes up from 90 to 95 per cent of all cardiac affections seen in pregnancy and probably an even larger proportion of the fatal cases. Historically, and still in nation-wide statistics, the leading causes of maternal death are sepsis, toxemia and hemorrhage. These have been brought under a large measure of control in areas where good prenatal care is available and generally sought and where most women are delivered in hospitals. Simultaneously, there has been a reduction in the death rate for pregnant women with heart disease, but it has not been so dramatic as the decrease in mortality from the "big three." While fewer women die of heart

TABLE 25. DISTRIBUTION OF MOTHERS WITH SPECIFIC COMPLICATIONS ACCORDING TO THE METHOD OF ADMINISTERING ANESTHESIA

Complications	Total	No Anesthesia	Intravenous	Inhalation	Caudal	Spinal	Local	Combination of Methods
				Per cent				
Heart disease	100.0	7.1	5.1	15.7	43.2	22.8	2.5	3.6
Diabetes	100.0	13.8	6.9	13.8	31.0	31.0	—	3.5
Tuberculosis	100.0	18.0	8.3	12.2	37.8	21.8	1.3	.6
Obesity	100.0	19.1	9.3	35.0	8.8	20.6	2.1	5.1
Toxemia	100.0	13.4	9.6	24.5	20.5	23.6	3.3	5.1
Hemorrhagic conditions	100.0	10.6	12.8	27.4	19.3	19.6	4.6	5.7
Breech	100.0	6.4	4.4	46.4	20.0	13.3	2.2	7.3
Cesarean section	100.0	—	10.8	3.0	13.5	50.2	—	22.5
				*Number**				
Heart disease	197	14	10	31	85	45	5	7
Diabetes	29	4	2	4	9	9	—	1
Tuberculosis	156	28	13	19	59	34	2	1
Obesity	194	37	18	68	17	40	4	10
Toxemia	974	130	93	239	200	230	32	50
Hemorrhagic conditions	368	39	47	101	71	72	17	21
Breech	315	20	14	146	63	42	7	23
Cesarean section	400	—	43	12	54	201	—	90

* Excludes mothers of twins.

disease in pregnancy, the relative position of this affection is changing in the lethal list.

As often happens, the maternal mortality in heart disease reflects a dichotomy between what can be done and what is done. Jensen's review of the literature* showed that prior to 1925 the maternal mortality for such women was about 10 per cent. It is interesting to note that this still is the level of mortality for neglected pregnant women with heart disease. The work of Burton E. Hamilton,† of the Boston Lying-in Hospital, was largely responsible for alerting clinicians to the seriousness of the problem and for showing that the great majority of such deaths were preventable.

* Jensen, J.: The Heart in Pregnancy, St. Louis, Mosby, 1938.

† Hamilton, B. E., and Thomson, K. J.: The Heart in Pregnancy and the Childbearing Age, Boston, Little, 1941.

According to the American Heart Association, it has been found useful in clinical care of patients to classify heart disease functionally:

Class 1. Patients with cardiac disease and *no limitation of activity.* Ordinary physical activity does not cause discomfort. Patients in this class do not have symptoms of cardiac insufficiency, nor do they experience anginal pain.

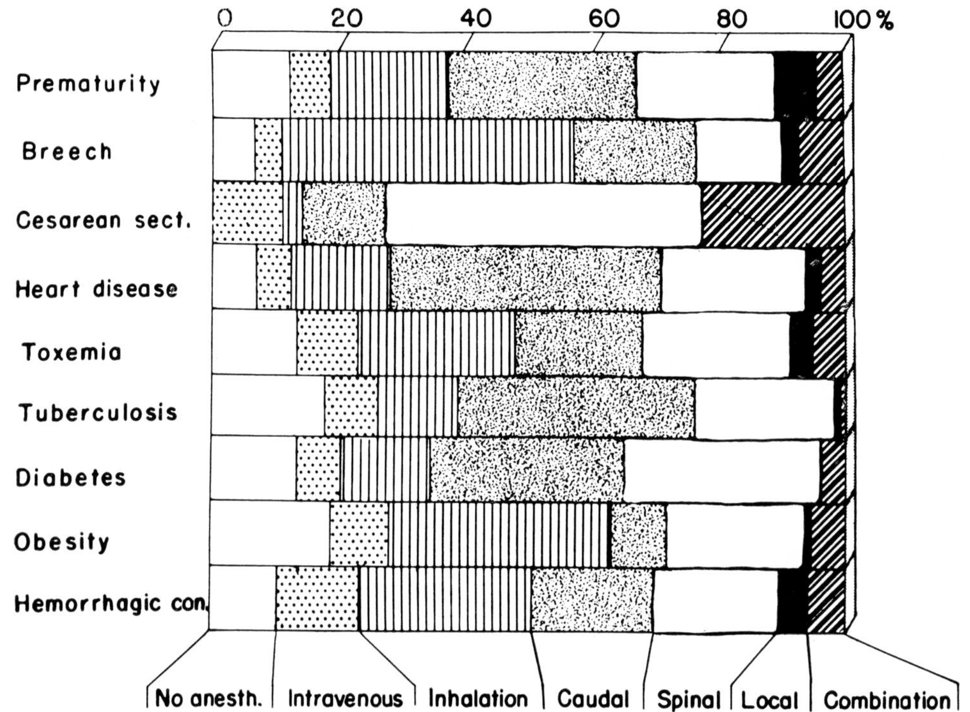

Fig. 85. Mothers with specific complications by method of administering anesthesia. Information is based on the Baltimore Obstetric Anesthesia Study.

Class 2. Patients with cardiac disease and *slight limitation of physical activity.* They are comfortable at rest. If ordinary physical activity is undertaken, discomfort results in the form of undue fatigue, palpitation, dyspnea or anginal pain.

Class 3. Patients with cardiac disease and *marked limitation of physical activity.* They are comfortable at rest. Discomfort in the form of undue fatigue, palpitation, dyspnea or anginal pain is caused by less than ordinary activity.

Class 4. Patients with cardiac disease who are *unable to carry on any physical activity without discomfort.* Symptoms of cardiac insufficiency or of anginal syndrome are present, even at rest.

Undeniably, pregnancy imposes a burden upon the heart. If the cardiac reserve is impaired significantly, congestive failure is very likely to occur in pregnancy unless preventive measures are taken. Although several investigators have tried to define quantitatively the magnitude of the burden imposed by pregnancy, the final answer still is unknown. Attempts to measure the cardiac output in pregnancy go back to the 1915 publication of Lindhard who, with Krogh, devised the first method for the estimation. Measurements with the nitrous oxide, the acetylene, the cardiac catheterization and the Hamilton dye methods all agree that the cardiac output is augmented during pregnancy. Nearly all published data are open to serious criticism. When the method has been adequate, almost no serial measurements have been made. The nitrous oxide and the acetylene methods were so conducted that some recirculation of blood had occurred, with the result that the calculated outputs were too low; this error possibly was magnified in pregnant women because of the accelerated circulatory rate. (Curiously, the acetylene method seems to have been validated in man by simultaneous measurements using arterial blood and mixed venous blood obtained by direct cardiac puncture.)

The results obtained at cardiac catheterization by Hamilton and by Palmer and Walker hardly can be accepted. They did not control the location of the catheter tip through which "mixed venous" blood was withdrawn. They probably used right auricular blood, which may or may not be fairly representative of mixed venous blood; in fact, there is suggestive evidence in their data that it sometimes was not mixed venous blood.

Werkö catheterized the pulmonary artery, and his work cannot be faulted, except that his patients were either in early or in late pregnancy. He found good agreement in simultaneous measurements with pulmonary artery catheterization and the Hamilton dye method. Using the latter method, he then made about 130 measurements in nearly 100 patients distributed throughout pregnancy. The average increase in cardiac output was about 16 per cent, and the maximum was attained in the first month of the second trimester. Thereafter the output decreased gradually.

Adams, using the Hamilton dye method, reports that the increase amounts to 32 per cent; the peak output was seen at the twenty-eighth week (in agreement with Hamilton), with a return to the nonpregnant level in the last weeks of pregnancy. Unfortunately, he gives very few data; the graph for cardiac output, plotted against the time of gestation, looks like the teeth of a crosscut saw, and the maximum increase might be based on one or a very few observations.

Rose, Bader, Bader and Braunwald studied 46 normal women distributed throughout pregnancy. By catheterization of the pulmonary artery, they found the peak output to be at the twenty-fifth to the twenty-seventh week. There was a rather rapid drop, almost to the nonpregnant level by the thirty-second week, and in the last month the output was at the nonpregnant level. At the peak, the mean output was 6.8 L. per minute, as compared with the nonpregnant mean of 4.9 (a rise of 39%).

In brief, the cardiac output increases during pregnancy. The increase occurs early, before an apparent metabolic need for it. It falls back toward or to the nonpregnant level in the last weeks of pregnancy, when one might think logically that the greatest need existed. Simultaneous measurements of cardiac output and oxygen consumption indicate that in early pregnancy the tissues do not extract the usual proportion of oxygen from the blood. In late pregnancy, the oxygen extraction increases, and this compensates for the falling cardiac output. The average increase in output, at its peak, has been estimated at from 16 to about 40 per cent.

The actual increment in work done by the heart in pregnancy undoubtedly falls short of the increase in output. The work is a function of 2 major factors: (1) the volume output and (2) the resistance against which the heart works. In pregnancy the blood viscosity is diminished by about 15 per cent, and the mean arterial pressure is decreased somewhat. Thus, the resistance to blood flow is lessened from the standpoint of cardiac work. This offsets in some degree the increase in output.

Nearly all investigations have been concerned with the cardiac output in healthy pregnant women, but Werkö has published a significant study of women with heart disease. He concludes that pregnant women in functional Classes 1 and 2 have essentially normal hemodynamics:

> The only difference between pregnant and nonpregnant patients with mitral valvular disease seems to be the slightly higher cardiac output and lower pulmonary vascular pressures in the pregnant patients.

In functional Class 3 (and 4) the situation is somewhat different. In nonpregnant patients the cardiac output varies inversely, more or less, with the degree of mitral stenosis and the height of the pulmonary vascular pressure. With the supervention of pregnancy, however, the cardiac output rises to normal, thus upsetting the balance between cardiac output and the vascular pressure in the lungs. This makes the pregnant woman with tight mitral stenosis especially susceptible to pulmonary edema, and explains in some measure the marked improvement resulting from the relaxation of the peripheral vascular resistance produced by major conduction anesthesia. The difficulty is that the pulmonary vascular pressure increases as a mechanical consequence of the stenosed valve, not because the myocardium is inadequate to carry the load of pregnancy; in fact, the myocardium functions too well, especially during tachycardia.

There are several other blood and hemodynamic changes in pregnancy that probably are of lesser importance. The red blood cell count and the hemoglobin typically decrease, the circulation rate is accelerated, and the blood volume is increased. The augmentation in blood volume is chiefly, but not entirely, in the plasma fraction. This increase begins in the first trimester and progresses steadily until the ninth lunar month, when the curve levels off or possibly falls somewhat. Some hours postpartum there is an acute rise in the blood volume and in the cardiac output. These changes may predispose to the cardiac failure or acute pulmonary edema observed clinically to be common at this time.

The diagnosis of rheumatic heart disease often is made for the first time when pregnant women seek prenatal care. For instance, at the New York Lying-in Hospital, one half of such women had no prior knowledge of their heart disease. In pregnancy, the diagnosis is sometimes difficult, for normal pregnancy has some features that mimic mitral valvular disease. There is a mild tachycardia. Edema of the lower extremities is common, and dyspnea and even orthopnea may be present. The rising diaphragm displaces the heart and often gives a distinct impression of cardiac enlargement by palpation, percussion or x-ray examination. In the x-ray picture the heart may have a mitral contour, and the barium-filled esophagus may be displaced. Then, too, a systolic murmur is very common in pregnancy. These signs, symptoms and x-ray findings in conjunction may lead to a false diagnosis of heart disease, and about 10 per cent of women so diagnosed in pregnancy prove, at follow-up examination, not to have heart disease. The majority of such mistakes are made when mitral insufficiency is thought to be the sole lesion. A history of rheumatic fever or its equivalent may be helpful, but such a history cannot be elicited from 30 to 50 per cent of women with rheumatic heart disease. Conversely, nearly half the women who do give such a history have no demonstrable heart disease.

The vast majority of pregnant women with rheumatic heart disease have mitral stenosis, occasionally in combination with aortic or other valvular lesions. The characteristic diastolic or presystolic murmur of mitral stenosis is not present invariably, but one should be reluctant to make the diagnosis of heart disease in its absence unless there are other strong indications of abnormality. Occasionally, the murmur cannot be heard outside a very small area over the valve, and then only after exercise and with the patient lying on her left side with the arm extended. The murmur can easily be missed, with fatal consequences.

Once the diagnosis is made, a strict enforcement of certain rules is necessary to prevent disaster. The principles of management are derived chiefly from the work of Hamilton and of Gorenberg.

1. Remembering that pregnancy increases the work load upon the heart, an effort is made to reduce other demands imposed by physical activity. Such patients should spend at least 8 or, better, 10 hours in bed every night and should lie down for an hour or two in the middle of the day. Strenuous activity should be avoided. Additional restrictions should be imposed between the twentieth and the thirty-fourth weeks when the cardiac output is highest.

2. Inasmuch as the older patients are more likely to decompensate in pregnancy, women aged 25 or older should be seen at weekly intervals.

3. If a patient has ever decompensated before, the burden of pregnancy is likely to cause failure again. Therefore, such patients should be hospitalized and kept at bed rest until after delivery.

4. The functional capacity of the heart is of paramount importance in the prognosis. Any patient in Class 3 or 4 (American Heart Association classification) prior to pregnancy should be hospitalized and kept at bed rest for the duration of the pregnancy.

5. At the least suspicion of decreasing cardiac reserve, the patient should be hospitalized for study. Experience has taught that upper respiratory infections are exceedingly dangerous. What is so diagnosed may be beginning cardiac failure, and, if it is not, the infection may precipitate decompensation. Any cough, nosebleed, hemoptysis and the like demand close investigation. If, in the hospital, the clinical course is that of a respiratory infection, and if the vital capacity, the circulation time and the venous pressure all are normal, the patient may be discharged after the infection has cleared.

6. Cesarean section is done for obstetric indications only. In the era when patients with heart disease were delivered by cesarean section, it was found that the maternal mortality was several times higher than in comparable cases delivered by vagina.

In addition to these 6 basic rules, there are a number of other working principles. The weight gain should be restricted; salt should be restricted; anemia should be prevented or treated promptly; any intercurrent disease should be prevented insofar as possible and treated actively if it occurs. Unfavorable complications include diabetes, hypertension, toxemia of pregnancy and, of course, auricular fibrillation.

The susceptibility to acute pulmonary edema can be countered in some degree. Any factor causing a sudden rise in the heart rate may precipitate this syndrome within a few minutes. Excitement and apprehension may prove fatal; therefore, the physician must establish good rapport with his patient and prepare her for what to expect in labor, delivery and other situations that may arise. One of the authors remembers a patient with mitral stenosis who went through pregnancy, labor and delivery uneventfully. In the puerperium her physician ordered a blood transfusion, but said nothing about it to the patient. The transfusion was started by the house officer with no explanation. To the patient, a blood transfusion seemed to be a dramatic, perhaps almost desperate lifesaving, measure and she became excited. Before receiving more than 20 cc. of blood she was in near-fatal acute pulmonary edema.

The principles of mangement outlined above, with local variations, have proved to be successful in a number of clinics. For instance, Gorenberg, at the Margaret Hague Maternity Hospital, has managed more than 600 Cardiac Clinic patients with only 2 deaths; in the same period the maternal mortality in private and nonregistered patients in the same hospital was far higher. No therapeutic abortions were done in this hospital. Fitzgerald and his co-workers, of the Cook County Hospital, report only 3 deaths in 460 Cardiac Clinic patients—all 3 deaths occurring after therapeutic abortion, which was done in 7 cases. In nonregistered patients the mortality was 9 per cent. Ullery, formerly of the Philadelphia Lying-in Hospital, reported 156 consecutive cases with 1 death. This death occurred in a nonregistered patient who was first seen in terminal cardiac failure. The most dramatic series was reported from the Dublin National Maternity Hospital, by Drury and his co-workers. In 220 consecutive "booked" cases there was not a single death, while the mortality in nonregistered cases was 20 per cent. These 220 women did not practice birth control, and they had been pregnant half their married lives. No therapeutic abortions, sterilizations or cesarean sections were done. Two thirds of the patients were aged 30 or more, 38 per cent were in Class 3 or 4, and 10 cases had auricular fibrillation. Obviously, there were many "unfavorable" cases in the series.

Therapeutic abortion for heart disease still is practiced widely. The indications given are history of decompensation, auricular fibrillation and low cardiac reserve (Class 3 or 4). Those who advocate therapeutic abortion in such cases advise that the operation be done by curettage, and that after the end of the first trimester it is safer to allow the pregnancy to continue than to do a hysterotomy. The experience of the Jersey City, the Chicago and the Dublin Clinics, recorded above, would seem to indicate that if the patient has been seen early enough to abort, she has been seen early enough to be given good prenatal care and carried through pregnancy successfully.

Finally, there is no evidence that pregnancy shortens the life expectancy, provided the patient survives the pregnancy. Indeed, further pregnancies, even with their hazards, do not increase the annual death rate.

TABLE 26. TOTAL LOSS AND INFANT MORTALITY FOR PREMATURE AND FULL-TERM INFANTS AMONG MOTHERS WITH HEART DISEASE ACCORDING TO METHODS OF ADMINISTERING ANESTHESIA

METHODS	Number*			Rate per 1,000 total births		
	TOTAL INFANTS	STILL-BIRTHS	NEONATAL DEATHS	TOTAL LOSS	STILL-BIRTHS	NEONATAL DEATHS
				Total Infants		
All methods	191	1	4	26.2	5.2	21.0
No anesthesia	12	1	—	83.3	83.3	—
Intravenous and inhalation	38	—	—	—	—	—
Caudal and spinal	129	—	4	31.0	—	31.0
Local	5	—	—	—	—	—
Combination of methods	7	—	—	—	—	—
				Prematures		
All methods	24	1	2	125.0	41.7	83.3
No anesthesia	2	1	—	—	—	—
Intravenous and inhalation	3	—	—	—	—	—
Caudal and spinal	17	—	2	117.6	—	117.6
Local	1	—	—	—	—	—
Combination of methods	1	—	—	—	—	—
				Full Term		
All methods	167	—	2	12.0	—	12.0
No anesthesia	10	—	—	—	—	—
Intravenous and inhalation	35	—	—	—	—	—
Caudal and spinal	112	—	2	17.9	—	17.9
Local	4	—	—	—	—	—
Combination of methods	6	—	—	—	—	—

* Twins, infants who died before onset of labor and analgesia and infants with congenital malformations incompatible with life, are excluded.

ANESTHESIA FOR ORGANIC HEART DISEASE

The diseased heart in obstetrics at the time of delivery presents certain problems over and above that presented during general surgery. Both labor and delivery produce additional strain upon the cardiac patient. It is interesting to note that of the cardiac obstetric patients who die, three quarters survive the immediate effects of labor and succumb in the puerperium. The factors of labor that add to the burden of the diseased heart are:

1. Emotional tension and fatigue from long hours of severe pain
2. Fear of what the next few hours will bring forth
3. Tachycardia resulting therefrom
4. Hypoxia attending actual decompensation or drug depression
5. Voluntary straining

Digitalis, oxygen and sedation in adequate doses are of primary importance in the management of prodromal and early labor. Table 26 presents the various anesthetic technics for the delivery of cardiac patients managed in the Baltimore study. In our opinion, conduction anesthesia with continuous caudal, continuous spinal or saddle block, which managed 129 of these cases, offered a very happy solution to many of the problems presented by the cardiac patient, since all survived. Under this form of management the patient is at ease and does not need her voluntary expulsive efforts. The rhythmic contractions of the uterus will expel the presenting part into the birth canal and usually will deliver it to the point of perineal bulging. From this point, outlet forceps and episiotomy will deliver the baby without adding to the already taxed circulatory system. Throughout labor and delivery the patients remain relaxed and keep up fluids, oxygen and nourishment. Through the mechanism of bloodless phlebotomy a distended right heart in mitral disease often is relieved of the taxing load of an overwhelming venous return. As a second choice, local anesthesia for delivery offers pharmacologic and toxicologic safety, provided there is adequate and satisfactory control of emotional stress. This can be established through a good "training for childbirth" program, which properly conditions the parturient in the understanding of the problems of labor and delivery. Since most women with serious heart disease are in the hospital weeks prior to delivery, the anesthesiologist should join the obstetrician in planning with the patient the management of labor and delivery. Certainly, one or more prelabor visits by the anesthesiologist to the patient are invaluable.

The contraindicated anesthesias in heart disease are those requiring hypoxic atmospheres or the use of those agents that depress ventilation through pharmacologic action.

DIABETES

Without hormonal supplementation diabetes and pregnancy are mutually incompatible. Prior to the advent of insulin in 1921, most diabetic women were sterile. So rarely did pregnancy complicate diabetes that Williams, in 1909, was able to collect only 65 cases from the entire literature of the world.

Occasionally, when diabetic women did become pregnant in the preinsulin era, some 25 per cent of the mothers

TABLE 27. CLASSIFICATION OF DIABETICS*

A	Glucose tolerance test diabetics
B	Onset over 20 years Duration less than 9 years Vascular disease: 0
C	Onset 10-19 years Duration 10-19 years Vascular disease: 0
D	Onset under 10 years Duration 20 years Vascular disease calcification in legs, retinitis
E	Patients with calcified pelvic vessels
F	Patients with nephritis

and 50 per cent of the infants died. The majority of these women died in acidosis and coma. Then, even as they are today, these factors were responsible for the loss of most of the infants. This disastrous consequence of the coexistence of pregnancy and diabetes is of much more than historical interest. It serves to bear out the mutual incompatibility of the two conditions that still operates today. No longer is sterility a factor, but we still see a high spontaneous abortion rate, a high premature rate and a perinatal loss rate of from 15 to 30 per cent.

The diagnosis of diabetes in the pregnant woman is not always easy. The presence of reducing substance in the urine may indicate lactosuria, lowered renal threshold or actual diabetes. Particularly in very mild cases, the fasting blood sugar may be normal. Postprandial blood and urine sugars may be of much more significance. The glucose tolerance test should be employed freely in pregnancy whenever sugar in the urine, obesity (180 lbs. +), a history of large infants, a history of stillbirths or congenital malformations and a family history of diabetes exist. Preferably, the

* Modified from Nelson *et al.*: Obst. & Gynec. 1:220, 1953.

test should be done during the last 2 trimesteis. It may be abnormal then but normal early in pregnancy and in the immediate puerperium. These slightly abnormal tests may not bespeak clinical diabetes, but they do indicate prediabetes and carry with them the same sort of fetal hazard, and, unless treated with careful dietary control, they foreshadow eventual frank clinical disease.

Some method of separating diabetics according to the duration and the severity of the disease is necessary, if only for comparison of results. Dr. Priscilla White has offered the classification shown in Table 27.

Such classification is not of great value in estimating the chances of infant survival as indicated in Figure 86. However, it does enable one clinic to compare its material with another and, as such, is of value until a better one is devised.

Success in the care of pregnant diabetics is in direct proportion to the meticulousness of prenatal care and the conscientiousness of the patient. The patients must be under rigid control. As pointed out by Pedowitz and Shlevin, keto-acidosis is the major factor in infant loss. If this can be prevented and early delivery obtained, the perinatal loss of viable infants will be less than 15 per cent. Of course, this is still 5 to 6 times the rate for nondiabetic mothers. White and her co-workers have been convinced that there is a steroid hormone imbalance in pregnant diabetics manifest by high urinary chorionic gonadotrophin and low estrogen and pregnanediol. They postulate that this situation can be improved by the administration of stilbestrol. While their basic work remains to be substantiated, there can be no question as to the excellence of their clinical results. However, the results without hormone therapy in many clinics are quite similar.

Hurwitz and Higano found a sudden upswing in culminative fetal deaths, from 38 per cent at 35 weeks to 81 per cent at 37 weeks. Most obstetricians now believe that diabetics are best delivered between the thirty-sixth and the thirty-seventh week. This may be by artificial induction of labor or by cesarean section. Of course, the rate for the latter will be high because of the high probability of unfavorable cervices at this time.

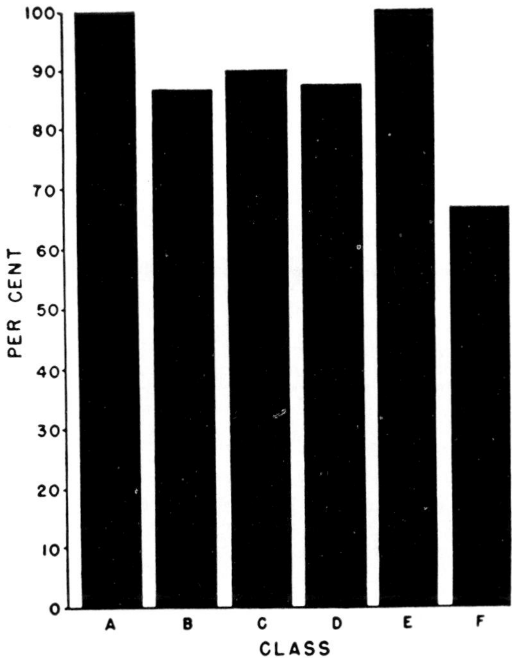

Fig. 86. Survival rate by class of the 128 viable pregnancies. (Nelson, Gillespie & White: Obst. & Gynec. 1:219-225)

Anesthesia for Diabetes

Table 25 presents our experience in the Baltimore study of the management of maternal diabetes from 1948 through 1951. Although 29 is a small number of cases, it is obvious that our choice for this condition is conduction anesthesia for the following reasons:

1. It does not alter the functional activity of the pancreas.

2. In both mother and baby the problem of acidosis is controlled more easily.

3. Many infants born of diabetic mothers are in poor condition and should be protected from the hazards of systemic narcosis. In a recent American Medical Association exhibit on the management of diabetes during labor, Joslin listed his choices of anesthesia as major vertebral conduction anesthesia and local anesthesia, and no other.

The administration of caudal anesthesia does not add the factor of narcosis to the already endangered baby. Our present policy in regard to delivery of these patients consists of vaginal delivery for those in whom labor can be induced and cesarean section from 2 to 3 weeks before term in those in whom induction presents difficulty. Spinal anesthesia has been our choice in this latter category.

TUBERCULOSIS

For some time now, phthisiologists and obstetricians have been convinced that pregnancy exerts no deleterious effect upon properly cared for pulmonary tuberculosis. Provided these patients can be kept under proper surveillance, there is no indication for therapeutic abortion. In a recent report based on 100 consecutive abortions for this disease, Schaeffer documents this nicely by showing that from 1932 to 1937, 23 per cent of the patients admitted to the New York Lying-in Hospital with tuberculosis were aborted, while from 1948 to 1951 this figure had fallen to 3.7 per cent. All these patients were treated with streptomycin, para-aminosalicylic acid and isoniazid in varying combinations, with good results in the control of the tuberculous lesions and no apparent un-

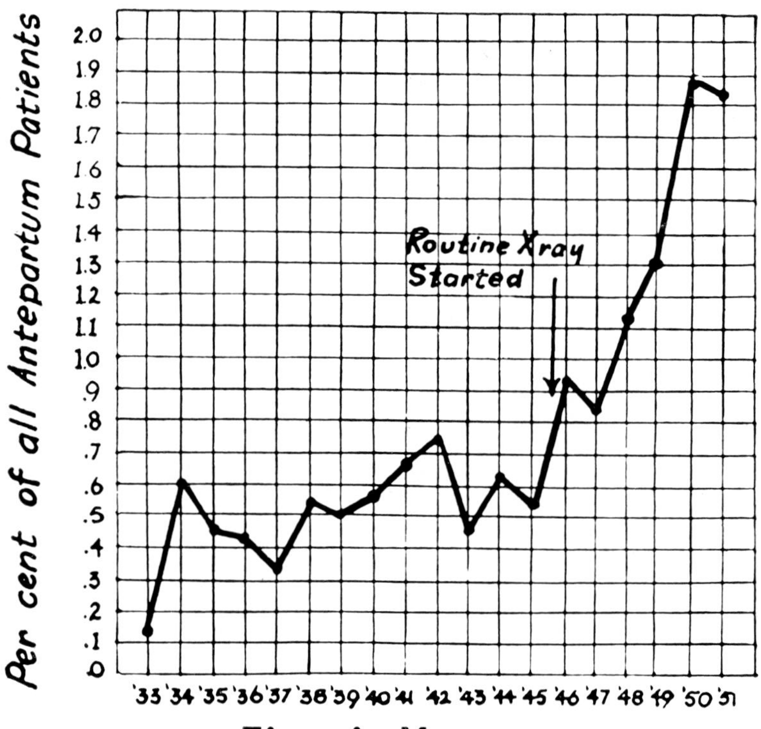

FIG. 87. Incidence of pulmonary tuberculosis at the New York Lying-in Hospital for the period 1933 to 1951. (Schaeffer, Douglas & Dreishpoon: Obst. & Gynec. 1:246)

TABLE 28. ANALGESIA IN TUBERCULOUS PATIENTS*

ANALGESIA	INACTIVE	ACTIVE
Meperidine and scopolamine	111	18
Morphine	93	15
Pentobarbital sodium, meperidine and scopolamine	50	7
No analgesia	46	6
Meperidine	32	6
Morphine and scopolamine	30	8
Pentobarbital sodium and meperidine	15	1
Pentobarbital sodium	12	0
Morphine plus another drug	39	3
Other drugs	11	3
TOTAL	439	67

* Schaefer, Douglas and Dreishpoon: Obstetric management of tuberculous patient, Obst. & Gynec. 1:248, 1953.

toward effect on their offspring. During the past 5 years, not a single patient at the Kings County Hospital has been aborted for tuberculosis. The same author has shown that equally good results can be obtained in pregnancy complicated by extrapulmonary tuberculosis. This appears to be valid with the exception of those rare cases of genital tuberculosis complicated by pregnancy. Studdiford has indicated that these do very poorly, and here perhaps there is an indication for artificial termination.

Case finding in the prenatal period is of great importance if good control of the disease is to be obtained. At the New York Lying-in Hospital there has been a threefold increase in the diagnosis of pulmonary tuberculosis concomitant with the initiation of routine chest roentgenograms for all prenatal patients. In this hospital the disease occurs twice as often as syphilis.

Delivery of patients with pulmonary tuberculosis presents few problems. Schaeffer and his colleagues believe that the encephalic approach to analgesia can be employed with safety, as indicated in Table 28. We have been somewhat averse to use routinely such drugs as morphine or Demerol in combination with scopolamine, and prefer in their place caudal analgesia and anesthesia (Table 29). While we have restricted the use of inhalation anesthesia, it is only proper to point out that Schaeffer has employed it with no untoward results in his very large experience.

Delivery should be as atraumatic as possible and labor not unduly prolonged. In this respect the indications for cesarean section in face of inertia should be liberal.

OBESITY

While obesity is not considered to be a major obstetric complication, it is associated often with complicating factors, such as hypertension, toxemia and certain other metabolic diseases. These add to both the maternal and the infant hazards. In addition, the babies of fat women are likely to be larger than nor-

TABLE 29. NUMBER OF PREMATURE AND FULL-TERM INFANTS AMONG MOTHERS WITH TUBERCULOSIS ACCORDING TO THE METHOD OF ADMINISTERING ANESTHESIA (BALTIMORE OBSTETRIC ANESTHESIA STUDY)

METHODS	TOTAL INFANTS*	PREMATURE†	FULL-TERM
All methods	156	18	138
No anesthesia	28	3	25
Intravenous	13	—	13
Inhalation	19	3	16
Caudal	59	8	51
Spinal[2]	34	4	30
Local	2	—	2
Combination of methods	1	—	1

* Twins, infants who died before onset of labor and analgesia and infants with congenital malformation incompatible with life, are excluded.

† One neonatal death among prematures delivered by spinal. No stillbirths.

TABLE 30. STILLBIRTH AND NEONATAL LOSS FOR PREMATURE AND FULL-TERM INFANTS AMONG OBESE MOTHERS ACCORDING TO METHODS OF ADMINISTERING DRUGS

Methods	Premature: Total Infants	Premature: Still-births	Premature: Neonatal Deaths	Full-Term: Total Infants	Full-Term: Still-births	Full-Term: Neonatal Deaths
			*Number**			
All methods	14	1	—	173	—	1
No anesthesia	5	—	—	27	—	—
Intravenous and inhalation	4	—	—	81	—	—
Caudal and spinal	3	1	—	53	—	1
Local	1	—	—	3	—	—
Combination of methods	1	—	—	9	—	—
			Rate per 1,000 total births			
All methods	71.7	71.4	—	5.8	—	5.8

* Twins, infants who died before onset of labor and analgesia and infants with congenital malformations incompatible with life, are excluded.

mal, or if premature are more apt to be stillborn. The incidence of inertia may be increased. In fact, every little complication that would go unnoticed in women of average weight becomes magnified in their obese sisters.

Table 30 shows the incidence of the various types of anesthesia administered to women weighing over 200 pounds in the Baltimore study. The high infant loss rate is due largely to an increase in the number of stillborn prematures. The difficulties in anesthesia are attested to by the large number of mothers receiving none.

Anesthesia in Obesity

In the fat patient, the hazard of anoxia from a partially blocked airway is increased. In such cases, the use of general anesthesia is an added risk. If operative delivery is anticipated, the anesthetist should be ready to use intratracheal anesthesia so that the patient's ventilation may be under constant control.

One of the arguments for spinal and caudal analgesia in these cases is that excessive dosage of the local anesthetic drugs is not required, whereas the quantity of general anesthesia used would be proportional to the body weight of the patient.

Obesity presents technical difficulties in any type of regional nerve block because of the physical obliteration of the topographic landmarks upon which the patient is dependent. Intravenous anesthesia definitely is contraindicated. Because of the reduced respiratory volume of the obese patient through the enlargement of the uterine tumor and the fatty collection in the adipose depots, the use of 100 per cent oxygen by inhalation during delivery is indicated in patients under regional nerve block.

Because of the large collection of fat throughout the body, the enormous quantities of general anesthetics required to produce equilibrium narcosis may produce a profound anesthesia of the fetus.

If general anesthesia is required, either cyclopropane or intravenous barbiturate-nitrous oxide with succinylcholine drip is preferred.

TOXEMIAS OF PREGNANCY

As now defined by the American Committee on Maternal Welfare:

Table 31. Toxemias of Pregnancy*

	Normal Non-pregnant Women	Normal Pregnancy: Maximal Change	Normal Pregnancy: Last Weeks of Pregnancy	Acute Toxemia Compared with Last Weeks of Normal Pregnancy
Plasma volume cc./Kg.	43.5	56	56	Decreased in severe cases
Red cell volume cc.	1,285	1,780	1,780	Decreased
Thiocyanate space cc./Kg.	230	310	300	Increased
Sodium space cc./Kg.	240	240	240	Increased
Total body water cc./Kg.	496	527	527	Increased
Capillary filtration cc./100 Gm., forearm/min.	0.111	—	0.160	Decreased
Cardiac output 1/min.	4.9	6.8	5.2	Increased (?)
Cerebral blood flow cc./100 Gm./min.	54	54	54	Normal
Liver blood flow cc./min.	1,550	1,620	1,420	Increased (?)
Skin (hand) blood flow cc./100, cc./min.	1	13	13	Increased
Forearm blood flow (musculoskeletal) cc./100, cc./min.	2	3.5	3.5	Increased (?)
Renal blood flow cc./min.†	940	1,360	960	Decreased
Glomerular filtration cc./min.	120	180	125	Decreased
Diodrast Tm mg./min.	42	—	46	Normal
Uterine blood flow				
cc./min.	—	—	600	Decreased
cc./100 Gm./min.	—	—	15	Decreased

* Eastman, N. J.: Williams Obstetrics, ed. 11, New York, Appleton, 1956.
† Corrected to body surface area of 1.73 sq. M.

Toxemia of pregnancy comprises some of the disorders encountered during gestation, or the early puerperium, which are characterized by one or more of the following signs: hypertension, edema, albuminuria, and in severe cases, convulsions and coma.

One disease not related specifically to pregnancy is included, namely, essential hypertension. Forms of renal disease, such as nephritis, and general metabolic disturbances, such as pernicious vomiting, or infectious processes, such as hepatitis, are not included. The classification is as follows:

1. Acute toxemia of pregnancy (onset after the twenty-fourth week): (A) pre-eclampsia—(a) mild, (b) severe; (B) eclampsia (convulsions or coma, usually both, when associated with hypertension, proteinuria or edema).

2. Chronic hypertensive (vascular) disease with pregnancy: (A) without superimposed acute toxemia (no exacerbation of hypertension or development of proteinuria)—(a) hypertension known to have antedated pregnancy, (b) hypertension discovered in pregnancy (before twenty-fourth week and with postpartum persistence); (B) with superimposed acute toxemia.

3. Unclassified toxemia (data insufficient to differentiate the diagnosis)

The criteria for diagnosing toxemia are:

1. **Hypertension.** Systolic pressure of 140 mm. Hg or more, or diastolic pressure of 90 or more, or an increase in the systolic pressure of 30 mm. or more, or an increase in the diastolic of 15 or more. These readings must be observed on at least 2 occasions at least 6 hours

apart. The specified increases in hypertensive patients make the diagnosis of superimposed acute toxemia.

2. **Edema.** The diagnosis of toxemia on the basis of edema alone can be made only when there is edema of the hands or the face, present in the morning and clinically evident.

3. **Proteinuria.** The diagnosis of toxemia on the basis of proteinuria can be made when clean or catheterized urines, on 2 or more successive days, show an unequivocal cloud of protein precipitated by any recognized test, or the excretion of 0.5 Gm. or more of protein per 24 hours, for at least 2 consecutive days.

Preeclampsia is classified as "severe" if any one of the following signs and symptoms is present. If none is present, the preeclampsia is classified as "mild":

1. Blood pressure of 160 or more systolic, or 110 or more diastolic, on at least 2 occasions 6 hours or more apart, with the patient at bed rest.
2. Proteinuria of 5 Gm. or more in 24 hours (3 or 4 plus on qualitative examination).
3. Oliguria (400 cc. or less per 24 hours).
4. Cerebral or visual disturbances.
5. Pulmonary edema or cyanosis.

The superimposition of acute toxemia upon hypertensive disease is diagnosed if the systolic pressure increases by 30 mm. or more, or if the diastolic pressure increases by 15 mm. or more, or if a significant degree of proteinuria appears.

Unfortunately, there is no stipulation as to what base line is to be used in determining the increase in blood pressure. About one third of women who begin pregnancy with hypertension show significant drops in the blood pressure throughout most of pregnancy. As they approach term, the blood pressure rises characteristically, often to about the prepregnant level. If the usual level in pregnancy is taken as the base line, many such patients may be classified as having superimposed preeclampsia, probably erroneously.

Another troublesome aspect posed by the hypertensive woman's behavior in pregnancy is that an appreciable proportion of them have drops of blood pressure into the normal range during most of the gestational period. Prepregnancy blood pressures seldom are known, and, when such a hypertensive patient shows the typical rise in blood pressure late in pregnancy, after a series of normal readings, she is likely to be misclassified as having preeclampsia.

The classification necessarily is arbitrary. Very occasionally preeclampsia appears before the twenty-fourth week, and hypertensive disease may first become manifest after the twenty-fourth week. Recurrent toxemia may be an entity, or it may be preeclampsia, or it may be a sign of vascular disease. Many believe that hypertensive disease predisposes to preeclampsia, but Dieckmann thinks that the syndrome represents an exacerbation of the hypertensive disease and is not preeclampsia. Finally, there are those who believe that all these subgroups are merely the spectrum of hypertensive disease as colored by pregnancy.

The toxemias of pregnancy are of common occurrence; they are seen in approximately 7 per cent of all gravidas. Together with infection and hemorrhage, they constitute the great triad of diseases responsible for the majority of maternal deaths. Between 20 and 25 per cent of the maternal mortalities occurring in the United States each year are accounted for by the toxemias. In addition, Chesley has presented evidence that, at least in the group designated as hypertension with superimposed toxemia, there is an increase in the remote death rate. As a cause of fetal wastage, the toxemias assume even greater importance. Conservatively, at least 30,000 stillbirths and neonatal deaths are attributable to this cause.

The discussion of classification is of some importance because the prognosis of both mother and child differs with the various categories; it is not only an attempt to limit the conditions under consideration. As has been indicated, the life expectancy of women with toxemias superimposed upon already pre-existing hypertension is decreased. In addition, not only is the infant mortality increased in all forms of toxemia, but it is influenced considerably more by some forms than others, as in Table 32.

TABLE 32. PERINATAL MORTALITY IN TOXEMIA (KINGS COUNTY HOSPITAL)*

	Number of Patients	*Per cent Perinatal Mortality*
Preeclampsia	586	5.97
Chronic hypertension	101	4.95
Chronic hypertension with superimposed preeclampsia	132	19.70
*Total perinatal mortality: 1,000 Gm. and over	819	7.94

It is fruitless in a text of this type to attempt a detailed discussion of the toxemias of pregnancy. Those who wish to pursue the subject are referred to the following publications:

Smith, G. V., and Smith, O. W.: Internal secretions and toxemia of late pregnancy, Physiol. Rev. **28**:1, 1948.

Chesley, L. C.: Kidney function in the normal and toxemic pregnant woman, M. Clin. North America **35**:699, 1951.

Chesley, L. C.: Weight changes and water balance in normal and toxic pregnancy, Am. J. Obst. & Gynec. **48**:565, 1944.

Dieckmann, W. J.: *The Toxemias of Pregnancy,* ed. 2, St. Louis, Mosby, 1952, and, finally, the superbly concise and comprehensive monograph:

Page, E. W.: *The Hypertensive Disorders of Pregnancy,* Springfield, Ill., Thomas, 1953.

By and large, the prophylactic treatment of the toxemias involves the obstetrician rather than the anesthetist. It is he who must decide whether pregnancy is to continue in the face of pre-existing hypertension. During the prenatal period he must be on the alert for the very first sign of preeclampsia, he must watch for sudden weight gain or other prodromata, and institute proper treatment. He must be ready to admit the patient to the hospital when necessary and determine the proper treatment and the optimum time of delivery. Often, it is in this latter stage that the anesthesiologist is called upon to play a role. Because of the multiple drugs used and the altered mechanisms in physiology of the toxemic woman, he must have some basic understanding of the processes involved.

Toxemia is one of the most protean of diseases and the most puzzling. In spite of much high caliber research directed at this problem, almost all of what we know today awaits reinterpretation tomorrow. In spite of the rather rigid criteria listed above, undoubted instances of toxemia are seen that are so at variance as to be hardly recognizable. In all probability, morphologic changes thought to be pathognomonic of this syndrome are largely the result of rather profound illness and not the basic causative factors. No doubt this is true of the specific pathologic changes in the liver and the kidney, as well as certain alterations in the chemical content of the blood.

Although many competent observers are of opinion that preeclampsia and essential hypertension are closely related, not only as to basic etiology, but also as to temporal occurrence — one being merely an acute and possibly premature manifestation of the other — the most thoughtful opinion available today would seem to indicate that such is not the case. Preeclampsia and essential hypertension are two different diseases. The problem has been to obtain means of differentiating one from the other by specific tests. In general, the author of each test has been able to differentiate the "hypertensions of pregnancy" into dissimilar syndromes and to have his results corroborated by other investigators. By and large, such tests have been used singly, although Govan and his coworkers have employed three in conjunction. If a battery of such tests pointed consistently to a single diagnosis, perhaps we could be more sure that we were dealing with different disease entities. On the other hand, if a patient were preeclamptic by one and hypertensive by the other, we might suspect "toxemia" to be a single disease with varying manifestations. Of course, one of the major stumbling blocks has been the wide variations in criteria used in the classification of toxemia. The first table in Dieckmann's book compares the relative frequencies of the subgroups of toxemia in 8 large hospitals: of all toxemias, preeclampsia makes up anywhere from 39 per cent in one hospital to 90 per cent in another.

Briefly, the following tests have been employed to differentiate preeclampsia from chronic hypertension:

Pitressin Test. Dieckmann and others found that patients with preeclampsia were extremely sensitive to Pitressin and Pituitrin. In normal pregnant women, a dose of Pitressin gives a negligible change in blood pressure. It also has no significant effect on patients having hypertensive disease. A similar dose given to patients with preeclampsia results in a marked rise in blood pressure, a decrease in urine volume output and subjective reactions.

Cold Pressor Test. Most of the studies made with the cold pressor tests in pregnancy were concerned with the prediction of the later development of toxemia. Opinion is divided as to its prognostic accuracy. Some observers have found that if the patient's hand or arm were immersed in iced water for a specific period of time, patients with chronic hypertensive disease would respond with an abnormal elevation in blood pressure, while those with preeclampsia would not. The results in this respect have not been conclusive either.

Tetraethyl Ammonium Chloride Test. Assali and his co-workers have found that normal pregnant women respond to intravenous TEAC with marked drops in blood pressure. Pregnant women with hypertensive disease also show considerable drops in blood pressure. In contrast, patients with preeclampsia show negligible decreases. Assali also claimed that the effect of high selective spinal anesthesia was similar to tetraethyl ammonium chloride and made the same differentiation among normal pregnancy, preeclampsia and hypertensive disease. Although in general the results of these tests have been in agreement with Assali's findings, in our hands they have not shown the consistency one would desire.

Sodium Tolerance Test. Dieckmann and his co-workers have made extensive studies of salt tolerance in normal pregnant and toxemic women, giving as much as 36 Gm. of salt a day for many consecutive days. They have proposed as a diagnostic test the rapid infusion of 1 L. of 2½ per cent sodium chloride. The bladder is emptied 15 minutes after the end of the infusion and two 1-hour urines then are collected and analyzed for sodium (or chloride). In normal pregnancy, they found a mean urinary sodium concentration of 240 mEq./L. ($\sigma = 40$). In 28 pregnant women with hypertensive disease, the mean was 196 ($\sigma = 52$), and in 20 women with preeclampsia, the mean was 101 with a standard deviation of 65 mEq./L. They set the urinary sodium concentration to be used in differential diagnosis as less than 144 mEq./L. for preeclampsia, 144 to 220 for hypertensive disease and over 220 for normal pregnancy. About 20 per cent of "mild" preeclamptics are not affected adversely as judged by blood-pressure response and degree of proteinuria, and they are able to concentrate sodium above 144. These are called pseudopreeclamptics by Dieckmann. The other 80 per cent of preeclamptics often react with increased proteinuria, aggravated hypertension, progression of edema and appearance of various symptoms.

However, it would seem that preeclampsia-eclampsia is a different disease entity from essential hypertension. The various tests listed above lack specificity, probably because they measure the effects of the disease and these effects vary widely from patient to patient.

Of particular interest to the anesthesiologist should be the effects of toxemia upon the vascular system, upon water metabolism, upon the central nervous system and upon certain elements in the blood.

A popular concept of preeclampsia-eclampsia is that, basically, it is a vascular phenomenon. This suggestion was made by Volhard many years ago, and it was popularized in this country by Irving. Hertig considered that vascular spasm led to a precapillary arteriolitis and was responsible for many of the pathologic changes seen in the liver and the kidney in the final stages of the disease.

Numerous observers, including Hallum and Landesman, have described retinal and bulbar arteriolar spasm in toxemia. It is altogether probable that the hypertension that exists in preeclampsia is caused by such vascular spasm. However, the question can be raised as to whether the vascular spasm is the fundamental causative agent of the disease or whether it is the result of some other factor. Before accepting vascular constriction as fundamental in the toxemic picture, one has to determine whether or not it precedes all other signs and whether or not, by compromising circulation, it impairs organ and tissue function. If the latter can be proved, at least on a theoretical ground, certain changes in kidney and placental function could be explained. However, at the present time, evidence is lacking that the function of these specific organs is influenced materially by a decrease in blood flow.

An equally important aspect of preeclampsia-eclampsia is the abnormality in water metabolism and distribution. This not only involves abnormal metabolism of water but electrolytes and probably hormones as well. Somewhat similar deviation in water metabolism occurs in normal pregnancy and possibly in some premenstrual women. Whether the situation in preeclampsia really represents a marked exacerbation of this phenomenon or is an entirely new situation is not known.

The problem of water retention may be approached in several ways. Rapid weight gain, representing edema, has been accepted almost universally as a precursor of preeclampsia. Some question has been raised by Siddall and Mack, who showed that 45 per cent of their nontoxic gravidae gained twice or more the average weight gain sometime during the last trimester of their pregnancies.

Another approach to the problem is the investigation of the compartmentation of fluid. Chesley, thinking erroneously that he was measuring the extracellular fluid, determined that the thiocyanate space was increased prior to the development of preeclampsia in many patients. This observation has been confirmed by Freis and Kenney. Although it is known now that the thiocyanate does not measure the extracellular fluid, it does approximate a measurement of the sodium space, which may be of greater importance in preeclampsia.

The third possible approach to this aspect of the problem is that of kidney function. Oliguria always accompanies severe preeclampsia, although probably it is not present in the milder forms of the disease. The urine of preeclamptic women long has been known to be low in sodium. However, Assali found that under osmotic diuresis the kidneys handled sodium normally, and, although such diuresis constitutes an abnormal situation, probably there is no basic defect in the preeclamptic's renal handling of sodium. The role of the kidney still has to be assessed. Normally, sodium excretion appears to depend on a balance between glomerular filtration and tubular reabsorption. In normal pregnancy there must be a substantial readjustment of the glomerulotubular balance, for glomerular filtration is increased by 50 to 100 per cent. In contrast with the filtration rates prevailing throughout normal pregnancy, nearly every preeclamptic has a depression of glomerular filtration amounting to almost 30 per cent. Unless there is an accompanying reduction in tubular reabsorption, there must be sodium retention. However, it has not been shown that the glomerular filtration rate falls at the incipience of acute toxemia.

As has been mentioned before, the evidence is good that there is a retention of sodium in preeclampsia. Salt-retaining steroids have been found in the urine of toxemic patients. However, the isolation of the particular steroid involved has not been accomplished, nor has there been found a correlation between the severity of "symptoms" and salt-retaining activity.

Of some interest is the hemoconcentration which has been emphasized by Dieckmann. Usually this is a characteristic of severe preeclampsia and eclampsia. Not only is there severe hemoconcentration but there are abrupt changes in its degree. Furthermore, from our own observations it would seem that the hemoconcentration becomes alleviated prior to remission of other signs and symptoms of the disease. The hemoconcentration probably is related to abrupt changes in plasma volume. These, however, are unexplained, but speculatively they may be related to ferritin. Shorr and Zweifach have found marked increase in both VEM and VDM in toxemia.

Very frequently, neither preeclampsia nor eclampsia is accompanied by any significant degree of nitrogenous retention, but in eclampsia there is an increasing uric acid concentration of the blood that is observed almost universally. Chesley has shown that this probably is related to a decrease in urate clearance.

The CO_2 combining power of the blood usually is unchanged in preeclampsia. However, in eclampsia it is not uncommon to see values below 30 vols. per cent. In 1929, Stander, Eastman, Harrison and Cadden demonstrated that the period immediately following an eclamptic convulsion was associated with a true acidosis, due to an uncompensated alkali deficit. They concluded that usually the eclamptic patient overcame the true acidosis by means of lowering the carbonic acid through deepened breathing. These authors concluded from their previous work on lactic and other organic acids in the blood that it was probable that the period of acidosis resulted from accumulations of these acids following muscular work incident to the convulsions.

Following the report of Rosenbaum and Maltby, who indicated that 65 per cent of posteclamptic women had abnormal electroencephalograms, there was a great deal of interest in this aspect of the disease. It was suggested that preeclamptic women who went on to convulsions might have a constitutional predisposition that would be manifest in the electroencephalogram. This has not been borne out by subsequent studies. Furthermore, no significant alteration in cerebral blood flow in preeclampsia has been found (McCall).

Treatment of the toxemias is directed essentially at combating signs and symptoms because the basic etiology of the disease is unknown. However, certain concepts are accepted as axiomatic in our present-day thinking. These concern the prophylactic approach, directed at prevention of the disease or, at least, the prevention of convulsions. However, it should be understood that although prophylactic treatment usually is efficacious, in some instances the disease proceeds willy-nilly to convulsions in spite of the best efforts of the physician to control blood pressure by sedation and the relaxation of vasospasm and the attempted correction of water and electrolyte imbalance by bed rest and adequate and appropriate fluid intake. Finally, the obstetric handling of these cases essentially is conservative. This does not mean that the obstetrician lets nature take its course, but it does mean that he does not intervene actively to terminate labor during periods of acute illness of the patient, such as during the period of convulsions in eclampsia. However, even in mild preeclampsia he should seek to terminate labor at the optimum time compatible with the safety of mother and child. Termination of pregnancy would seem wise should the cervix be favorable and the head in the pelvis. As the severity of the symptoms increases, a more radical approach to the termination of pregnancy is advantageous to both mother and child. It is well to remember, although we do not mean in any sense to preach therapeutic nihilism, that, like so many other diseases, both eclampsia and preeclampsia show a tendency toward spontaneous amelioration with the simplest types of therapy.

Prophylactic (Prenatal Care)

1. A schedule of prenatal care that increases the frequency of visits until patients are seen once a week in the last month or two of pregnancy
2. Observation of blood pressure, urine and weight at each visit
3. Limitation of salt intake after midpregnancy
4. The control of sudden weight gain by adequate dietary adjustment or even hospital admission — hospital admission when signs or symptoms of toxemia are present

Mild Preeclampsia

1. Hospitalization with bed rest
2. Measurement of intake and output
3. Fluid intake approximately 3,000 cc. a day
4. Salt-poor diet
5. Delivery when indicated and compatible with infant survival; rarely by the abdominal route

   A. Analgesia choice for labor: (a) anatomic approach: caudal or peridural last half of labor; (b) encephalic approach: barbiturate with Demerol sedation without scopolamine

   B. Anesthesia choice for delivery: (a) conduction anesthesia; (b) intravenous; (c) inhalation: ether

   C. Postpartum sedation with Demerol, barbiturates or both advisable

Severe Preeclampsia

Treatment as above, but if reflexes are hyperactive, or in the presence of symptoms of impending eclampsia, magnesium sulfate 50 per cent may be given as follows: 5 Gm. in each buttock and

5 Gm. every 4 hours, the precautions cited below being observed. Other anticonvulsant agents listed below may prove equally satisfactory.

In preeclampsia a foremost consideration is the question of when and how to deliver the patient. If a sterile vaginal examination gives evidence that the cervix is favorable for induction of labor, this obviously is the method least harmful to the patient and her child. However, in the event of an unfavorable cervix, rupture of the membranes may yield unfortunate results. Should the induction of labor be desirable, it can be accomplished by simple rupture of membranes or by the administration of dilute intravenous Pitocin (see uterine inertia) or both. Apparently, in many instances an unfavorable cervix can be converted to a favorable one by a daily course of intravenous Pitocin. There appears to be a crystallization of thought in the leading centers in this country that temporizing in the face of severe preeclampsia is unjustified. In summarizing the management of preeclampsia at the Margaret Hague Hospital, Cosgrove and Chesley state:

> Progressively severe pregnancy toxemias, whether grafted on pre-existing hypertensions or not must not be temporized with. Ruthlessly radical termination of pregnancy serves alike the interest of mother and fetus; the convulsive toxemias should be treated wholly along conservative medical lines without artificial interference with the pregnancy; recovered convulsive toxemia should have pregnancy terminated exactly as in severe progressive non-convulsive type.

In the eleventh edition of Williams' *Textbook of Obstetrics,* Eastman writes:

> If severe preeclampsia . . . does not improve with medicinal therapy after one or two days, termination of pregnancy is usually advisable from the viewpoint both of the mother and the infant. If the cervix is favorable for induction, rupture of membranes should be carried out but if it is not favorable, cesarean section is the procedure of choice.

Anesthesia for Abdominal Delivery. CONDUCTION. (1) Continuous spinal; (2) spinal; (3) epidural: lumbar or caudal.

Eclampsia

1. Absolute rest in bed with a minimum of disturbing procedures
2. Constant nursing attendance
3. Side rails on bed
4. Blood pressure taken hourly, cuff being left on arm
5. If patient is comatose, tongue blade between teeth for protection of tongue and bulb at hand for aspirating mucus from throat; tracheotomy equipment at hand if ineffective suctioning permits accumulation of mucus
6. Nothing by mouth during the acute stage
7. Oxygen administration at least 10 minutes after convulsions
8. Insertion of indwelling catheter and measurement of urinary output
9. Determination of 24-hour output of urinary protein
10. Limitation of intake of sodium chloride to 1 Gm. daily
11. Limitation of fluid intake to 1,500 cc. for the first 24 hours and then 1,500 cc. plus the amount of urinary output for the previous day. In calculating the intake, all parenteral fluid except blood and plasma included.
12. From 500 to 1,000 cc. of 5 per cent dextrose and water begun intravenously, the solution being allowed to drip slowly.

The anticonvulsant agent may be given in this tubing.

Anticonvulsant Agents and Their Use

A moderate degree of general sedation is desired usually. One of the following methods may be selected:

Sodium Amytal 0.3 Gm. intramuscularly every 8 hours as needed

Pentobarbital sodium 0.1 Gm. orally every 4 to 6 hours

Paraldehyde 20 cc. in 30 cc. of oil given rectally every 8 hours

Magnesium sulfate 6 to 8 Gm. to 1,000 cc. of 5 per cent dextrose given at the rate of 60 drops a minute

Magnesium sulfate 10 Gm. (50% solution) in ½ per cent procaine 5 Gm. in each buttock and 5 Gm. repeated in 4 to 6 hours. Magnesium sulfate is excreted by the kidneys. In cases of oliguria the dosage should be regulated with care. Fortunately, the deep reflexes disappear at a blood level of approximately 10 mg. per cent. Respiratory depression occurs at a slightly higher concentration, so that some warning is given.

Veratrum viride (Veratrone) 0.2 cc. intravenously, followed in 1 hour by an intravenous infusion of 5 per cent dex-

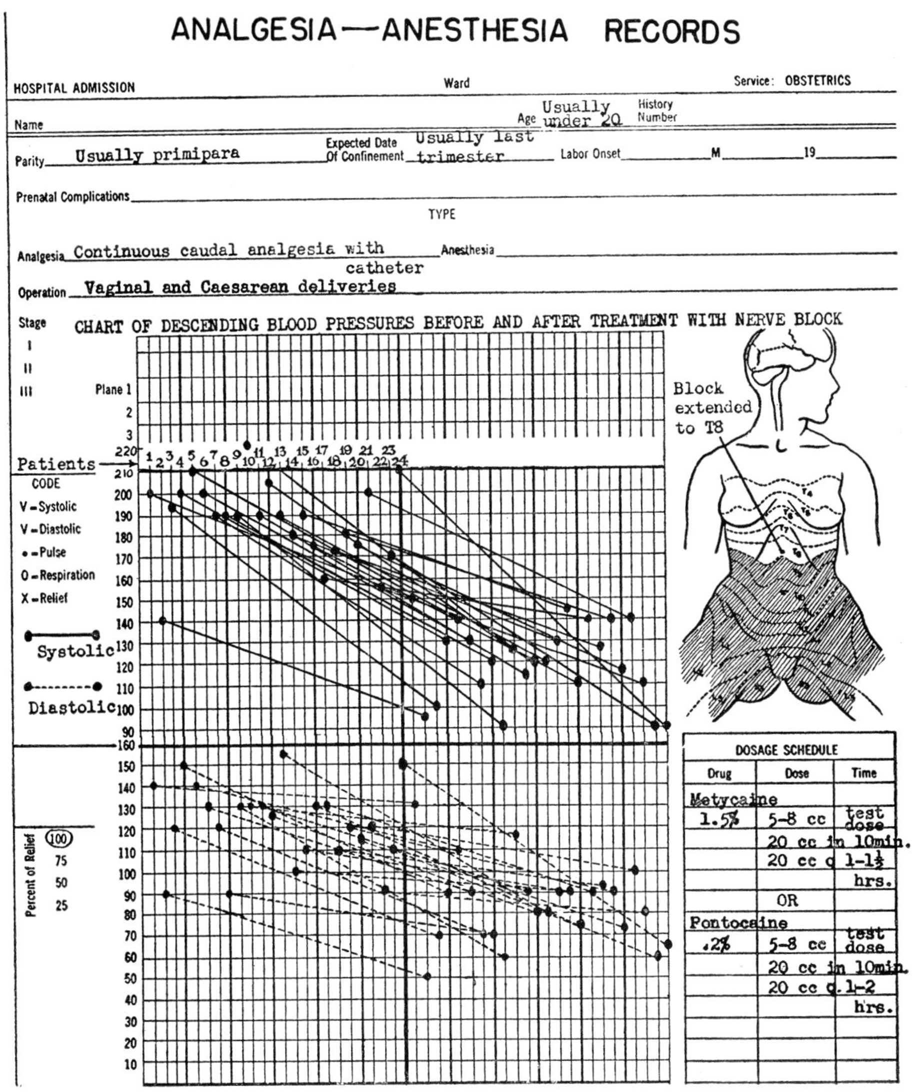

FIG. 88. The effect of continuous caudal on the blood pressure in acute toxemia.

trose, a sufficient amount of Veratrone being added so that the patient receives 0.2 cc. per hour

Apresoline 15 to 40 mg. (average dose 20 mg.) intravenously, repeated as often as necessary to maintain lowered blood pressure

Although the Cincinnati group has published splendid results with the use of Veratrum viride in combination with magnesium sulfate we have seen convulsions continue in spite of the lowering of blood pressure with Veratrum viride and with Apresoline. In addition, several recent reports have indicated that Apresoline may cause kidney tubular damage, and in some instances after prolonged use it may be responsible for lupuslike lesions. Also, we have seen convulsions occur with blood magnesium levels in excess of 7 mg. per cent.

In view of these observations it may be necessary to use the anticonvulsant agents synergistically.

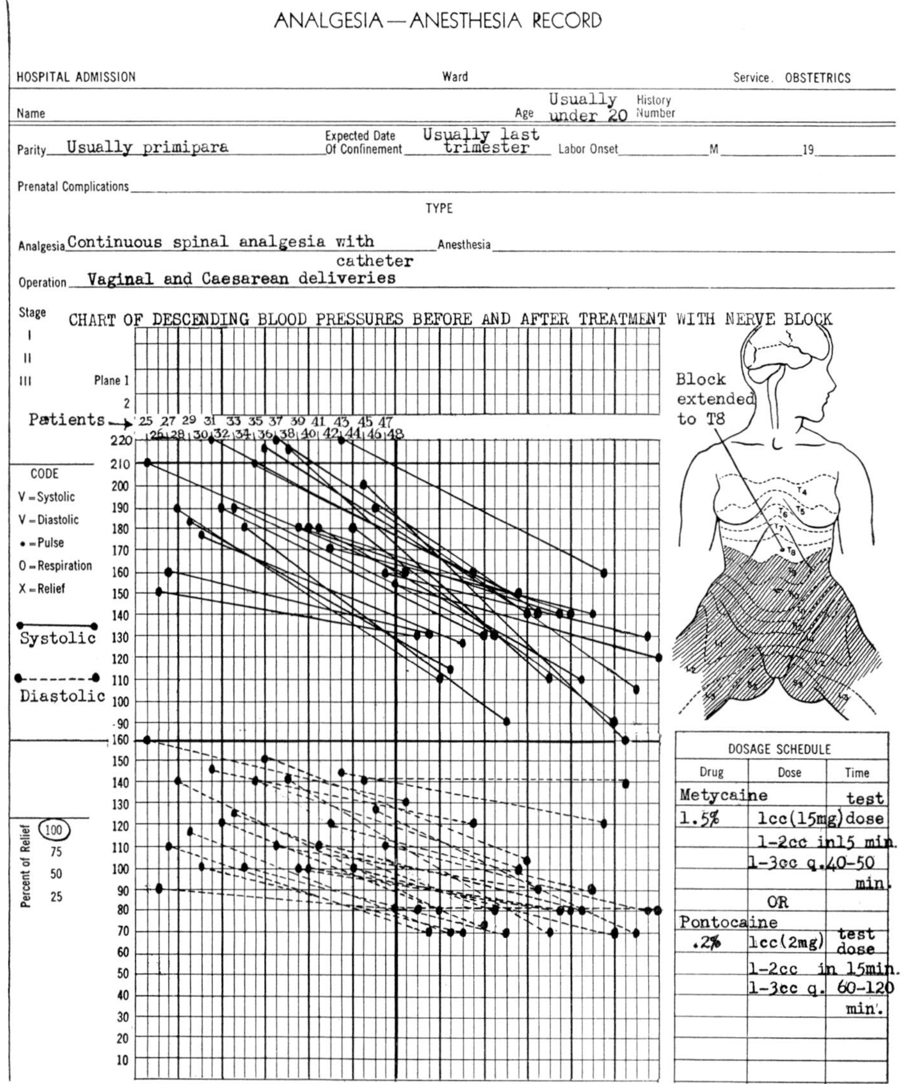

FIG. 89. The effect of continuous spinal on the blood pressure in acute toxemia.

Anesthesia for the Management of Eclampsia

Continuous Regional Block

This method was advocated by Whitacre, Hingson and Turner. They have reported 74 cases of eclampsia treated by continuous high caudal or spinal anesthesia with only 3 maternal deaths (see Figs. 88 and 89). McElrath, Ware, Winn and Schelin prefer continuous spinal and report good results. Whether the effects of caudal or spinal are due to an improved circulation of the kidneys or of the uterus or to the autonomic blockade of the entire splanchnic area is unknown. The procedure carries with it some risk, and it should be done only under the supervision of an anesthesiologist. The choice as to which of these methods is desirable will depend upon the available facilities and upon the experience and the judgment of the clinician.

In eclampsia on the basis of the mechanisms described, conduction nerve block of the deranged sympathetic nervous system can be established and maintained by (1) continuous caudal analgesia, (2) continuous lumbar epidural

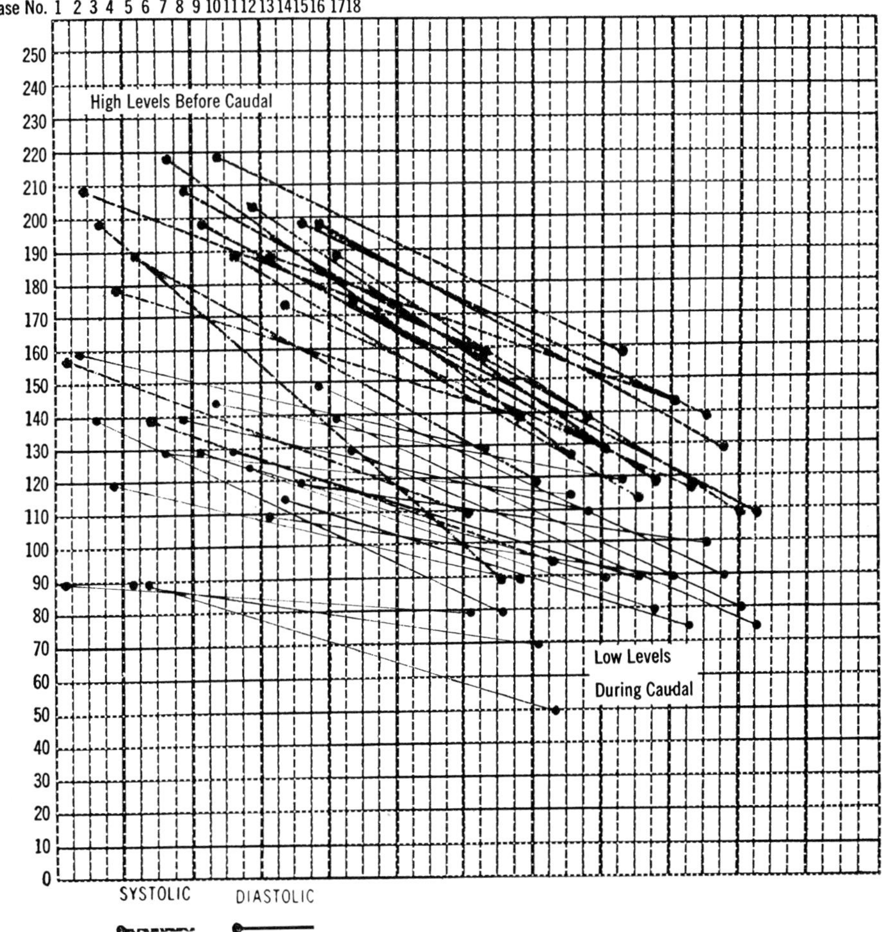

Fig. 90. Blood pressure levels before treatment and after control with continuous caudal analgesia in 18 consecutive cases of eclampsia with convulsions treated at the John Gaston Hospital, Memphis, Tenn. There was 1 death in this group.

analgesia and (3) continuous spinal anesthesia. All three methods, which also provide relief of pain for labor and delivery, produce a block of the small unmyelinated sympathetic nerve fibers. With the level of block extended through the lumbar plexus, a bloodless phlebotomy is produced with a vasomotor expansion of the vascular bed of the pelvis and the lower extremities. With the level of block extended to the eighth thoracic segment, the kidneys and the suprarenal glands are essentially denervated.

Since patients in eclampsia are comatose, semicomatose, irrational, un-co-operative or convulsant, the ureteral or the plastic catheter technics of one of the three nerve block procedures is preferred to the indwelling needle technic.

In our selection of one of the three methods we are influenced in our decision by anatomic factors that facilitate or impede a specific method. These are:

1. Palpability of the sacral hiatus or a lumbar interspinous space
2. Disproportionate obesity or edema obscuring the sacral hiatus or the lumbar interspinous space
3. Local infection of overlying skin

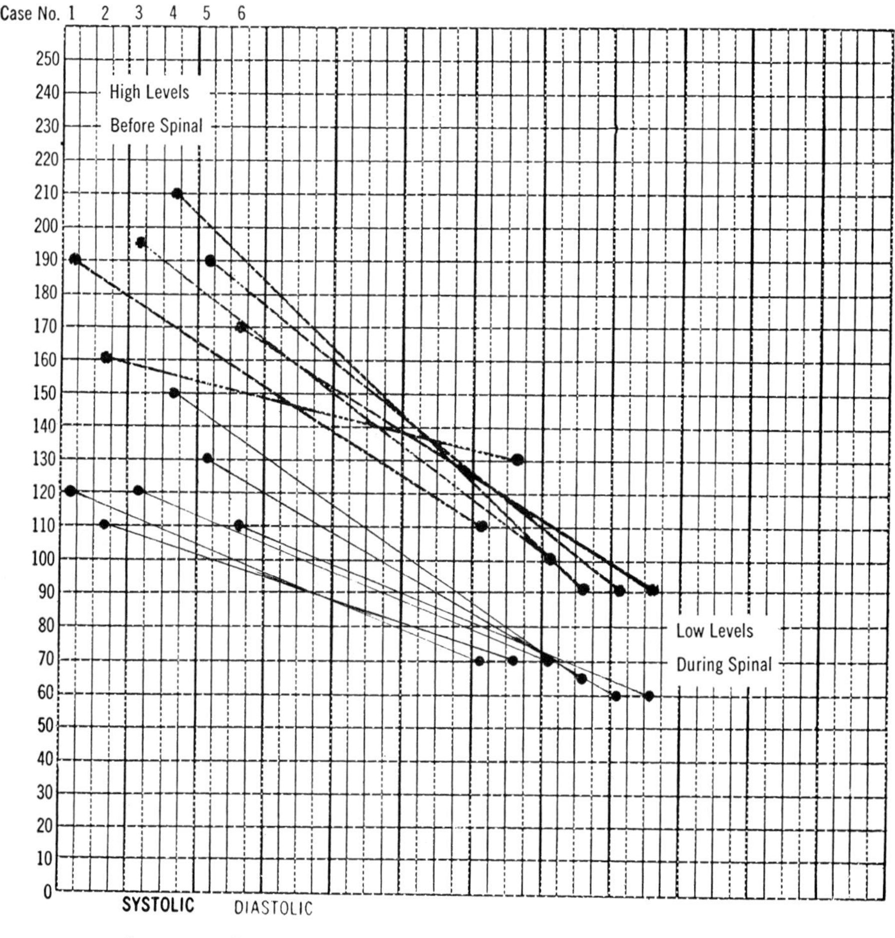

FIG. 91. Blood pressure levels before treatment and after control with continuous catheter (Tuohy) spinal anesthesia in 6 cases of eclampsia with convulsions treated at the John Gaston Hospital, Memphis, Tenn. In this group there were no deaths.

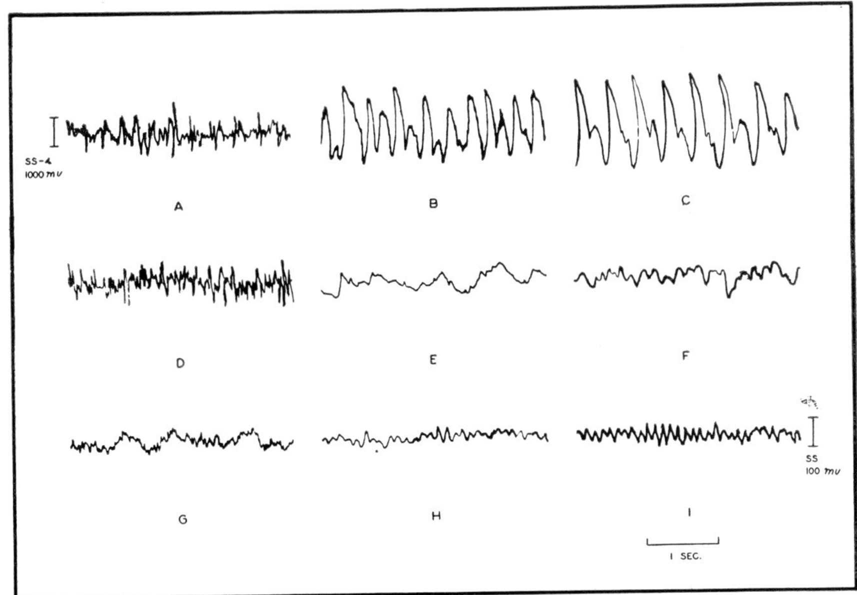

FIG. 92.* Presents samples of the electro-encephalographic tracings made on an eclamptic patient during a convulsion and as the patient improved coincident with, and following, the administration of a continuous caudal analgesia. These tracings were recorded and are herewith described by Dr. Hudson Jost, Director of the Psychophysiological Laboratories of the Department of Psychiatry at the University of Tennessee Medical School. In comparing the abnormal tracings with the normal, reference should be made to Tracing I, which represents the only essentially normal tracing obtained on this patient.

Tracing	*Date*	*Time*	*Medication*	*B.P.*	*Sensitivity*
A	4-10-46	11:48 A.M.		170/120	SS-4
		11:55 A.M.	30 cc. Metycaine		
B	4-10-46	11:56 A.M.		150/120	SS
		12:05 P.M.	15 cc. Metycaine		
C	4-10-46	12:15 P.M.		140/90	SS
		12:20 P.M.	15 cc. Metycaine		
D	4-10-46	12:21 P.M.		150/120	SS-4
E	4-10-46	12:25 P.M.		60/10	SS
F	4-10-46	12:37 P.M.		100/55	SS
G	4-11-46			136/110	SS
H	4-17-46			108/64	SS
I	4-22-46			100/75	SS

Tracings A through F are samples of recordings taken at intervals during the administration of Metycaine from 11:48 A.M. to 12:37 P.M., April 10, 1946. The tracing marked A was recorded during a generalized eclamptic convulsion immediately prior to the administration of Metycaine, when the blood pressure was 170/120. Tracing D was taken during a tonic convulsion that appeared before the blood pressure was lowered by the caudal analgesia. The amplitude of both

* The use of electro-encephalographic tracings to detect the abnormal functioning of neurons in the cerebral cortex during the convulsive and the preconvulsive stages of eclampsia, as well as the evidences of improvement in cortical function in relationship to treatment, was suggested by Dr. T. S. Hill, Professor of Psychiatry, at the University of Tennessee Medical School, and utilized by Dr. Frank Whitacre, Professor of Obstetrics and Gynecology, of the same university, who reported these observations.

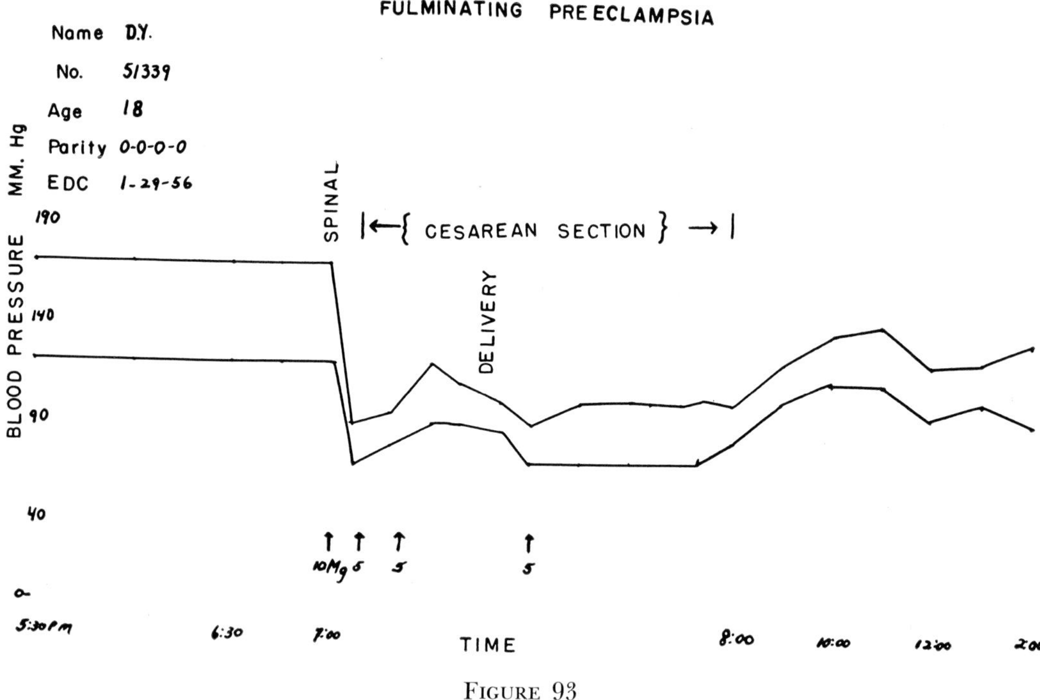

FIGURE 93

Spinal anesthesia and extradural block are always treacherous in preeclampsia because of the lability of the blood pressure. This is especially marked if magnesium sulfate has been used. Figures 93 and 94 show precipitous falls with both spinal and caudal. Fortunately, these infants both survived. These falls in blood pressure can be prevented by maintaining the pressure at a constant level with a carefully regulated drip of neosynephrine diluted 1 cc. in 1,000 cc. of dextrose. The use of routine standard doses of vasopressor at the induction of the block cannot be too strongly condemned in these cases. Figure 95 shows moderate blood pressure elevation in such an instance with subsequent eclampsia.

---

of these is 97 per cent normal when compared with the standard sensitivity wherein 1 cm. equals 100 mv. as shown in the other samples. The calibration for A and D is given in the upper left-hand corner of the chart. The standardization for the remaining tracings is shown in the lower right-hand corner of the figure. Tracings B and C depict the interconvulsive pattern, which is similar to the wave forms found in petit mal epilepsy. Tracing E shows the electro-encephalographic tracing after the blood pressure had dropped to 60/10 and the patient was comatose. Tracing F was obtained when the blood pressure was re-established at 100/55. It will be noted that the cortical potential pattern is not completely normal, although the amplitude of the waves had decreased and their frequency had increased, producing a somewhat less abnormal pattern.

Tracings G, H and I depict samples of recordings made at intervals of 1, 7 and 12 days, respectively, following the administration of caudal analgesia. Tracing G represents an electro-encephalographic tracing taken on April 11, 1946, the day following delivery, when the blood pressure was 136/100. Tracing H was obtained 7 days later, at which time the blood pressure was 108/64 and the electro-encephalographic tracing was almost normal. The final sample, Tracing I, was taken 12 days after delivery, at which time the tracing was essentially normal.

FULMINATING PREECLAMPSIA

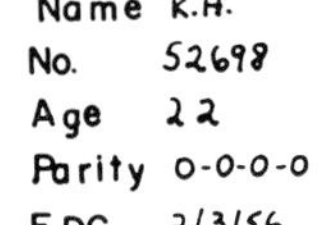

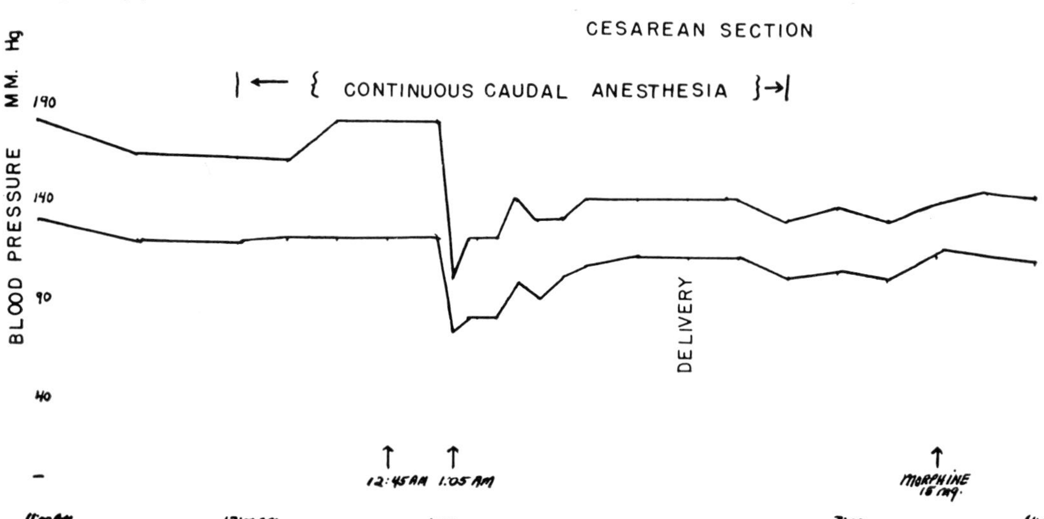

FIGURE 94

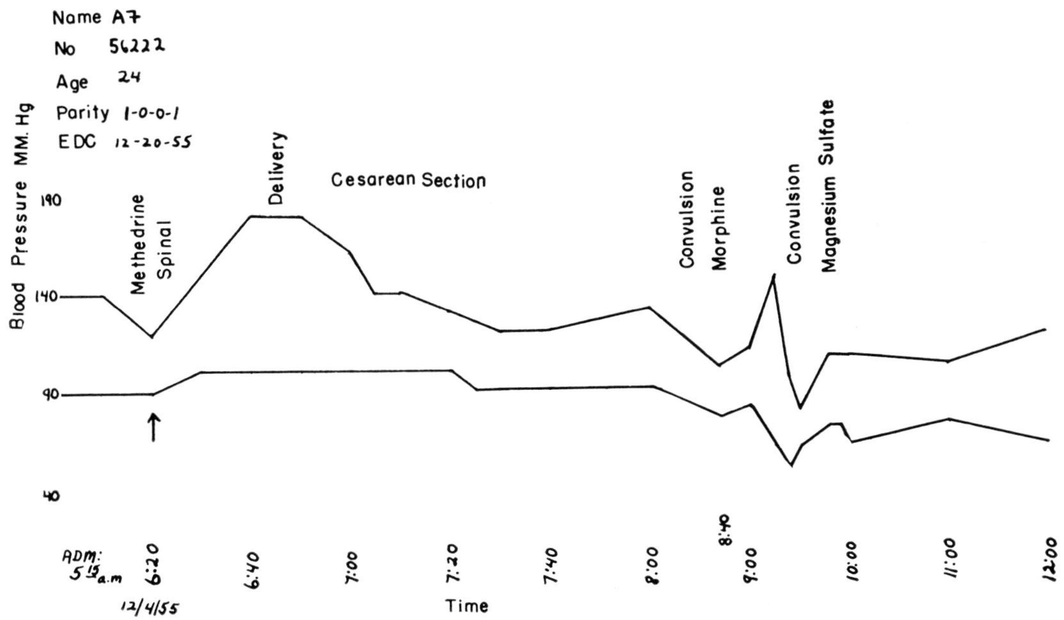

FIGURE 95

Summary

Seventy-four consecutive cases of eclampsia that occurred chiefly in the hospitals of Memphis, Tenn. are presented. All were treated with conduction anesthesia nerve blocks as a measure useful in the control of the hypertensive crises attended by convulsions and nervous irritability. In 6 instances, because of edema over the vertebral column and/or uncontrolled muscular movements of patients in semicoma, these technics could not be instituted after several attempts at needle and catheter insertion. However, they are included to maintain the sequence of the series. Some of these cases had been treated for several hours with magnesium sulfate sedation, intravenous glucose and distilled water, and oxygen. The conduction nerve block was reserved as a last-resort measure. Some of the cases were managed with conduction nerve blocks alone from the onset of symptoms for a period of from 12 to 48 hours after the last convulsion or hypertensive crisis. Only 2 of these patients had any convulsion after the institution of an effective nerve block, and both had single convulsions within the first 30 minutes which later were controlled as the nerve blocks became intensified. It is our opinion that obvious improvement resulted from the nerve blocks in all cases except that in which the patient succumbed immediately after a spinal injection of 30 mg. of Metycaine. However, autopsy in this case revealed irretrievable damage from interventricular hemorrhage.

Finally, even though the further development and standardizations of these technics offer much in the active treatment of eclampsia, we wish to emphasize the fact that they are powerful remedies that should not be used by those who have had little or no experience with them. The meticulous adjustment of dosage for the individual, the maintenance of slowly and evenly reduced blood pressure, the preservation of optimum circulating fluid volumes, the administration of oxygen-enriched atmospheres and the understanding of the effect of altered vascular physiology superimposed on both mother and baby during the period of therapy, require an understanding that can be gained only through experience.

Physicians lacking this background who are confronted with an occasional case of eclampsia will have better results in treating it with the procedures described above.

In cases requiring general anesthesia or anesthesia supplement to conduction anesthesia for delivery, intravenous barbiturates with 100 per cent oxygen represent the method of choice.

The procedures contraindicated in eclampsia are as follows:

1. Ether, which diminishes markedly the excretion of urine through the kidney after 10 minutes of anesthesia
2. Chloroform, which may accentuate the underlying pathology in the liver
3. Avertin, which is not recommended because of its toxic effect upon both liver and kidney

Warning!

All anesthesiologists not accustomed to the synergistic vasodepression produced by a combination of major vertebral conduction anesthesia, or even deep planes of barbiturate and ether anesthesia, and large doses of magnesium sulfate, should use conservative doses and have readily at hand the vasopressors in intravenous drip plus oxygen.

Anesthesia in Hypertensive Disease

Parturients with hypertension present a definite anesthetic hazard during labor. Not infrequently, the emotional strain of labor, the associated pain and the generalized vasoconstriction tend to bring about a rise in blood pressure. Thus, any agents that can submerge the emotional tension, as do the barbiturates, Demerol and paraldehyde, are of distinct value. It has been our experience that the extremes of hypertension will diminish in the process of adequate sedation with these drugs. In the presence of hypertension, the use of nitrous oxide is questioned by Lundy because of the possible development of anoxemia with the consequent elevation of blood pressure.

It has been our experience that continuous caudal and continuous spinal analgesia reduce markedly the blood pressure of patients with hypertension to more normal limits, irrespective of whether they were pregnant or not. Some of these patients showed a blood pressure fall of 100 mm. of mercury without demonstrating an adverse pharmacologic effect. In fact, not infrequently such unpleasant symptoms as blurred vision, headache and nausea during the hypertensive episodes were relieved completely by the hypotension produced by caudal analgesia.

Nevertheless, we emphasize the need for caution in managing a patient by any method that produces so marked and rapid a blood pressure fall. The patient should be surrounded by the safeguards of available oxygen for inhalation, vasopressor drugs for intramuscular or intravenous injection, and facilities for raising the lower extremities to right angles with the body in sudden emergencies that may require an autotransfusion from the pooled reservoirs of the dilated vessels of the extremities.

No patient who normally has a hypertension should have her pressure fall to 100 mm. of mercury systolic and below without the institution of supportive treatment.

Essential hypertension and recent coronary thrombosis do not necessarily contraindicate the use of spinal or caudal analgesia. When one of these methods has been chosen in the presence of hypertension and thrombosis, the blood pressure should be supported in such a way that further thrombosis will be unlikely to result from further stasis of blood.

In the establishment of the level of analgesia, it is our purpose to proceed more slowly and cautiously than in the uncomplicated case. In such cases it may be wise to take an hour or more to provide total relief from pain.

The patient should be made to understand that the so-called "pilot" pains remaining can be controlled completely at the proper time, that, in effect, they are left as an indicator of the progress of labor, with the added assurance that the vasomotor block has not ascended to a dangerous level.

In the presence of hypertension, should any chosen agent initiate a further blood pressure rise, that agent should be withheld and the patient managed in some other manner. For this type of case one should consider the so-called "balanced" anesthesia of Lundy, or the "anoci" association anesthesia of Crile, in which the emotions are controlled by one of the forms of sedation or general anesthesia, and the pain is controlled by the anatomic approach, as with caudal, spinal, pudendal, presacral or perineal block.

Anesthesia for Renal Disease

Certain of the general anesthetics—ether, chloroform, ethyl chloride and divinyl ether—exert an irritating effect upon the tubular epithelium of the kidney, as manifested by the presence of red blood cells and epithelial casts in the urine during the postoperative state. These 4 anesthetics also produce a temporary anuria during anesthesia and for the few hours thereafter a later compensatory polyuria.

Nitrous oxide, cyclopropane and paraldehyde also produce a moderate suppression of the renal excretory function but no irritation phenomena. These drugs are a better choice than the volatile agents listed above.

In the presence of serious disease of the kidneys, the use of Pentothal Sodium or Avertin is complicated by the possible development of coma. In the presence of coma, the use of these drugs may intensify this condition.

Spinal and continuous spinal analgesia and anesthesia, caudal and continuous caudal analgesia and other forms of regional nerve block usually are satisfactory for pain relief measures in parturients with renal disease. We have found that an extension of the regional nerve block to include the sympathetic components of the ninth and the tenth thoracic segments sometimes will produce an increase in the flow of urine. A notable example was a patient with pre-eclampsia and cardiovascular disease who, in the state of semicoma, had produced only 400 cc. of urine in 24 hours. In order to relieve her pains in labor, continuous caudal analgesia was instituted. During the next 6 hours her measured output of urine was 1,400 cc. This may be explained on the basis of a vasomotor block of the afferent arterioles of the kidneys.

We believe that one of these regional blocks would be indicated in cases presenting evidence of anuria from any cause.

Cyclopropane probably is the best general anesthesia supplement.

CONTROL OF PAIN IN OBSTETRIC COMPLICATIONS

Hemorrhagic Complications

Obstetric hemorrhage, along with toxemia and infection, constitutes a third of the great triad of abnormalities that account for the major portion of maternal deaths in the United States. The yearly fetal wastage associated with this syndrome, if abortion is included, cannot be estimated accurately, but certainly it approaches half a million lives. The major conditions responsible for significant hemorrhage during gestation along with the fetal wastage are indicated in Table 33.

Table 33. The Incidence of Various Entities Responsible for Obstetric Hemorrhage

Entity	Incidence Per 1,000 Births	Per Cent Fetal Wastage
Abortion*		
Spontaneous	100	100
Induced	Unknown	100
Therapeutic	2.8	100
Ectopic	2.2	100
Placental Separation†		
Previa	3.8	14.2
Abruptio	13.0	54.5
Marginal Sinus Rupture	6.9	21.0
Rupture of Uterus	1.2	35.8
Miscellaneous	21.0	15.7
Postpartum Hemorrhage		
Early	43.5	—
Late	0.3	—

* Spontaneous abortion data from Hertig. Therapeutic data from New York City Health Department, 1953, figured per 1,000 live births. Ectopic data from New York City Health Department, 1953.

† Data from the Kings County Hospital for years 1951-54: 10,951 deliveries.

Frequently, the well-being of the fetus can be ignored and attention directed solely to the treatment of the situation at hand. This is particularly true for abortion and those instances of obstetric hemorrhage in which the fetus either is dead or has been delivered already. From the point of view of anesthesia, this simplifies the situation, although when there is some chance of fetal salvage the nicest judgment is required. In general, in the face of hemorrhage, an encephalic type of anesthesia, as free from induction difficulties as possible and giving adequate relaxation for the operative procedure, is desirable. In order to make the most advantageous selection, it is important that the anesthesiologist have some idea of the possible alterations in physiology, the various general forms of obstetric treatment and possible complications.

Abortion

Spontaneous abortion can be threatened, imminent, incomplete or complete.

Threatened abortion is indicated when there are cramps and/or bleeding and when an examination shows that the cervix is long and closed and the membranes are intact. The majority of these occur somewhere between the eighth and the twelfth week of pregnancy. Medical forms of therapy in this condition are legion, and no surgical treatment is required.

Imminent abortion is merely the next step in this process. The cervix shows effacement and some dilatation, and frequently the membranes are ruptured.

In incomplete abortion, part of the fetus or the placenta will have been passed. Inasmuch as there is no chance of saving the pregnancy, treatment consists of emptying the uterus. There are 2 schools of thought as to when and how this should be done. In one, every effort is made to accomplish this spontaneously with the use of pituitary extract or merely the employment of time. In the other, the uterus is emptied as soon as possible except in the face of parametritis or peritonitis. Although both types of therapy are completely acceptable, our own not inconsiderable experience indicates that immediate therapy is much more satisfactory to the patient and offers as good, if not better, results. Treatment consists of emptying the uterus of the products of conception manually or with a sponge forceps, or by acutal dilatation and curettage. The means employed to empty the uterus will depend upon the judgment of the operator.

In general, fatal hemorrhage from abortion is rare, and in cases of true spontaneous abortion infection is not common. However, in those instances in which the fetus has been dead some time, spontaneous abortion can be associated with a rather marked febrile episode. Of course, the difficulty is to distinguish between the purely spontaneous abortion and induced abortion. This cannot be done by any known diagnostic method, and as patients almost invariably will deny interference, the operator should always suspect it. Inasmuch as induced abortion cannot be differentiated from spontaneous abortion, the treatment for both, if they are incomplete or imminent, is in general the same. The contraindications to immediate emptying of the uterus are infection, as indicated above, and possible perforation from attempted induction. Adequate supportive therapy should be given before and during the operative procedure. In some instances of badly infected abortion, acute renal failure occurs. Both the infection and accompanying shock play an etiologic role. The latter should be prevented by adequate replacement of blood. Occasionally, shock occurs from sepsis alone without blood loss, due to dilatation of the vascular bed. In these cases, care must be exercised not to overload the vascular system with transfusion or infusion. Here the blood pressure may be maintained with a continuous intravenous drip of noradrenalin (4 cc. in 1,000 cc. 5 per cent dextrose). However, it cannot be emphasized too strongly that vasoconstrictors never are the treatment for shock due to hemorrhage.

Therapeutic abortion is the termination of pregnancy prior to the period of viability for the purpose of saving the life of the mother or safeguarding her health, including her mental health. This procedure is governed by statutes or common law in all the states, but the wording of the regulations varies widely. Therapeutic abortion never should be performed without the written approval of at least 2 consultants. Many hospitals now have Abortion Boards that study the indications in every case. As the years have passed and a better understanding of the physiology of pregnancy and the care of the patients has been obtained, the medical indications for therapeutic abortion have been reduced consistently. Perhaps today the best medical indication is chronic hypertensive vascular disease with a history of previous superimposed toxemia. Here, as indicated in the preceding section, Chesley has shown a definite increase in the remote annual death rates. Severe rheumatic heart disease with a previous history of decompensation formerly was considered to be one of the major indications for this operation. However, recently some doubt has been cast upon the validity of this indication. Another possible indication is carcinoma of the cervix. Also, there are certain psychiatric situations and rare acute disease in which abortion may offer a solution.

Therapeutic abortion may be performed either vaginally or by the abdominal route. The decision as to which approach is to be used is based on the duration of pregnancy (the vaginal route should not be used if pregnancy is of more than 10-12 weeks' duration) and the desirability of tubal ligation. In general, therapeutic abortion is performed for severe and chronic illness, and, therefore, should be accompanied by tubal ligation. This may not be true for mental illness, although insufficient information is available on this point.

The type of anesthesia chosen will depend upon the condition of the patient. The encephalic approach can be used in those patients with mental illness, carcinoma of the cervix, or possibly hypertensive disease. The anatomic approach can be reserved for those individuals in whom inhalation anesthesia in particular would be detrimental.

Anesthesia for Completion of Abortion

Inhalation—1. Cyclopropane
2. Intravenous Barbiturate

Occasionally, in some busy institutions, abortions are completed under analgesia using morphine or Demerol and a barbiturate and scopolamine, the theory being that this sort of therapy carries a certain amount of safety with it, and that a large amount of anesthesia is not necessary for the procedure. We cannot subscribe to this.

Ectopic Pregnancy

Although ectopic pregnancy is a type of abortion, it requires more extensive therapy and presents certain complex anesthesia problems. By ectopic pregnancy is meant any gestation located outside the uterine cavity. It includes not only those pregnancies in the tube but those situated in the interstitial portion of the uterus and in the ovary. For the purpose of this book, a discussion of tubal gestations will suffice, as these constitute 95 per cent of all ectopic pregnancies, and, roughly, the problems are similar to those of the rarer types of extra-uterine gestation.

Ectopic pregnancy occurs once in 177 pregnancies in white women; in Negresses it is slightly more common. This differential is believed to be due to the higher incidence of pelvic inflammatory disease in the latter, although any process that interferes with the progress of the fertilized egg down the oviduct can cause extra-uterine nidation, and inflammatory disease is by no means a sole causative agent.

An oviducal pregnancy may terminate in 3 possible ways. The products of conception may be aborted from the end of the oviduct or into the uterine cavity; the oviduct may rupture into either the abdominal cavity or the broad ligament; the fetus may die, and the products of conception may be absorbed. In all 3 processes, the possibility of hemorrhage that will necessitate immediate treatment is real.

In the so-called "typical" case of ruptured oviducal pregnancy, the diagnosis is made easily. After a month or two of amenorrhea, there are slight vaginal bleeding, a sudden onset of severe abdominal pain with shock and/or syncope, and various signs and symptoms of blood in the peritoneal cavity. Unfortunately, however, more than half the cases are atypical. In these, according to Lavell and Marchetti, amenorrhea and vaginal spotting or bleeding occur only 75 per cent of the time, while pain is present from 90 to 98 per cent of the time. Syncope and shock are of variable occurrence, being reported in from 29 to 47 per cent of cases. In most instances of ectopic pregnancy, the physical findings are extremely variable. By far the most common finding is extreme tenderness on palpation of the uterus or the vaginal vault or upon movement of the cervix. This sign is present at least three quarters of the time. A mass has been found in only a quarter of our own cases, while changes in uterine size are present in only a small minority of the patients.

Hormonal tests are without value if they are negative and point merely to the existence of living chorionic tissue if they are positive.

There are diagnostic procedures that may be of some value should the presence of an oviducal pregnancy remain in doubt. These are vaginal examination under anesthesia, culdoscopy and puncture of the posterior cul-de-sac. If the patient is difficult to examine and the differential diagnosis rests between pelvic inflammatory disease and ectopic pregnancy, examination under anesthesia often is helpful. The anesthetic required is necessarily of short duration, but it should supply enough relaxation to permit the procedure to be carried out adequately.

For a detailed description of the technic of culdoscopy, the reader is referred to the articles of Decker and TeLinde. This procedure is carried out with the patient in the knee-chest position. Although the patient can be held in this position while she is unconscious, the whole procedure is easier if the patient is able to co-operate. Thus, the anatomic approach giving a localized anesthesia or infiltration of the posterior cul-de-sac with procaine is more satisfactory. Once the area has been anesthetized, the culdoscope, which is merely an endoscope with an angulated mirror, is passed into the posterior cul-de-sac, and the oviducts and the pelvic organs are visualized easily.

The third diagnostic procedure of value is puncture of the posterior cul-de-sac. This can be done with a long needle, in which case either no anesthesia or simple local infiltration of the area is needed, or the posterior cul-de-sac can be opened, in which case some local infiltration will suffice. These are blind procedures, and, although sometimes they serve to differentiate a collection of pus from blood in the posterior cul-de-sac, they have led to some unfortunate diagnostic errors.

Treatment consists of laparotomy with the appropriate operation to control hemorrhage.

Anesthesia for Ectopic Pregnancy

Diagnostic Procedures

Vaginal Examination:

ENCEPHALIC. *Inhalation — Cyclopropane (Reserve Midget). Intravenous — Pentothal Sodium.*

Culdoscopy:

ANATOMIC. *Spinal—Lucaine. Caudal. Local.*

Posterior Cul-de-sac Puncture:

LOCAL.

Operative Procedures

Encephalic:

INHALATION—CYCLOPROPANE.

Anatomic:

SPINAL. Rarely indicated.

TOPICAL AND LOCAL. Supplemented with 400 mg. 2% Xylocaine in peritoneal cavity in poor-risk cases.

PLACENTA PREVIA

Placenta previa and abruptio placenta both are causes of bleeding in the last trimester of pregnancy, and both are due to separation of the placenta. However, because of the different location of the placenta at the time of the accident, the character of the bleeding and its resultant complications are quite different.

Placenta previa occurs once in 200 labors. It varies in degree, according to the location of the placenta in relation to the internal os. Three degrees are recognized.

Total Placenta Previa. The internal os is totally covered by the placenta.

Partial Placenta Previa. The internal os is partially covered by the placenta.

Low Implantation of the Placenta. The placenta encroaches upon the internal os and can be palpated when the examining finger is introduced through the cervix.

These degrees are only relative, as it is apparent that they may change with the dilating cervix.

Two factors favor the appearance of placenta previa — multiparity and atrophic changes in the endometrium. It occurs comparatively rarely in primigravidae, but it increases directly with the number and the frequency of children.

The bleeding with placenta previa usually occurs quite unexpectedly and without pain. Hardly ever is the initial hemorrhage severe enough to cause mortality, and, in fact, it rarely causes even shock, unless the patient has had a previous low hemoglobin.

On admission to the hospital the patient usually has ceased to bleed. She is not in shock, although her hemoglobin level may be low. Palpation of the abdomen shows frequently that the presenting part is unengaged. These patients should not be examined rectally or vaginally unless preparation is made to combat blood loss and to effect delivery. The patient should be grouped and matched for transfusion. The diagnosis of placenta previa can be made indirectly from the patient's story, but directly only by introduction of a finger through the cervix. This type of examination may cause severe bleeding and may make it necessary for the obstetrician to terminate pregnancy directly following the examination.

Formerly, this type of immediate treatment was considered to be good procedure, placenta previa being considered an emergency. However, in recent times, it has been pointed out by Macafee, Johnson and Williams that the high infant mortality associated with placenta previa was due largely to prematurity, and that if delivery could be postponed, a reduction in the infant mortality could be obtained.

Furthermore, it was pointed out independently by these investigators that the first hemorrhage rarely was fatal unless there had been previous interference. If the hemoglobin is maintained at a level of 10 Gm., subsequent hemorrhages also are not fatal. Thus, the currently practiced expectant type of treatment with the patient remaining under surveillance, preferably in the hospital, until the fetus has reached such a size that its life expectancy is favorable. Once the fetus has reached adequate size, vaginal examination can be carried out in the operating room and delivery effected in the most desirable manner.

There are 2 general methods of treating placenta previa—by compression and by cesarean section. The former should be reserved only for the mildest degrees of low implantation. The compression methods consist of rupture of the membranes and allowing the head to tamponade the placenta and the lower uterine segment. Occasionally, additional pressure is applied by scalp traction. Two additional methods of applying pressure to the placenta and the lower uterine segment formerly were in favor, but they now are becoming obsolete. They consist of the Braxton-Hicks version with the fetal thigh as a tamponade, or the use of a bag for this purpose. The Braxton-Hicks version now is considered to be dangerous, due to the extremely soft and friable character of the lower uterine segment and the real danger of rupture during any sort of manipulation, because of the danger of infection and the accompanying high infant loss rate. The bag has fallen into disuse.

Vaginal examination to determine the type of placenta previa can be carried out without anesthesia. If the placenta merely is low implanted, simple rupture of the membranes will suffice. However, in the primigravida, all types but low implantative should be treated with cesarean section. In multiparas, too, cesarean section is becoming a more accepted type of treatment for most degrees of placenta previa. If the patient is bleeding actively and the situation is more or less one of emergency, the anesthesia should be selected without regard for fetal survival and with strict attention to the mother. In general, inhalation forms will be selected. However, if the patient has been in the hospital for many weeks, and if there is no bleeding, the life of the fetus is one of the primary concerns, and the conduction type of anesthesia obviously is superior. More than average attention should be paid to maintenance of blood pressure and replacement in cases so managed.

Warning!

In the case of suspected placenta previa, no vaginal examination should be done without full anesthesia coverage and complete preparation for cesarean section.

Anesthesia for Placenta Previa

Diagnostic vaginal examination: None.

In face of hemorrhage (cesarean section): Encephalic—inhalation (cyclopropane).

No hemorrhage (cesarean section): Anatomic. Spinal. Caudal. Lumbar extradural.

Vaginal delivery: Analgesia — light plane. Anesthesia—anatomic—pudendal block.

Eastman reports the fetal mortality from placenta previa to be in the neighborhood of 25 per cent, with some of the higher figures ranging up to 55 per cent. It will be noted from Table 24 that the infant mortality from placenta previa in the Baltimore Study was only 13.3 per cent for all babies, and that it reached a low of 8.5 per cent for term infants. Similar results are seen in Table 33. This vastly lowered infant mortality can be attributed to the expectant treatment of placenta previa, the increased use of cesarean section and proper and wise selection of anesthesia for delivery.

Abruptio Placenta

Abruptio placenta is the sudden complete or partial separation of a normally implanted placenta. Its etiology is obscure, but in many instances it is preceded by hypertension.

In 20 per cent of the cases the bleeding is concealed, and in the remainder it is overt. Fortunately, in most instances neither the blood loss nor the degree of separation is marked. However, this accident is accompanied sometimes by sudden severe abdominal pain and shock out of proportion to blood loss. This is especially true if there is no obvious hemorrhage.

In mild cases, diagnosis is made by exclusion of placenta previa and other causes of hemorrhage. In the rare severe form, shock is present, the uterus is lignous, and fetal heart frequently is absent.

Treatment. Frequently the separation is mild and occurs during labor. No treatment is necessary other than rupture of the membranes and perhaps the administration of intravenous pituitary extract. In severe cases, particularly when the hemorrhage is concealed, the treatment must be expeditious and well planned. There are 2 complications which, although rare, make the time required to effect delivery of importance. These are (1) blood clotting deficits and (2) acute renal failure.

Apparently, in a very few cases of placental separation with hemorrhage into and injury to the decidual plate and the uterine muscle, there is a release of thromboplastin that rapidly depletes the maternal blood of its fibrinogen. A thrombolytic enzyme also may be released. The result, of course, is a failure of the blood to clot adequately. This always should be watched for in placental separation and combated, if it is found, by the administration of fibrinogen, or, if this is not available, by freshly drawn blood. For more details the reader is referred to the exhaustive writings of Reid and his co-workers. More frequently is renal depression associated with abruptio placenta. Apparently, it is related to shock, plus the presence of either free hemoglobin or myoglobin in the blood stream. The association of abruptio placenta with hemorrhage into and damage to the uterine muscle sets the stage for this possibility. In many instances, there results only a mild and temporary oliguria, but in others, true renal failure occurs. We are indebted to the classic work of Oliver for a clear understanding of this complication. He believes that a suppression of blood flow to the kidneys causes sufficient hypoxia to account for the damage seen not only in the tubular cells but in the underlying basement membrane.

With these complications in mind, the treatment of premature separation of the placenta becomes more logical and does not necessarily divide itself into either conservative or radical schools. The type of therapy selected depends upon the number of estimated hours necessary to accomplish delivery and the severity of the abruption. This is a matter of judgment requiring considerable experience on the part of the obstetrician. However, if the patient is a multigravida, and the cervix already is effaced partially and is dilated somewhat and if the uterus is not contracted too firmly but shows some contraction and relaxation, then simple rupture of the membranes, with the intravenous administration of dilute pituitary extract, should accomplish delivery within a short time, possibly in 3 or 4 hours, in an entirely satisfactory manner.

On the other hand, if the patient is a primigravida, in shock, with the uterus contracted firmly and the cervix long and closed, then delivery from below will be a long-drawn-out process, and, despite supportive therapy, one or both of the forementioned complications may eventuate. In this latter instance, therefore, delivery should be accomplished by cesarean section. In a conservative clinic, this philosophy will result in approximately a 15 to 20 per cent cesarean section rate in cases of abruption of the placenta. In either event, the obstetrician and the anesthesiologist should realize that this is an extremely serious situation for the patient, and that not only does one border continually on the possibility of severe shock but other more complex complications may occur. Therefore, the analgesia and the anesthesia should be selected accordingly.

Anesthesia for Abruptio Placenta

Vaginal delivery: Analgesia (encephalic—light plane). Anesthesia (encephalic—cyclopropane. Anatomic—pudendal block).

Cesarean section: Encephalic (inhalation—cyclopropane).

Rupture of Marginal Sinus

Another cause of last-trimester bleeding, which has received some attention lately, is rupture of the marginal sinus of the placenta. The human placenta has a circular sinus that is more or less complete round its whole periphery. This contains maternal blood and constitutes one of the sources of venous drainage of the placenta. It is bounded on its inferior surface by the decidual plate, laterally by the junction of the decidual and the chorionic plates, superiorly by the chorionic plate, and medially by the placenta proper. Any marginal separation of the placenta will rupture the sinus, and maternal bleeding will ensue. Unfortunately, the diagnosis of rupture of the marginal sinus must be made after the delivery of the placenta, and it can be presumed only if bleeding occurs prior to, or during, labor. Even after delivery of the placenta, the pathologic diagnosis is made with some difficulty, due to the fact that the marginal sinus always ruptures when the placenta separates normally.

Fish and co-workers, and Harris have written rather extensively on this subject. In our own experience, rupture of the marginal sinus has an incidence of about 15 to 20 per cent of cases of antepartum hemorrhage and a fetal loss rate of 20 per cent. However, inasmuch as the diagnosis is only a presumptive one prior to delivery, there is no specific treatment, nor is any specific type of analgesia or anesthesia to be recommended. In the face of antepartum bleeding not associated with placenta previa, or slightly excessive bleeding during labor, the minimum amount of analgesia and conduction or infiltration anesthesia should be used.

Dystocia

Dystocia means difficult labor. It can be related to relative disproportion between the fetal head and the pelvis, dysfunction of the uterus or malposition of the fetus. Except in the face of unpredictable accidents, such as prolapsed cord in a transverse lie, dystocia need not yield materially higher maternal mortality or morbidity or an increase in perinatal loss. However, such utopian results can be obtained only with the full employment of modern diagnostic and therapeutic tools, impeccable obstetric judgment, and the proper selection and timing of obstetric pain relief and anesthesia. Unfortunately, no one of us can quite measure up to these requirements at all times, thus the perinatal loss in dystocia is doubled or trebled perhaps, while now and then an occasional mother still loses her life or, perhaps worse, is made either a physical or an emotional cripple as a result of dystocic labor.

Pelvic Contraction

The commonest cause of cephalopelvic disproportion is pelvic contraction.

TABLE 34. TOTAL LOSS AND INFANT MORTALITY FOR PREMATURE AND FULL-TERM INFANTS AMONG MOTHERS WITH HEMORRHAGIC CONDITIONS ACCORDING TO METHODS OF ADMINISTERING ANESTHESIA

METHODS	*Number**			*Rate per 1,000 total births*		
	TOTAL INFANTS	STILL-BIRTHS	NEONATAL DEATHS	TOTAL LOSS	STILL-BIRTHS	NEONATAL DEATHS
				Total Infants		
All methods	335	8	20	83.6	23.9	59.7
No anesthesia	31	—	4	129.0	—	129.0
Intravenous and inhalation	131	2	5	53.5	15.3	38.2
Caudal and spinal	140	5	8	92.8	35.7	57.1
Local	16	1	3	250.0	62.5	187.5
Combination of methods	17	—	—	—	—	—
				Prematures		
All methods	113	4	18	194.7	35.4	159.3
No anesthesia	11	—	4	363.6	—	363.6
Intravenous and inhalation	36	—	5	138.9	—	138.9
Caudal and spinal	50	4	7	220.0	80.0	140.0
Local	10	—	2	200.0	—	200.0
Combination of methods	6	—	—	—	—	—
				Full Terms		
All methods	222	4	2	27.0	18.0	9.0
No anesthesia	20	—	—	—	—	—
Intravenous and inhalation	95	2	—	21.1	21.1	—
Caudal and spinal	90	1	1	22.2	11.1	11.1
Local	6	1	1	333.4	166.7	166.7
Combination of methods	11	—	—	—	—	—

* Twins, infants who died before onset of labor and analgesia and infants with congenital malformations incompatible with life, are excluded.

Its frequency exceeds that of many other serious obstetric complications such as placenta previa, abruptio placenta, diabetes, heart disease, etc. The only major obstetric complication that is more frequent is toxemia.

The diagnosis of pelvic contraction depends primarily upon measurement of all the planes in both their anteroposterior characters and in their transverse diameters. As has been indicated previously, this can be accomplished with accuracy only by the x-ray. However, fortunately in gross contraction of the inlet and, perhaps, the mid-pelvis, certain indications of difficulty can be obtained by clinical measurement and examination of the pelvis. These can be reinforced by failure of labor to progress satisfactorily. Rarely does the skilled obstetrician fail to diagnose even borderline contractions on this basis. However, his judgment is much more certain, particularly if there is a question of stimulation of labor if he has accurate x-ray measurements of the pelvic diameters. The critical* measurements of the pelvis by x-ray are shown in Table 35.

A pelvis may be contracted in either the anteroposterior or the transverse diameter in any one, two or all three of the planes. Inlet contraction is most common in ward practice, while mid-pelvic difficulties are encountered more frequently among private patients.

The simplest contraction of the inlet to recognize is that of the anteroposterior diameter. In the past this was caused most commonly by rickets and perhaps

* *Critical* is used here to define the borderline of pelvic contraction. It is not necessarily an indication for cesarean section.

TABLE 35. PELVIC PLANES AND "CRITICAL" MEASUREMENTS

PLANES	Diameters in Centimeters		
	ANTERO-POSTERIOR	TRANS-VERSE	POSTERO-SAGITTAL
Inlet	10.0	12.0	—
Mid-plane	11.5	9.5	4.0
Outlet	11.0	10.0	7.5

it is so even today. In such a pelvis, if there is a compensating increase in the transverse diameter and labor is forceful, the head frequently can negotiate the inlet by molding and tilting one or the other parietal bones through first. Prolonged labor in face of insurmountable pelvic contraction can damage an infant seriously. Furthermore, premature rupture of the membranes may be followed by prolapse of the cord. Such pelvic contractions, if unrecognized and neglected, may end in rupture of the uterus.

More recently recognized transverse contractions of the inlet are equally serious, although they are harder to diagnose clinically. Data from Kaltreider show that contraction of the inlet in either diameter leads to an equal amount of difficulty, while contraction of both diameters increases the difficulty threefold.

Frequently in inlet contraction the remainder of the pelvis is normal. Such is not the case in mid-plane contractions, which most often are accompanied by contractions of the outlet. Furthermore, inlet contractions often are announced by failure of the head to engage. Not so with contractions of the deeper planes of the pelvis, where the occiput may present at the outlet before the difficulty is evident. These mid-plane and outlet contractions are treacherous. Operative interference should be avoided and delivery accomplished as far as possible by natural forces.

Much has been said about absolute mensuration. If the shape of the pelvis is wrong, even though the diameters may be adequate sufficient space may not be available for the fetal head. Thus, in the classic android pelvis the angulation of the fore pelvis makes this whole anterior segment unavailable and may be the seat of surprising difficulty. Furthermore, in this type of pelvis the greatest transverse diameter recedes toward the sacrum. Thus, an entirely false impression is given by knowing the mere numerical diameters of this pelvis. Configuration of the pelvis determines to what extent the measureable diameters are utilizable. No student of pelvimetry can fail to ignore the import of pelvic morphology.

The final test of any pelvis is the passage of the fetal head through it. Inasmuch as the head cannot be measured, nor can the forces be foretold, the eventual decision rests frequently upon a trial of labor. Such a trial need not be long. In fact, if all the data discussed above have been obtained, the obstetrician should be able to determine in a very few hours the chances of success. During this period the morale of the patient should be sustained by encouragement and by the actual presence of the obstetrician. The peak of the pains can be dulled by Demerol, but deep sedation or anatomic block probably is contraindicated.

UTERINE INERTIA

This term commonly is employed to indicate uterine dysfunction. It is mis-

TABLE 36. PER CENT DIFFICULTY IN EFFECTING DELIVERY

		Anteroposterior	
		<10	>10
Transverse	>12	0.34	11.4
	<12	10.94	30.8

leading, difficult to define exactly, and includes a number of different entities springing from a multiplicity of causes.

The observations made earlier in this book on normal labor are of considerable importance in understanding the rationale of treatment of uterine dysfunction. We indicated that in normal labor there were regularly occurring contractions and a progressive and continuous dilatation of the cervix. This was accomplished (1) by the presence of a decreasing gradient of activity from the fundus to the lower uterine segment, (2) by an increasing disparity between the work done by the fundus and that by the lower uterine segment as labor progresses, (3) by good synchronization between the various parts of the uterus during contraction and (4) by an amniotic fluid pressure level that exceeds 15 mm. of mercury during contraction. Failure of the uterus to contract with sufficient vigor and co-ordination in order to effect continuous cervical dilatation stems from a distortion of the above-mentioned patterns and results in prolongation of labor. Clinically, two types of inertia exist. In some instances, labor is desultory from the onset, with pains occurring at more or less infrequent intervals and with irregular intensity. Sometimes these contractions are painful, out of proportion to their palpated force, and significant cervical dilatation does no ensue. In these instances, labor may last for several days. On other occasions, labor begins normally, and cervical dilatation progresses to a point at which the pains become ineffective and the force of the uterine contractions decrease to a point at which cervical dilatation no longer occurs. These two clinical types have been named *primary* and *secondary* uterine inertia, respectively. While these terms defy exact definition, and some confusion exists regarding their meaning, they do serve to differentiate two clinical conditions whose treatment and physiologic bases are quite different.

Little or nothing is known regarding the etiology of primary uterine inertia. It may be associated with developmental defects of the uterus, malposition of the fetus or cephalopelvic disproportion. While it does not occur in any particular body type, it is apt to be found in nervous, high-strung, worrisome individuals. The placid, mature parturient rarely has primary uterine inertia. Also, there can be little doubt that premature use of sedatives or, especially, block analgesics can, and do, cause cases of primary uterine inertia. However, in our experience, this is not a major causative factor. Endocrine imbalance and, in particular, insufficient estrogen may play a role, although efforts to counteract this abnormality with large doses of estrogen have failed to produce uniformly satisfactory results.

The patient with primary uterine inertia frequently complains of pains that are out of proportion to their severity on palpation. At the height of the contractions the uterus still can be indented readily, in spite of vigorous protestations from the patient. Furthermore, the cervix does not dilate progressively, although some effacement and perhaps slight dilatation may take place after long hours. This process can be differentiated from false labor by the fact that it continues, whereas false labor terminates spontaneously. Tracings with the multichannel strain gauge tokodynamometer do not establish a very clear differentiation between these two entities. The contraction patterns have no rule as to regularity, either in frequency or in force. The fundal waves are sharp in both ascent and descent, and no plateau exists. Frequently the midzone contraction equals, or is of greater intensity than, those in the fundus, and there is no absolute fundal dominance. It is this reversal of fundal dominance that produces the feeling of pain out of proportion to the severity of the contraction. Also, numerous contractions fail to exert a pressure in excess of 15 mm. of mercury, which is the critical level, below which cervical dilatation will not occur.

At the present state of our knowledge, the therapy of choice is time and sedation. While tempting, active interference is of little avail. Even such mild agents as frequent enemas or large doses of castor oil serve only to exhaust the patient and to increase her discomfort and her mental anguish. In most instances, artificial rupture of the membranes will not alter or increase the abnormal contraction pattern. Furthermore, this procedure may interject the danger of infection on an already trying situation. Usually, the stimulation of labor with pituitary extract in the face of true primary inertia is unsuccessful; in fact, pre-existing abnormal patterns of contractility may be worsened by such treatment, and the fetal oxygenation may be jeopardized. Often it happens that some cervical dilatation can be obtained with oxytocic therapy, but the drug becomes ineffective before full dilatation can be achieved, and cesarean section may be necessary. In time, mild sedation and liberal use of antibiotics usually will eventuate in a successful outcome. The dose in sedation chosen should be adequate to inhibit the ineffective uterine contractions and to give the patient adequate sleep and rest. For this purpose we use 16 mg. (1/4 gr.) morphine or 100 mg. of Demerol plus 0.1 to 0.2 Gm. (1 1/2 to 3 gr.) of a short-acting barbiturate. These patients frequently eat poorly during this period. The urine should be watched for acetone, and adequate supportive therapy in the form of dextrose and saline infusion should be given. Unfortunately, primary uterine inertia is accompanied frequently by spontaneous premature rupture of the membranes. This is of bad prognostic import. The obstetrician should assure himself that no cephalopelvic disproportion exists. Even if such disproportion is not present, in view of the real hazard to the infant in primary inertia, the abnormality should not be allowed to become unduly prolonged. If the patient begins to show evidence of infection, the uterus should be emptied promptly by cesarean section. The anesthesia chosen in this case should be of the anatomic type.

Occasionally, the cervix will dilate slowly with primary uterine inertia. In the primigravida, if it attains a dilatation of 3 cm., or in the multipara, of 4, it can be anticipated that intravenous pituitary extract will bring labor to a successful termination.

Secondary uterine inertia also is difficult to define precisely. In general, it includes labor that starts normally but

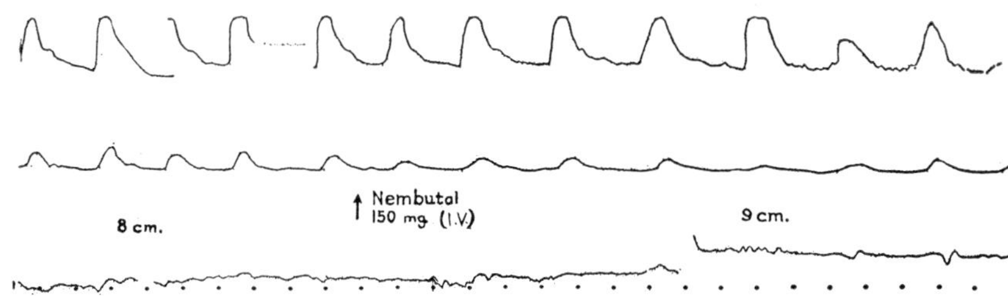

Fig. 96. Tokodynagraph showing lack of effect of intravenous Nembutal on uterine contractions. (Hellman, L. M.: M. Clin. North America 35:791)

falters in mid-course, regardless of the etiology. This implies naturally that there is some prolongation of labor, and that there is a period of delay in cervical dilatation. Prolongation of labor over 20 hours should bring about a considered re-evaluation of the causes and the expected outcome. The delay in cervical dilatation necessary to make the diagnosis of secondary uterine inertia is subject to some disagreement. Actually, inasmuch as normal labor implies a continuous dilatation, any delay may be pathologic. The more astute the obstetrician and the sooner he is aware of this delay, the sooner he can initiate therapy, and the better his results will be. Not only is there disagreement about the exact terms of the definition, but there is also a divergence of opinion as to the type of therapy advocated.

Custom decrees two main types of treatment: (1) rest–sedation and support; (2) uterine stimulation by enemas, change of position, rupture of the membranes and oxytocics. The first is based on the concept that the uterus becomes tired and requires rest in order to resume its task in a satisfactory manner. The second is based upon the theory that in normal labor there is no exhaustion of smooth muscle provided the general condition of the mother is good. It employs an ascending scale of stimulation, beginning with the relatively innocuous enema and progressing through more definitive measures to oxytocics. A better and a more thorough understanding of the etiologic and the physiologic bases of secondary uterine inertia might indicate a more rational approach to therapy.

In an analysis of 10,000 labors at the Kings County Hospital, secondary uterine inertia occurred in 3.0 per cent of cases with an infant mortality of 4.7 per cent. No common etiologic condition was found. In the absence of fetal malposition or pelvic or uterine abnormalities, it may be that some form of analgesia, particularly spinal and caudal, does contribute to inertia of this type. However, this is not the rule, and, once labor is established definitely and sedation is started, even anatomic blockade causes only a momentary delay in labor. The drugs used in the anatomic approach to pain relief can cause complete cessation of labor in some cases if the level becomes higher than thoracic 9.

Studies with the multichannel tokodynamometer have delineated three types of abnormality in secondary uterine inertia.

1. The contractions are few, irregular and far apart. The uterine pressure is less than 15 mm. of mercury, and fundal dominance is not absolute. The patient feels few, if any, pains, and the uterus is not contracted readily on palpation.
2. The contractions are more or less regular, rather firm and extremely painful. While the uterine pressure is adequate, there is a reversal of the contraction pattern with the mid-segment doing more work than the fundus.
3. Rarely, there is asynchronism between the right and the left sides of the fundus or between the upper and the lower segments. When this persists, cervical dilatation will not occur.

While these three highly different patterns exist singly in secondary uterine inertia, there are instances in which combinations of all three are present. Therapy should be directed toward correction or, at least, amelioration of these pattern abnormalities and toward the resumption of strong and effective uterine contraction.

In the face of a reversal of gradient where the pain complained of by the patient is greater than one would suppose on palpation, rest and sedation may be expected to give better results than stimulation. The use of morphine or Demerol plus short-acting barbiturates, as indicated above, should produce from

4 to 5 hours of adequate rest. The additional administration of 5 to 10 per cent dextrose is a helpful supportive adjunct. If one is fortunate, good labor will begin spontaneously or with the stimulation of an enema when the patient awakes. When this does not occur, the lapse of time adds greatly to the possibility of uterine infection and fetal exodus. Even with the proper antibiotic therapy, intra-uterine infection does occur although the maternal temperature may be normal. This not only presents a definite hazard to the fetus, but it makes more doubtful the successful termination of labor with Pitocin stimulation.

There is no question that uterine stimulation, if successful, presents a far more satisfactory answer to the problem. Usually, the simple remedies of enema and walking are tried before more radical therapy, such as rupture of the membranes and pituitary extract. Frequently, rupture of the membranes is successful alone. It commits the obstetrician definitely and implies that delivery must be accomplished within the near, foreseeable future. Failure to achieve this goal may result in fetal death and in grave danger to the mother. Either at the time of rupture of the membranes or within a short period, the uterus should be stimulated with pituitary extract. Present knowledge would seem to indicate that while there is little difference in the oxytocic effect between pituitrin and Pitocin, since the latter lacks the pressor substance, it is the drug of choice. In recent times, most Pitocin in labor has been given by the continuous intravenous drip technic. This is a more physiologic method of administering the drug, and apparently it yields more satisfactory and safer results. It was first suggested by Page, but more recently it has been the subject of intense study with reports appearing in many publications. In general, Pitocin is mixed thoroughly with 5 per cent dextrose at a concentration of 1 min., or frequently less, per 100 cc. of solution. At this concentration, 50 cc. of solution will contain 0.5 min. of Pitocin. If it is desired to give this amount over a 30-minute period, it will be necessary to administer the solution at the rate of 1.7 cc. per minute.

The glucose solution containing the Pitocin is placed in an intravenous bottle, with a Murphy drip apparatus interposed in the rubber tubing and an adjustable clamp placed above the Murphy drip device. This should be tested prior to administering the solution to the patient in order to determine the number of drops per minute necessary to give 1 cc. With the needle flow entirely shut off, the needle is inserted into an arm vein and the number of drops per minute slowly increased in order to yield from 0.25 to 0.5 min. per half hour. The usual rate is about 25 to 30 drops per minute, although this can be reduced considerably and adequate therapeutic results still obtained. It is very important not to have the solution flowing when the needle is inserted, because in this way dangerous amounts of Pitocin may be given before the rate of flow is regulated properly. The number of drops per minute always should be built up from 0 slowly and the therapeutic result observed. The patient never should be left alone for a single moment while the solution is running, because the best of clamps slip sometimes, and occasionally the patient exhibits untoward reactions or titanic contractions. Occasionally, also, the fetal heart tones may show alterations. If this does occur, the drip should be discontinued until the cause of the abnormality has been determined. This has happened rarely in our experience, and when it has occurred we have found that an immediate stopping of the flow corrects these disturbances at once and that no harm has been done.

Several factors influence adversely the

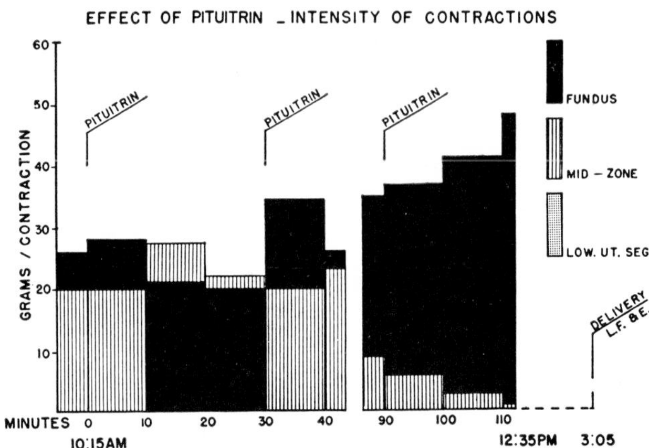

FIG. 97. The effect of intermittent administration of ½ min. intramuscular Pituitrin. The reversal of work is shown at the 10-minute mark and lasts through the 30-minute mark. (Hellman, L. M.: M. Clin. North America 35:791)

success of intravenous Pitocin therapy in the treatment of secondary uterine inertia. These are intrapartum fever, long labor prior to the onset of therapy, high station of the head prior to the onset of therapy and prolongation of inertia before treatment.

Even the proper use of intravenous pituitary extract, employed without delay in diagnosis as soon as secondary uterine inertia has become apparent, meets with failure in some cases. Studies with the multichannel tokodynamometer have thrown some light on this failure rate. There is a tendency for pituitary extract to produce a reversal of fundal dominance in normal labor. In most instances, this reversal can be broken through if the dosage is repeated but not increased. The occurrence of reversal seems to be related to the magnitude of the dose, as indicated in Figure 97, which shows the loss of fundal dominance and breakthrough with single intramuscular doses of pituitary extract in normal labor. In the following charts, the degree of fundal dominance is measured numerically by the work index, which is the work done by fundus divided by that of the mid-zone. The larger the number, the more efficacious the contractions. In Figure 98, while the contractions increased in force and frequency, there was no increase in the work index. However, if the single-dose method was changed to the continuous intravenous method, quite the contrary situation prevailed, as indicated in Figure 99, where there was a very marked increase in fundal dominance. It is probable that instances of a reversal of fundal dominance occur even with the use of extremely infinitesimal doses by the intravenous method. This may account for the small but persistent cases of failure in treatment of secondary uterine inertia by this method.

Always in an inert labor, the patient is aware that some abnormality exists. She tends to be worried and disturbed. The occurrence of pain when the uterus is being stimulated does not add to her peace of mind. We have found that the anatomic control of pain, such as continuous caudal or continuous peridural, is a very satisfactory adjunct to the use of pituitary extract, and in no way does it decrease its efficacy. Furthermore, in inert labor, and especially in those instances in which oxytocics have been used, the fetus may have been subjected to episodes of hypoxia. In considering anesthesia for delivery, this always should be borne in mind. Thus it is far better to use some anatomic approach—either a continuation of the caudal or the peridural or the administration of low dosage spinal or local infiltration.

In most cases of secondary uterine inertia, when Pitocin stimulation works,

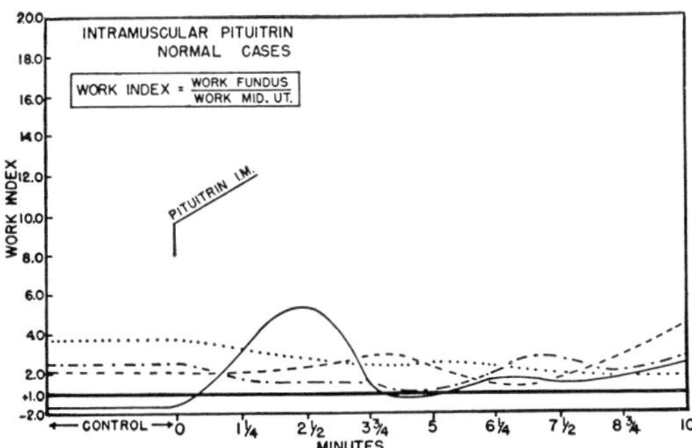

FIG. 98. The work index in 4 normal cases after the injection of 1/4 min. intramuscular Pituitrin. (Hellman, L. M.: M. Clin. North America 35:791)

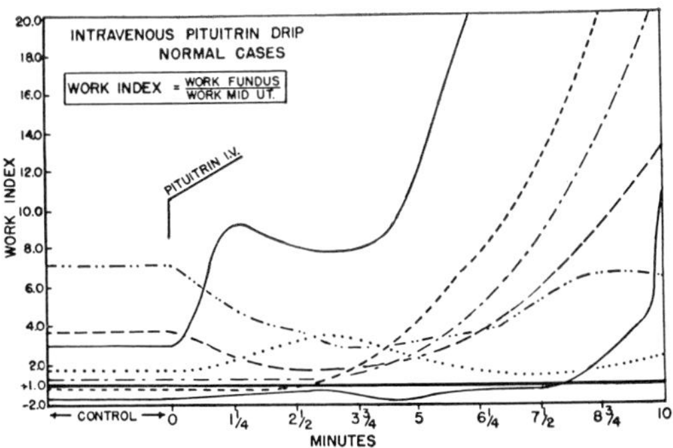

FIG. 99. The work index in 7 normal cases following the use of intravenous Pituitrin. (Hellman, L. M.: M. Clin. North America 35:791)

it is quickly successful. If one infusion of 500 cc. has been only partially successful in securing full dilatation, a short rest of 2 to 3 hours is advisable before the second infusion is begun. It is not wise to stimulate these patients beyond that point. Failure of stimulation is an indication for cesarean section.

A Safety Code for the Use of Pituitary Extract

1. Don't with borderline pelvic contraction
2. Don't with fetal malposition
3. Don't with parity greater than IV
4. Don't with age greater than 34
5. Don't leave the patient unattended
6. Don't when in doubt

MALPOSITIONS

Occiput Posterior and Extended Positions

The most minor of the abnormalities of position of the fetus is the presentation by posterior occiput. In the majority of instances, the posterior occiput will rotate to the anterior, and delivery will take place in a normal fashion. In at least 3 per cent of cases, the occiput remains in the posterior position. In these cases of persistent occiput posterior, one school of thought holds that the occiput should be rotated, either manually or by forceps, and delivered as an anterior occiput. Another is of the opinion that the persistent posterior occiput is the result of peculiar pelvic configuration, especially of the sacrum and the posterosagittal diameter. This latter effects delivery with a deep mediolateral episiotomy. In any event, no special attention need be given to analgesia or anesthesia in this abnormality, if indeed it can be termed such.

Extension of the fetal head rather than flexion during labor causes the fetus to present by either the face or the brow. Examination of Figures 101 and 102 will show quite readily that a normal-sized infant cannot be delivered vaginally by brow presentation, and this can be done in face presentation only if the chin is anterior and the occiput occupies a hollow of the sacrum. Diagnosis of these presentations is made by abdominal palpation when the cephalic prominence is found on the same side as the back, and by vaginal examination when the orbital ridges and other features of the face can be palpated.

The causes of these extended positions are manifold, but in most series contracted pelvis looms large. It is important to bear this in mind, for x-ray

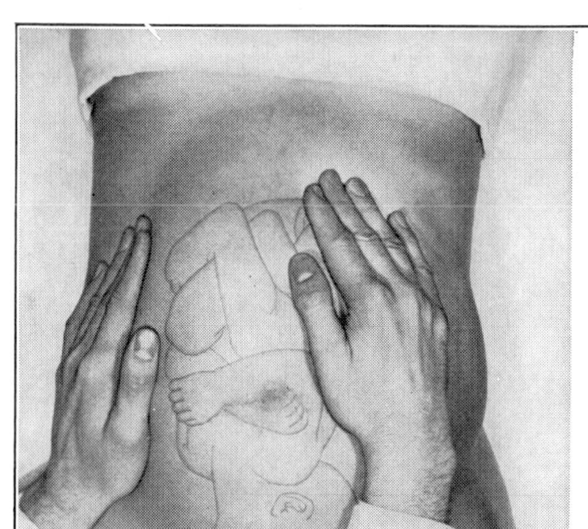

1st Maneuver

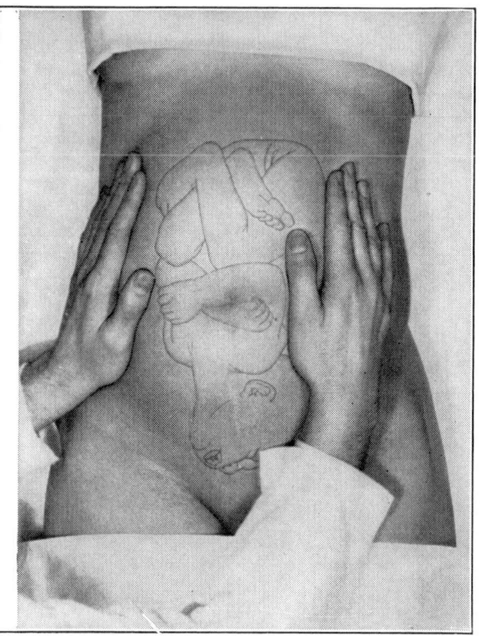

2nd Maneuver

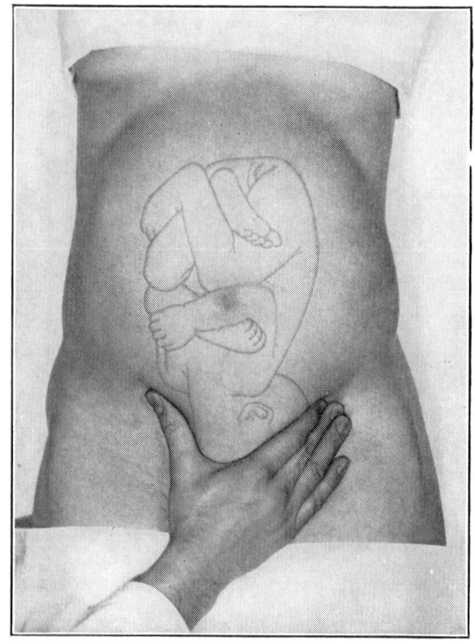

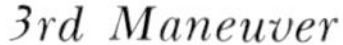

3rd Maneuver

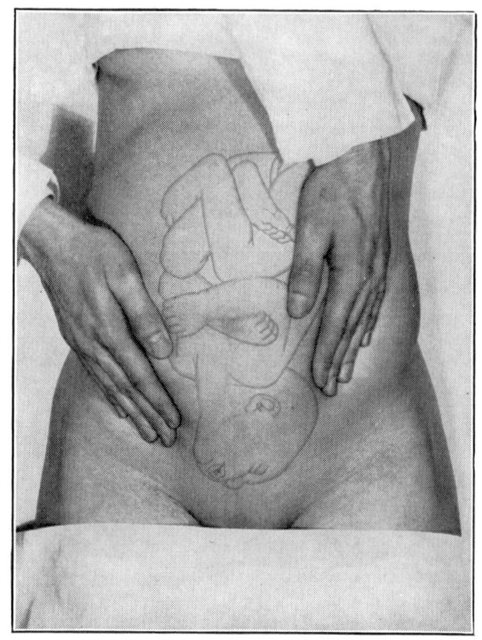

4th Maneuver

Fig. 100. Palpation in right mento-anterior position. (Eastman, N. J.: Williams Obstetrics, ed. 11, New York, Appleton)

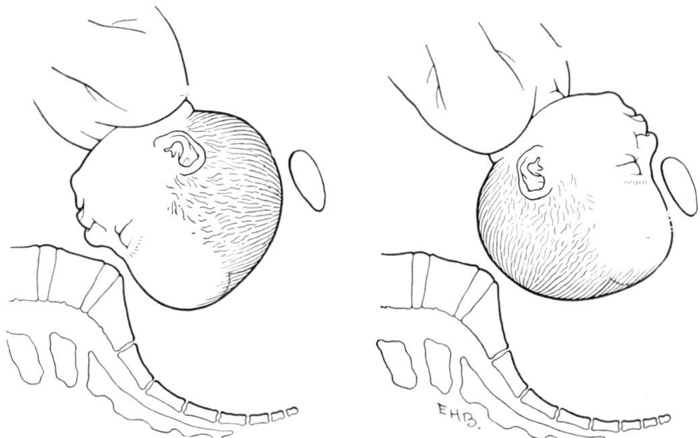

Fig. 101. Brow presentation. (*Left*) Posteriorly. (*Right*) Anteriorly. (Eastman, N. J.: Williams Obstetrics, ed. 11, New York, Appleton)

pelvimetry is always desirable and often indicates the type of delivery.

In the majority of face presentations with adequate pelvis, the chin will rotate anteriorly late in labor, and termination can be effected either spontaneously with deep episiotomy or by means of a simple forceps. However, the over-all fetal mortality in this condition is approximately 14 per cent, and any significant degree of pelvic contraction or persistence of the chin in the posterior position should be an indication for cesarean section.

Brow presentations are somewhat rarer than face presentations, although their etiology is the same. Often, they are transitory, being a stage in the spontaneous evolution of either face or occiput presentations. If the brow persists, cesarean section is the only means of terminating labor safely.

There are several recognized methods either of converting the extended positions of the head to flexed occiput presentation or rotating persistent posterior face presentations. These should be attempted only if the pelvis is normal. To be successful, such vaginal manipulations should be conducted under deep anesthesia with membranes either intact or very recently ruptured. These attempts

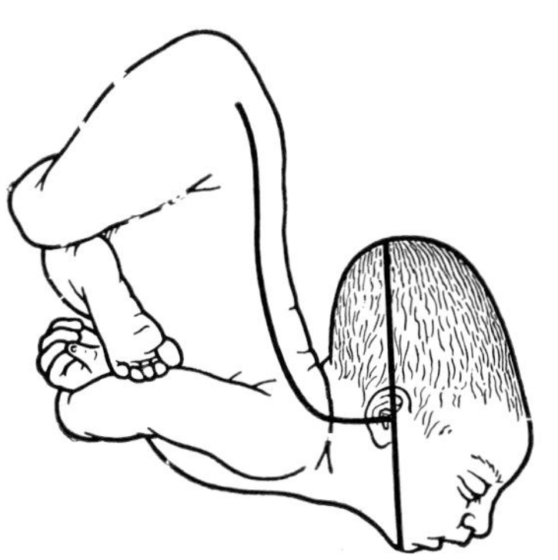

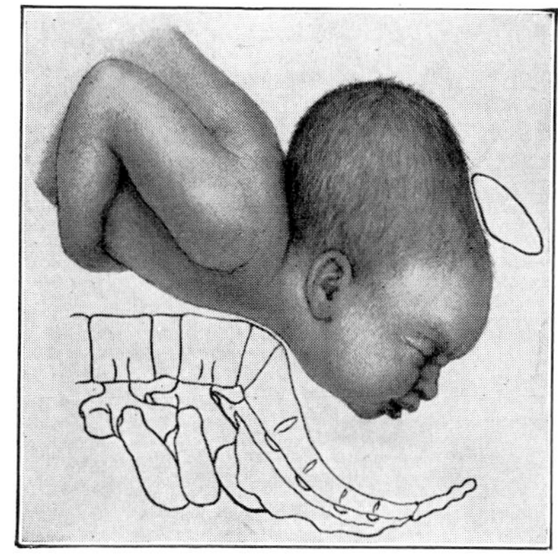

Fig. 102. Face presentation. (*Left*) Occiput on the long end of head lever. (*Right*) Chin directly posterior, showing impossibility of spontaneous delivery, unless rotation occurs. (Eastman, N. J.: Williams Obstetrics, ed. 11, New York, Appleton)

TABLE 37. TOTAL LOSS AND INFANT MORTALITY FOR PREMATURES AND FULL-TERM INFANTS AMONG MOTHERS WITH BREECHES ACCORDING TO METHODS OF ADMINISTERING ANESTHESIA

Methods	*Number**			*Rate per 1,000 total births*		
	Total Infants	Still-births	Neonatal Deaths	Total Loss	Still-births	Neonatal Deaths
			Total Infants			
All methods	297	5	15	67.3	16.8	50.5
No anesthesia	19	1	2	157.9	52.6	105.3
Intravenous and inhalation	147	2	3	34.0	13.6	20.4
Caudal and spinal	102	2	8	98.0	19.6	78.4
Local	7	—	1	142.9	—	142.9
Combination of methods	22	—	1	45.5	—	45.5
			Prematures			
All methods	68	2	11	191.2	29.4	161.8
No anesthesia	9	1	2	333.3	111.1	222.2
Intravenous and inhalation	24	—	3	125.0	—	125.0
Caudal and spinal	24	1	5	250.0	41.7	208.3
Local	6	—	1	166.7	—	166.7
Combination of methods	5	—	—	—	—	—
			Full Term			
All methods	229	3	4	30.6	13.1	17.5
No anesthesia	10	—	—	—	—	—
Intravenous and inhalation	123	2	—	16.3	16.3	—
Caudal and spinal	78	1	3	51.3	12.8	38.5
Local	1	—	—	—	—	—
Combination of methods	17	—	1	58.8	—	58.8

* Twins, infants who died before onset of labor and analgesia and infants with congenital malformations incompatible with life, are excluded.

at conversion are successful sometimes, but they require very adequate relaxation and the presence of a considerable amount of amniotic fluid.

Anesthesia for Extended Positions of the Fetal Head

For Vaginal Delivery:

Analgesia (encephalic, routine). Anatomic (not recommended because of late perineal rotation of face).

Anesthesia: Encephalic (routine). Anatomic (terminal saddle block). Local (infiltration).

For Vaginal and Intra-uterine Manipulation:

Anesthesia (encephalic—ether or chloroform, unless contraindicated, then cyclopropane).

For Cesarean Section:

See discussion of cesarean section anesthesia.

BREECH PRESENTATIONS

Breech presentation is one of the more frequent malpositions; it occurs in approximately 3 per cent of deliveries. In addition, it is one of the most important from the standpoint of both obstetrician and anesthesiologist, for it carries with it a fetal loss rate in term infants of nearly three times the expected rate (Table 38). In addition, it has an over-all fetal mortality rate of from 10 to 20 per cent. A recent report by Hall indicates that the gross fetal mortality rate is 9.9 per cent.

The etiology of breech presentation is obscure, but prematurity, as well as contracted pelvis and other abnormalities of the birth canal, may play a role.

Breech presentation is divided into three types as follows:

1. **Complete Breech.** The feet and the legs are flexed on the thighs, and the thighs are flexed on the abdomen, so that the buttocks and the feet present.

2. **Incomplete Breech** (Footling). One or both feet present through the cervix.

3. **Frank Breech.** The legs are extended and lie against the abdomen and the chest with the feet meeting the solars. The buttocks alone present.

This classification is important, because it has some bearing on the high fetal mortality. One of the factors in infant loss in breech presentation is prolapse of the cord. This accident occurs in 0.5 per cent of deliveries. Moore and Steptoe found its occurrence to be the same for frank breech, but 22 and 12 times higher in incomplete and complete breech, respectively.

The somber prognosis for the child is due to several additional factors. In the first place, when the buttocks are born, the umbilicus is at the pelvic brim, and the cord may be compressed. While the unjeopardized infant can endure this compression for some time, one that has been subjected to periods of anoxia during labor can stand this additional insult only for an exceedingly brief period. Furthermore, Holland and Capon have shown that the after-coming head is subject to additional strains, and that the possibility of tentorial tear and subsequent intracranial hemorrhage is twice as great in breech as in vertex presentation.

Breech deliveries may be of three types:

1. **Spontaneous breech delivery,** in which the entire infant is expelled by natural forces without any traction being applied and without any manipulation other than support of the infant. This is uncommon.

2. **A partial breech extraction,** in which the infant is extruded as far as the umbilicus by natural forces, but the remainder of the body is extracted by the attendant.

3. **A total breech extraction,** in which the entire body of the infant is extracted by the obstetrician.

Variations in the technic of breech delivery depend upon the type of presentation, the well-being of the infant and the skill of the surgeon. They need not be dealt with in detail here, but there are a few general principles that have a bearing on analgesia and in particular on anesthesia, and these should be discussed.

In the first place, it is of extreme importance that the measurements of the pelvis be known accurately by means of x-ray pelvimetry. This is of special importance in primigravidas, but it should not be neglected in the multipara, even though an adequate-sized infant has been delivered previously by vertex. The least degree of significant pelvic contraction should be an indication for cesarean section. In addition, particularly in primigravidas, in view of the extremely poor infant prognosis, cesarean section is indicated if any other abnormality occurs that jeopardizes the infant. While not wishing to be completely dogmatic on this aspect of the subject, the appearance of uterine inertia, in combination with breech presentation, is probably an indication for cesarean section. This is said in spite of the good results with Pitocin stimulation reported by some.

Labor in breech presentation may be somewhat prolonged. In addition, a fair degree of maternal co-operation may be necessary to expel the breech as far as the umbilicus. These two factors should be borne in mind in selecting a pain-relief program for a patient with this complication. Furthermore, one always should be alert to the fact that in breech, fetal distress may occur after full dilatation and may require quick action, for which anesthesia is necessary. Even in the more normal cases of partial breech extraction, there always is a little importance on the haste of the surgeon and hurry in the induction of anesthesia.

In the Baltimore study, some type of encephalic analgesia, plus terminal inhalation or intravenous anesthesia, was chosen in 50 per cent of the cases, and an additional 15 per cent had encephalic analgesia and terminal block or local infiltration. Only one fifth of the cases were conducted entirely under caudal analgesia. The reason for this is the difficulty in achieving spontaneous birth to the umbilicus under this form of pain relief and the resultant increase in complete breech extraction. This operation can be done under caudal anesthesia, but it requires patience and skill, and it is not a procedure for the occasional surgeon. Furthermore, it should not be attempted if the infant is excessive in size. Technically, complete extraction is easier if relaxation is more complete, as with inhalation anesthesia.

There is probably no ideal analgesia and anesthesia program for a patient with a breech presentation. Whereas the continuous block methods make it possible to intervene at any time and on short notice, they do not give sufficient relaxation in all cases to perform the operative procedure necessary. On the other hand, the encephalic forms of approach, particularly inhalation anesthesia, require some time for induction. Although in the Baltimore study intravenous anesthesia was not used too often, if the breech has been born spontaneously to the umbilicus, this furnishes one of the best methods of handling the remainder of the delivery. Similarly, particularly in multiparas, the conduct of labor under analgesia with terminal local infiltration furnishes a program of some merit.

Analgesia and Anesthesia for Breech Presentation

Spontaneous or Partial Extraction:

Analgesia (encephalic, routine).

Psychoanalgesia (anatomic, caudal).

Anesthesia: Encephalic (inhalation—cyclopropane with the Reserve Midget machine. Intravenous). Anatomic terminal block. Local infiltration. Caudal.

Breech Extraction:

Encephalic (inhalation—ether, cyclopropane).

Anatomic (not recommended for the inexperienced operator).

The infant mortality in breech presentation by various methods of anesthesia is shown in Table 35. In considering the full-term infants only, there is an apparent advantage in the encephalic approach, as indicated by the intravenous and the inhalation methods. However, the numbers are small, and the difference is not of statistical significance.

Transverse Presentation

In transverse presentation, the long axis of the fetus lies perpendicular to the long axis of the mother. It occurs approximately once in every 200 deliveries, more frequently in multiparas than in primiparas, and it carries with it an extremely high infant mortality. Not infrequently, labor is complicated by the prolapse of the cord or a small part. If the fetus is alive and if labor is not near termination, cesarean section offers the best method of solution. However, if the cervix is dilated almost fully, a bag can be placed through it, and version and extraction can be done at full dilatation. However, if the membranes have been ruptured for any length of time, this operation also becomes difficult. In neglected transverse presentations with the fetus dead and impacted into the pelvis, decapitation can be carried out with a sickle knife and subsequent delivery effected. Transverse lie is a serious complication of labor. In neglected forms, rupture of the uterus can occur, while even in unneglected cases there always is a much greater risk to the baby than with either vertex or breech presentation. In those cases in which vaginal manipulation is to be carried out, particularly if version and extraction are to be done, deep ether anesthesia is necessary to give adequate relaxation.

Multiple Pregnancy

According to Guttmacher, twinning occurs in the United States in 1.108 per cent of births. There is considerable variation in this figure according to racial stock. Thus, twins occur rather more frequently in the nonwhite than the white. If the twinning frequency in the population is expressed as $1/N$, then a mathematical approximation as to the occurrence of triplets will be $1/N^2$.

The infant mortality in twin gestation is at least twice that for single pregnancy. This is entirely understandable when one considers that toxemia, premature separation of the placenta, placenta previa and malformations are many times more frequent in multiple gestation. Perhaps, however, prematurity here also takes the greatest toll. Twin pregnancies terminate from 2 to 3 weeks prior to the expected date of confinement. The infant mortality also increases with the size of the litter, being cited by Record as 15.2 per cent for twins as against 30.9 per cent for triplets.

Table 38. Number of Stillbirths and Neonatal Deaths Among Multiple Births According to the Method of Administering Drugs

Methods	Total Infants*	Stillbirths	Neonatal Deaths
All methods	223	1	4
No anesthesia	15	—	2
Inhalation	69	—	—
Intravenous	4	—	—
Caudal	72	1	—
Spinal	35	—	1
Local	7	—	1
Combination of methods	21	—	—
	Total Loss	**Stillbirths**	**Neonatal Deaths**
Rate per 1,000 births	44.8	9.0	35.8

* Cesarean sections, infants who died before onset of labor and analgesia and infants with congenital malformations incompatible with life, are excluded. (Baltimore Obstetric Anesthesia Study)

Multiple gestation constitutes a real hazard to the mother. This is due largely to the combined occurrence of toxemia and postpartum hemorrhage. The best protection these mothers can have is meticulous prenatal care, spontaneous delivery and complete readiness to cover any postpartum blood loss.

Usually, labor in twin gestation is not prolonged. Due to the great distention of the uterus, the cervix often is effaced partially and dilated at the onset of labor. Spontaneous delivery is the most satisfactory. As soon as the first twin is born, the obstetrician ruptures the membranes of the second sac and, by combined abdominal and vaginal manipulation, attempts to arrange the second twin in longitudinal presentation. If this can be accomplished, the presenting part is eased into the birth canal and delivered.

TABLE 39. PERCENTAGE OF FIRST AND SECOND TWINS IN POOR CONDITION AS INDICATED BY THE BREATHING AND THE CRYING TIME

	Breathing Time		
	Per cent	*Number* *	
Twin	One Plus Minute	Total Known	One Plus Minute
1st twin	1.9	105	2
2nd twin	9.2	109	10
	Crying Time		
	Per cent	*Number* *	
	Two Plus Minutes	Total Known	Two Plus Minutes
1st twin	11.4	105	12
2nd twin	23.9	109	26

* Stillbirths, cesarean sections, infants who died before onset of labor and analgesia and infants with congenital malformations incompatible with life, are excluded.

There need be little delay between the 2 births. If the second twin cannot be manipulated properly, or if partial separation of the placenta occurs, prompt version and extraction should be done.

Table 38 shows that in the Baltimore study over half the multiple pregnancies were delivered by some form of anatomic anesthesia, caudal being the most popular. The advantages of this approach can be readily understood. It spares the small twin infants from the possible narcotic effects of general anesthesia. With the high infant mortality in plural gestation, any reduction in jeopardy may be worth while. Table 39 shows that this is no theoretic consideration. An analysis of breathing and crying times shows a significantly higher poor reaction in second twins. At Western Reserve University Hospitals we have determined cyclopropane blood levels in 3 mothers delivering twins as constant from 14 to 18 mg. per cent after 10 minutes of anesthesia at the time of birth of the first twin. The cord blood cyclopropane of the 3 first twins varied from 8 to 11 mg. per cent. The cord blood cyclopropane of the 3 second twins delivered 5 to 8 minutes later was 14 to 17 mg. per cent. These studies indicate increased hazard to the second twin, who is exposed to transplacental cyclopropane for a longer period of time than the first twin. The great disadvantage of this approach is the lack of sufficient relaxation to do easily a version and extraction, should such be necessary. With skill and training, this operation can be carried out under caudal; however, it is done more easily if a little general anesthetic is added. It takes only a short time to achieve sufficient relaxation with a little superimposed cyclopropane. Perhaps this is an area in which the newly introduced Reserve Midget might serve.

CESAREAN SECTION

Cesarean section is performed currently in about 4 to 6 per cent of deliveries in modern obstetric teaching clinics. This figure shows great variation, depending on the material and the number of complicated cases referred to the various clinics. However, there can be little doubt that the more liberal use of this procedure has resulted in the saving of many infant lives and the reduction of obstetric injuries to mothers. Nevertheless, even when performed electively, cesarean section does not yield 100 per cent infant survival. According to most recent figures, the fetal loss in elective cesarean section is slightly in excess of 1 per cent. Because cesarean section is performed in mechanically complicated obstetric cases, upon medically ill mothers or in an effort to save an already jeopardized infant, anesthesia for this operation should be selected with the greatest care and skill. Of course, the major consideration is the complication for which the cesarean section is done. A list of indications is

TABLE 40. RELATIVE INCIDENCE OF COMMON INDICATIONS FOR CESAREAN SECTION*

Pelvic contraction and mechanical dystocia	
Pelvic contraction	273
Uterine inertia	66
Malpresentations	44
Oversized baby	8
Tumor blocking birth canal	23
TOTAL	414
Previous cesarean section	240
Hemorrhagic complications	
Placenta previa	91
Abruptio placentae	49
TOTAL	140
Toxemias	
Preeclampsia	70
Chronic hypertensive vascular disease	26
TOTAL	96
Intercurrent disease	
Diabetes mellitus	14
Other	12
TOTAL	26
Miscellaneous	
Elderly primigravida	32
Other	52
TOTAL	84
GRAND TOTAL	1,000

* Eastman, N. J.: Williams Obstetrics, ed. 10, New York, Appleton, 1950.

shown in Table 40 for 1,000 consecutive cesarean sections.

Once one has selected the appropriate anesthesia for a given complication, then one can consider the fetus, its age and other factors that already have jeopardized its survival. A final consideration is the duration of the operative procedure.

There is a tendency to select complicated anatomic forms of anesthesia because they are supposed to give the infant the best chance of survival. Gordon, however, has pointed out that 25 per cent of the maternal deaths in Brooklyn still are related to cesarean section, and of these one fourth are related to anesthesia. The anesthesia selected never should be so complicated that it is beyond the capabilities of the staff to conduct it safely.

Taken all in all, when there is no contraindication, the anatomic methods of anesthesia offer both mother and infant the best opportunities for a satisfactory outcome. There are those who favor local infiltration; others prefer various methods of central vertebral block; still others prefer a combination of methods. In the Baltimore study, as indicated in Table 41, the anatomic methods of approach were used far more frequently than any others.

The infant mortality in these 401 cesarean sections is 59.6 per 1,000 total births. This is a satisfactory figure considering the complications involved. Again, because of the fact that there was individualization in the choice of anesthesia, there is little difference in the final infant results among the various methods.

TABLE 41. THE INCIDENCE OF VARIOUS TYPES OF ANESTHESIA FOR CESAREAN SECTION

METHOD	NUMBER*	PERCENTAGE
Anatomic		
Spinal	201	50.0
Combination†	91	22.8
Peridural	33	8.2
Caudal	21	5.2
Encephalic		
Intravenous	43	10.8
Inhalation	12	3.0
TOTAL	401	100.0

*Mothers of twins excluded.
†Usually, local infiltration or field block plus intravenous at the time of uterine incision.

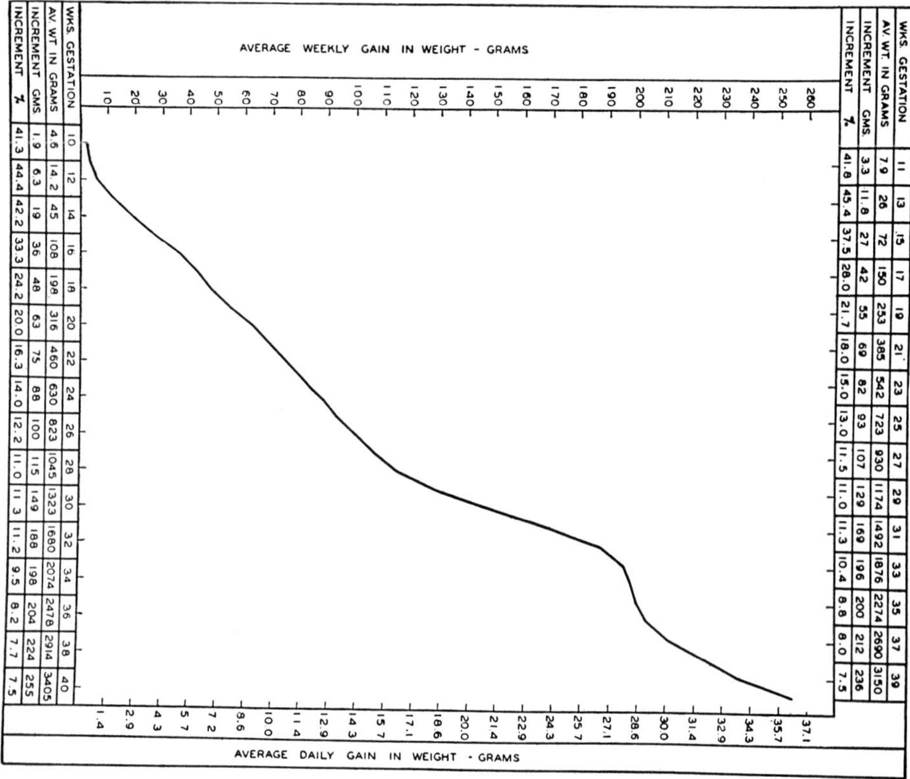

FIG. 103A. Average daily and weekly fetal gain in weight, with average weight of fetuses plotted with menstrual age of fetuses. (Streeter, G. L.: Contributions to Embryology, vol. 11, Carnegie Institution of Washington, Publication No. 274)

For more details concerning technics, see Chapter 4.

PREMATURITY

Prematurity accounts for almost half of the perinatal loss. There is no great mystery as to the cause of the deaths of these infants. Their organs are not fully enough developed for extra-uterine survival. Try as we may to create a satisfying artificial environment for them, we seem to have reached a point of diminishing returns in the improvement of nurseries and in the excellence of pediatric care. Were the causative factors in prematurity understood, then perhaps some prophylaxis could be undertaken to prevent its occurrence, with the resultant saving of many lives. Until such time we must do what we can in the care of the infant both during and after birth.

These premature births do not come unexpectedly. The anticipated date of delivery and the abdominal examination allow the obstetrician to guess pretty accurately the weight of the infant. Furthermore, roughly 40 per cent of these labors are related to obstetric causes such as placenta previa, premature separation of the placenta, toxemia, syphilis and heart disease. Certain labors are induced prematurely because the obstetrician feels that there is a better chance of extra-uterine survival than could be expected if the pregnancy were allowed to continue.

Many complicated classifications of

Table 42. Total Loss and Infant Mortality for Premature and Full-Term Infants Among Mothers Delivered by Cesarean Section According to Methods of Administering Anesthesia

Methods	Number* Total Infants	Number* Stillbirths	Number* Neonatal Deaths	Rate per 1,000 total births Total Loss	Rate per 1,000 total births Stillbirths	Rate per 1,000 total births Neonatal Deaths
				Total Infants		
All methods	386	1	22	59.6	2.6	57.0
Encephalic						
Intravenous and inhalation	47	—	3	63.8	—	63.8
Anatomic						
Caudal and spinal	252	—	14	55.6	—	55.6
Combination of methods	87	1	5	69.0	11.5	57.5
				Premature		
All methods	89	1	16	191.0	11.2	179.8
Encephalic						
Intravenous and inhalation	14	—	3	214.3	—	214.3
Anatomic						
Caudal and spinal	56	—	11	196.4	—	196.4
Combination of methods	19	1	2	157.9	52.6	105.3
				Full Term		
All methods	297	—	6	20.2	—	20.2
Encephalic						
Intravenous and inhalation	33	—	—	—	—	—
Anatomic						
Caudal and spinal	196	—	3	15.3	—	15.3
Combination of methods	68	—	3	44.1	—	44.1

* Twins, infants who died before onset of labor and analgesia and infants with congenital malformations, are excluded.

prematurity, such as combinations of weight, length and the duration of gestation, have been attempted. These have been replaced largely by the simple classification by weight. A premature infant is one who weighs less than 2,500 Gm. but more than 1,000 Gm. A glance at Figure 103 will show some justification for the selection of 2,500 Gm. as the upper limit. Above this weight the infant survival rate is nearly constant and almost equal to that of the term infant. The chances of survival below 1,000 Gm., although very poor, still are not zero. Infants weighing from this figure to 400 Gm. are classified as immature. Below 400 Gm. no known survival has occurred, and fetuses in this category are termed abortions.

In dealing with prematurity, the percentage chance of survival, as indicated in Figure 103, should be clearly understood. In addition, the data in Figure 104 give the weekly expected weight increment. These data have especial significance if the obstetrician contemplates early interruption of pregnancy.

A common error in handling premature labor is the administration of sedatives or narcotic drugs in a vain effort to halt the process. As has been indicated previously, these drugs traverse the placenta readily. In most instances, labor is not delayed by the administration of such drugs, and birth occurs within a short while at a time when the already feeble infant has received the maximum amount of drug. In general, patients undergoing premature labor should not receive in significant amounts any analgesic that crosses the placenta. This means that the encephalic approach to analgesia and to anesthesia is contraindicated. These patients are excellent candidates for anatomic forms of pain relief and for psychoanalgesia. At the time of delivery we prefer to use an episiotomy that can be performed easily under infiltration anesthesia, enabling the delivery to be completed spontaneously with properly directed and controlled fundal pressure. If this is not sufficient, an easy outlet forceps can be performed.

Analgesia and Anesthesia for Prematurity

Analgesia: Encephalic (contraindicated). Anatomic (all types). Psychoanalgesia for labor only.

Anesthesia: Encephalic (contraindicated). Anatomic (all types).

It will be noted from Table 41 that the anatomic approach to pain relief in prematurity was selected almost three times as frequently as any other in the Baltimore study. The figures for infant mortality are presented in Table 42. As could be anticipated, when the anesthesia and the analgesia were selected to fit the individual case, there was not a significant difference between conduction and encephalic methods in infant wastage. The apparent advantage enjoyed by intravenous anesthesia stems from the fact that this was used in heavier infants, while frequently no anesthesia was administered for the smaller and the less mature infants. The latter category yielded an anticipated disproportionate number of deaths.

TABLE 43. INCIDENCE OF VARIOUS TYPES OF ANESTHESIA IN PREMATURITY

METHOD	NUMBER		PERCENTAGE
Anatomic	431		60.6
Caudal		232	
Spinal		149	
Local		50	
Encephalic	174		24.5
Inhalation		139	
Intravenous		35	
Psychoanalgesia	87		12.2
Combination of methods	19		2.7

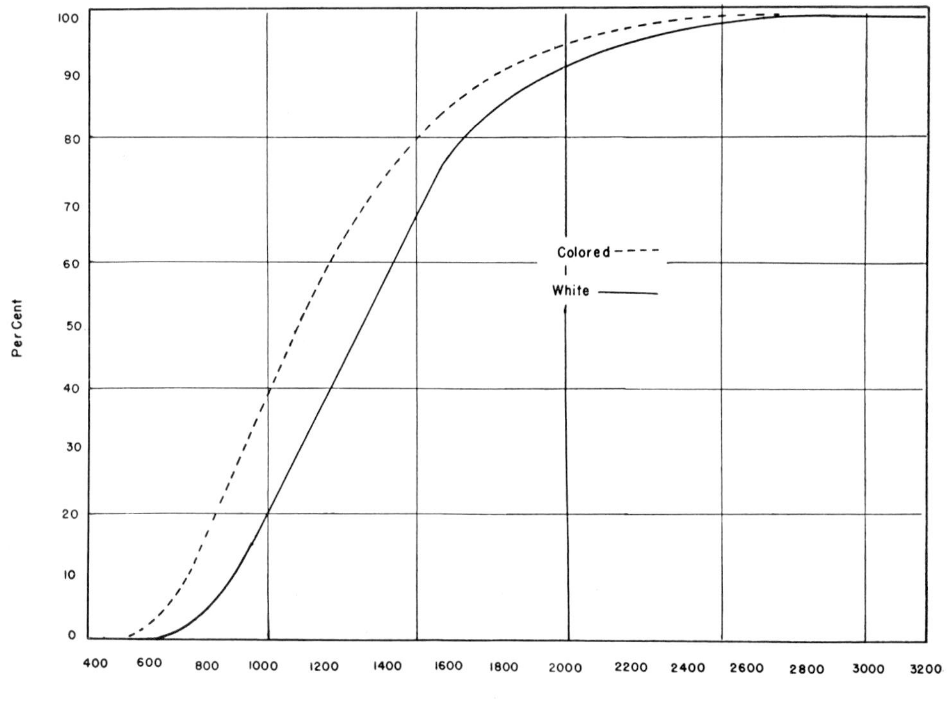

FIG. 103B. Infant survival by weight. (Kings County Hospital)

TABLE 44. TOTAL LOSS FOR PREMATURES* BY SPECIFIED BIRTHWEIGHT GROUPS ACCORDING TO METHODS OF ADMINISTERING ANESTHESIA

Method	*Number*†			*Rate per 1,000 total births*		
	Total Births	Still-births	Neonatal Deaths	Total Loss	Still-births	Neonatal Deaths
				1,000 to 1,999 Gm.		
Total	211	4	41	213.3	19.0	194.3
No anesthesia	34	1	10	323.5	29.4	294.1
Intravenous	6	—	1	166.7	—	166.7
Inhalation	35	—	6	171.4	—	171.4
Conduction:						
Caudal	69	3	8	159.4	43.5	115.9
Spinal	34	—	11	323.5		323.5
Local	31	—	5	161.3		161.3
Combination of methods	2	—	—	—	—	—
				2,000 to 2,499 Gm.		
Total	500	2	9	22.0	4.0	18.0
No anesthesia	53	—	1	18.9	—	18.9
Intravenous	29	—	—	—	—	—
Inhalation	104	—	5	48.1	—	48.1
Conduction						
Caudal	163	2	1	18.4	12.3	6.1
Spinal	115	—	1	8.7	—	8.7
Local	19	—	1	52.6	—	52.6
Combination of methods	17	—	—	—	—	—

* Prematures include all infants weighing 1,000 to 2,499 Gm. Sinai includes 4 live infants weighing less than 1,000 Gm.

† Twins, cesarean sections, infants who died before onset of labor and analgesia and infants with congenital malformation incompatible with life, are excluded.

BIBLIOGRAPHY

HEART DISEASE

Adams, J. Q.: Cardiovascular physiology in normal pregnancy: studies with the dye dilution technique, Am. J. Obst. & Gynec. **67**:741, 1954.

Drury, M. I., O'Driscoll, M. K., Hanrathy, T. D., and Barry, A. P.: Rheumatic heart disease complicating pregnancy, Brit. M. J. **1**:70, 1954.

Fitzgerald, J. E., Webster, A., Zummo, B. P., and Williams, P. C.: Evaluation of adequate antepartum care for the cardiac patient, J. A. M. A. **146**:910, 1951.

Gorenberg, H.: Rheumatic heart disease, Am. J. Obst. & Gynec. **45**:835, 1943.

Gorenberg, H., and Chesley, L. C.: Rheumatic heart disease in pregnancy: immediate and remote prognosis, Obst. & Gynec. **1**:15, 1953.

Hamilton, H. F. H.: The cardiac output in normal pregnancy as determined by the Cournand right heart catheterization technique, J. Obst. & Gynaec. Brit. Emp. **56**:548, 1949.

Linhard, J.: Über das Minutenvolum des Herzens bei Rukes und bei Muskelarbeit, Arch. ges. Physiol. **161**:233, 1915.

Palmer, A. J., and Walker, A. H. C.: The maternal circulation in normal pregnancy, J. Obst. & Gynaec. Brit. Emp. **56**:537, 1949.

Rose, D. J., Bader, R. A., Bader, M. E., and Braunwald, E.: Cardiac hemodynamics in pregnancy as studied by cardiac catheterization, Am. J. Obst. & Gynec. (In press)

Ullery, J. C.: The management of pregnancy complicated by heart disease, Am. J. Obst. & Gynec. **67**:834, 1954.

Werkö, L.: Pregnancy and heart disease, Acta obst. et gynec. scandinav. **33**:162. 1954.

———: Studies in the Problems of Circulation in Pregnancy. In Toxemias of Pregnancy, Ciba Symposium, Blakiston Co.. Phila., 1950.

Werkö, L., Bucht, H., Lagerlöf, H., and Holmgran, A.: Circulation vid graviditet, Nord. med. **40**:1868, 1948.

TOXEMIA

Assali, N. S., Kaplan, S. A., Foman, S. J., and Douglas, R. A., Jr.: Renal function studies in toxemia of pregnancy: Excretion of solutes and renal hemodynamics during osmotic diuresis, J. Clin. Invest. 32:44, 1953.

Assali, N. S., and Prystowsky, H.: Studies on autonomic blockade, J. Clin. Invest. **29**:1354, 1950.

Chesley, L. C.: Kidney function in the normal and toxemic pregnant woman, M. Clin. North America **35**:699, 1951.

———: Weight changes and water balance in normal and toxic pregnancy, Am. J. Obst. & Gynec. **48**:565, 1944.

Chesley, L. C., Annitto, J. E., and Jarvis, D. G.: A study of the interaction of pregnancy and hypertensive disease, Am. J. Obst. & Gynec. **53**:851, 1947.

Chesley, L. C., and Chesley, E. R.: An analysis of some factors associated with the development of pre-eclampsia, Am. J. Obst. & Gynec. **45**:748, 1943.

Cosgrove, S. A., and Chesley, L. C.: The clinical management of the late toxemia of pregnancy, Obst. & Gynec. Surv. **3**:769, 1948.

Dieckmann, W. J.: The Toxemias of Pregnancy, 2 ed., St. Louis, Mosby, 1952.

Freis, E. D., and Kenney, J. F.: Plasma volume, total circulating protein, and "available fluid" abnormalities in preeclampsia and eclampsia, J. Clin. Invest. **27**:283, 1948.

Govan, A. D. T., Mulherjce, C. L., Hewitt, J., and Harper, W. F.: The humoral origin of hypertension in toxaemia of pregnancy, J. Obst. & Gynaec. Brit. Emp. **58**:217, 1951.

Hallum, A. V.: Eye changes in hypertensive toxemia of pregnancy, J. A. M. A. **106**:1649, 1936.

Hertig, A. T.: Vascular pathology in the hypertensive albuminuric toxemias of pregnancy, Clinics **4**:602, 1945.

Irving, F. C.: The vascular aspects of eclampsia, Am. J. Obst. & Gynec. **31**:466, 1936.

Landesman, R., Douglas, R. G., and Holze, E.: The bulbar conjunctival vascular bed in the toxemias of pregnancy, Am. J. Obst. & Gynec. **68**:170, 1954.

McCall, M. L.: Cerebral blood flow and metabolism in toxemias of pregnancy, Surg., Gynec. & Obst. **89**:715, 1949.

McElrath, P. J., Ware, H. H., Jr., Winn, W. C., and Schelin, E. C.: Continuous spinal anesthesia in the treatment of severe preeclampsia and eclampsia: preliminary report of a study of 24 cases, Am. J. Obst. & Gynec. **58**:1084, 1949.

Rosenbaum, M., and Maltby, G. L.: Relation of cerebral dysrhythmia to eclampsia, Am. J. Obst. & Gynec. **45**:992, 1943.

Shorr, E., and Zweifach, B. W.: Pregnancy Wastage, Springfield, Thomas, 1953.

Siddall, R. S., and Mack, H. C.: Weight changes in the last four months of pregnancy, Am. J. Obst. & Gynec. **26**:244, 1933.

Smith, G. V., and Smith, O. W.: Internal secretions and toxemia of late pregnancy, Physiol. Rev. **28**:1, 1948.

Stander, H. J., Eastman, N. J., Harrison, E. P. H., Jr., and Cadden, J. F.: The acid-base equilibrium of the blood in eclampsia, J. Biol. Chem. **85**:233, 1929.

Volhard, F.: Die doppelseitigen hämatogenen Niereverkrankungen, Berlin, Springer, 1918.

Whitacre, F. E., Hingson, R. A., and Turner, H. B.: The treatment of eclampsia by means of regional nerve block, South. M. J. **41**:920, 1948.

THERAPEUTIC ABORTION

Chesley, L. C., and Jarvis, D. G.: A study of the interaction of pregnancy and hypertensive disease, Am. J. Obst. & Gynec. **53**:851, 1947.

Rosen, H.: Therapeutic Abortion, New York, Julian, 1954.

ECTOPIC PREGNANCY

Decker, A.: A simple technic to test tubal patency, Am. J. Obst. & Gynec. **50**:227, 1945.

Lavell, T. E.: Diagnosis of ectopic gestation from clinical analysis of 410 cases at Bellevue Hospital, Am. J. Obst. & Gynec. **18**:379, 1929.

Marchette, A. A., Kuder, K., and Kuder, A.: A clinical evaluation of ectopic pregnancy, Am. J. Obst. & Gynec. **52**:544, 1946.

TeLinde, R. W., and Rutledge, F. N.: Culdoscopy, a useful gynecological procedure, Am. J. Obst. & Gynec. **55**:102, 1948.

PLACENTA PREVIA

Johnson, R. A.: The Plan Most Likely to Succeed in the Cases of the Patient with Placenta Previa. Read before the American Association of Obstetrics & Gynecology, Hot Springs, Arkansas, 1955.

Macaffee, C. H. G.: Placenta previa — a study of 174 cases, J. Obst. & Gynaec. Brit. Emp. **52**:313, 1945.

Williams, J. T.: The expectant management of placenta previa, Am. J. Obst. & Gynec. **55**:169, 1948.

ABRUPTIO PLACENTA

Oliver, J., MacDowell, M., and Tracy, A.: The pathogenesis of acute renal failure associated with traumatic and toxic injury, J. Clin. Invest. **30**:1305, 1951.

Page, E. W., King, E. B., and Merrill, J. A.: Abruptio placenta: dangers of delay in delivery, Obst. & Gynec. **3**:385, 1954.

Weiner, A. E., Reid, D. E., and Roby, C. C.: Incoagulable blood in severe separation of the placenta: a method of management, Am. J. Obst. & Gynec. **66**:475, 1953.

RUPTURE OF MARGINAL SINUS

Fish, J. S., Bartholomew, R. H., Calvin, E. D., and Grimes, W. H.: The role of marginal sinus rupture in antenatal hemorrhage, Am. J. Obst. & Gynec. **61**:20, 1951.

MALPOSITION

Hall, J. E., and Kohl, S. G.: Breech presentation: a study of 1456 cases, Am. J. Obst. & Gynec. (In press)

Hellman, L. M., Epperson, J. W., and Connally, F.: Face and brow presentation, Am. J. Obst. & Gynec. **59**:831, 1950.

Moore, W. T., and Steptoe, P. P.: The experience of the Johns Hopkins Hospital with breech presentation, South. M. J. **36**:295, 1943.

Renke, T.: Face presentation, Am. J. Obst. & Gynec. **66**:1185, 1953.

PELVIC CONTRACTION

Kaltreider, F. D.: Criteria of inlet contraction, Am. J. Obst. & Gynec. **62**:600, 1951.

UTERINE INERTIA

Hellman, L. M.: Factors influencing successful posterior pituitary treatment of functional uterine dystocia with particular consideration of its intravenous administration, Am. J. Obst. & Gynec. **57**: 364, 1949.

Hellman, L. M., Harris, J. S., and Reynolds, S. R. M.: Intravenous pituitary extract in labor with data on patterns of uterine contractility, Am. J. Obst. & Gynec. **59**:41, 1950.

Page, E. W.: Response of human uterus to pitocin tannate in oil, Proc. Soc. Exper. Biol. & Med. **52**:195, 1943.

Reynolds, S. R. M., Harris, J. S., and Kaiser, I. H.: Clinical Measurement of Uterine Forces in Pregnancy and Labor, Springfield, Ill., Thomas, 1954.

MULTIPLE PREGNANCY

Guttmacher, A. F.: The incidence of multiple births in man and some of the other unipara, Obst. & Gynec. **2**:22, 1953.

CESAREAN SECTION

Gordon, C. A.: Cesarean section death, Am. J. Obst. & Gynec. **63**:284, 1952.

PREMATURITY

Dunham, E. C.: Premature Infants, New York, Hoeber, 1955.

TUBERCULOSIS

Schaffer, G., Douglas, R. G., and Dreispoon, I. H.: Tuberculosis and abortion, Am. Rev. Tuberc. **70**:49, 1954.

Studdiford, W.: Pregnancy and pelvic tuberculosis, Am. J. Obst. & Gynec. **69**:379, 1955.

DIABETES

Hurwitz, D., and Higano, N.: Diabetes and pregnancy, New England J. Med. **247**: 305, 1952.

Pedowitz, P., and Shlevin, E. L.: The pregnant diabetic patient, Am. J. Obst. & Gynec. **69**:395, 1955.

White, Paul: Symposium on diabetes mellitus; pregnancy complicating diabetes, Am. J. Med. **7**:609, 1949.

Williams, J. W.: The clinical significance of glycosuria in pregnant women, Am. J. M. Sc. **137**:1, 1909.

»» 7 «« Anesthesia Mortality

Mechanisms Involved in Anesthetic Deaths: A Survey of Operating Room and Obstetric Delivery Room Related Mortality in the University Hospitals of Cleveland for the Period 1944 through 1954*

For the period of 11 decades since the introduction of anesthesia, physicians, physiologists, pharmacologists, chemists and nurses have directed their attention to the protection of the patient whose natural defenses are obtunded through narcosis of brain or depolarization of nerves for the obliteration of surgical and obstetric pain. The consultations of the pathologist and the public health statistician are welcomed within the clinical team devoted to the task of the elimination of anesthetic deaths. In view of the fact that 8,000,000 people in the United States require surgical anesthesia in the nation's operating rooms; that another 4,000,000 mothers require either analgesia or anesthetic drugs, or both, during childbirth (not forgetting the 4,000,000 passive intra-uterine passengers who received the identical intravascular toxicologic dosage of drugs across the placenta through the umbilical veins); and that an even larger group received a local injection or an anesthetic gas in dental surgery—we agree with Beecher and Todd that "anesthesia might be likened to a Public Health Disease."

It is time for the state medical societies, the national public health facilities and the research foundations to survey not only the dramatic apex of the problem of anesthetic and operating-room mortality but also the much broader base of the pyramid of morbidity and the surveillance of recovery from both surgery and anesthesia of these substantial proportions of our population.

The present literature on the subject is both alarming and confusing. The journal *Anesthesiology* reported in 1946 that there was approximately 1 anesthesia-related death to each 1,000 anesthesias. Brown, of the Royal Adelaide Hospital, in Australia, analyzed 133 anesthesia-related deaths in 151,000 anesthesias in a 10-year survey (1941 through 1951) in that hospital. Lyford, Berger and Shumacker reviewed 75 deaths that occurred in the operating rooms during the administration of 51,392 anesthetics in the Johns Hopkins Hospital within the decade 1931 to 1941. Of these deaths 20 (26.7%) were attributed to a major anesthetic factor. A superficial comparison of these 2 reports, each covering a period of 1 decade, would seem to indicate that the death rate on the operating table in the Johns Hopkins Hospital, calculated as 1 in each 690 operations, was far more unfavorable than the death rate of 1 in each 1,135 operations in the Royal Adelaide Hospital.

---

* Reprinted from New York State Journal of Medicine, January, 1956. Robert A. Hingson, M.D., Professor of Anesthesia, William D. Holden, M.D., Professor of Surgery, and Allan C. Barnes, M.D., Professor of Obstetrics and Gynecology, School of Medicine, Western Reserve University, Cleveland, Ohio; Directors of Respective Departments, University Hospitals of Cleveland, Cleveland, Ohio.

ANALYSIS OF THE DEATHS UNRELATED TO THE ANESTHESIA IN THE JOHNS HOPKINS HOSPITAL

However, one gets a different picture upon closer analysis when it is determined that 29 of the 55 deaths thought to be unrelated to the anesthesia occurred during difficult craniotomies. Some of these patients died from hemorrhage, and all were in critical condition from increased intracranial pressure at the time of operation. These deaths included cases of hydrocephalus and tumors of the anterior and the posterior fossa, as well as traumatic cases in which the intracranial pressure had been increasing steadily during the preliminary period of conservative treatment. Sixteen deaths occurred during difficult intrathoracic operations, many of the patients being critically ill at the time of operation. Of these 16 deaths, 9 occurred during pneumonectomy or lobectomy; 1 during pulmonary plexectomy in a critically ill patient with asthma; 1 during repair of an esophagotracheal fistula in an infant 3 days old; 1 during resection of lower esophagus and cardia for carcinoma; and 3 resulted from obstruction of the respiratory tract by material from tuberculous or pyogenic cavities which emptied during operation.

On the other hand, the Royal Adelaide Hospital, with a much better record in the operating room, did not have such a high incidence of critically ill patients who had been referred from many hospitals for last-resort surgery. However, even here a lesson emerges if we as a surgical anesthesia team strive to avoid unnecessary operating-room mortality: *operations of necessity should be performed if the patient is not in extremis.* Through years of experience in many hospitals we are convinced of another axiom in the salvage of operating room life: *the greater the operative and the anesthetic risk, the more the prerequisite necessity of having the most skillful and experienced surgical and anesthetic team in the field, teaching by example rather than from the side lines.* Our third admonition is: *the nearer the patient is to an exodus lethalis, the shorter the time he must be subjected to either the trauma of surgery or the narcosis of anesthesia. Likewise, the quantity of both surgery and anesthesia must be reduced proportionately.*

The literature today on surgery, obstetrics and anesthesia very properly documents abundant data to assist us in defining the problem, ascribing a cause and making recommendations for elimination of anesthesia mortality. However, it is not a single hospital experience for a decade or longer or a comparison of the data from two or more that will give us the final answer, but rather the building of an educational program based upon the lessons learned from a survey of these abundant data in order that continually we may train ourselves and our residents to simplify our technics, eliminate unnecessary delays upon the anesthetized patient which prolongs his milligram toxicologic uptake, and surround him with the best physiologic cardiorespiratory balance possible through blood and fluid replacement therapy and adequate ventilation.

A survey is presented in the following tables of operating-room actual and related mortality in the University Hospitals of Cleveland for the period January 1, 1945, through December 31, 1954, in a total of 136,043 patients. These included 1,476 intrathoracic operations (more than 85% on the heart and the great vessels in critically ill patients) and 42,789 obstetric deliveries.

There were 127 fatalities either during anesthesia or within 24 hours from a determined cause associated with either anesthesia or surgery, or both. Cases in

TABLE 45. UNIVERSITY HOSPITALS OF CLEVELAND, OHIO,

Year	Total No. of Anesthesias Adminis- tered in Surgery and Obstetrics	Total No. of Anesthesias Adminis- tered for Intra- thoracic Operations	Deaths Dur- ing Intra- tho- racic Oper- ations	Gen- eral Sur- gery Deaths	Deaths Dur- ing Ob- stetric De- livery	Total Deaths	Total and **Com- bined** Rate: One Death In:	Anes- thesia Sole Factor	Sur- gery or Dis- ease Sole Factor	Anes- thesia Major Factor	Anes- thesia Minor Factor	Inde- ter- mi- nate
1945	10,648	99	3	6	2	11	**1,318** 968	2	4	2	3	0
1946	11,949	69	2	9	3	14	**990** 953	5	3	6	0	0
1947	13,304	85	1	8	2	11	**1,329** 1,209	3	3	2	2	1
1948	12,544	106	3	6	1	10	**1,777** 1,792	1	4	2	3	0
1949	12,932	92	2	7	2	11	**1,426** 1,394	3	4	1	3	0
1950	13,495	114	5	7	0	12	**1,911** 1,349	2	4	1	3	2
1951	13,482	154	8	7	0	15	**1,904** 890	2	12	0	0	1
1952	15,650	237	4	10	0	14	**1,541** 1,118	1	10	1	2	0
1953	15,877	267	9	4	1	14	**3,122** 1,134	3	7	1	1	2
1954	16,162	253	12	3	0	15	**5,303** 1,077	1	10	2	1	1
TOTALS	136,043	1,476	49	67	11†	127	Avg.: 1,188	23	61	18	18	7

* All patients who had a lethal crisis in surgery, such as cardiac arrest, major aspiration of vomitus, profound and prolonged shock and were resuscitated, but subsequently died on the division, are included in this analysis.

† Includes cesarean sections.

Boldface figures indicate combined death rate in general surgery and obstetrics.

OPERATING ROOM AND DELIVERY ROOM MORTALITY STUDY*

Year	*Anesthetic Agents Used*								*Age Groups*			
	Ether	Nitrous Oxide	Cyclo-pro-pane	Pento-thal	Spinal	Local	Curare	Avertin	0–4	5–13	14–49	50–80+
1945	**9** 6,102	**3** 3,827		**1** 1,296	438			**0** 729				
1946	**9** 6,315	**5** 5,599	**0** 63	**3** 2,362	**4** 23		**2** 83	**0** 654				
1947	**7** 6,820	**3** 6,098	**0** 329	**2** 2,653	**1** 1,767		**1** 287	**1** 402	8	3	27	31
1948	**5** 6,641	**2** 5,505	**1** 128	**1** 2,542	**1** 2,281	**0** 2,542	**1** 84	**0** 200				
1949	**5** 6,135	**2** 5,925	**1** 59	**1** 2,693	**0** 2,577	**0** 2,693	**1** 100	**0** 218				
1950	**8** 5,537	**7** 5,747	**0** 186	**0** 2,919	**0** 3,122	**1** 1,919	**6** 204	**1** 227				
1951	**12** 6,012	**5** 4,290	**1** 107	**3** 2,874	**0** 3,148	**2** 2,350	**5** 374	**0** 168				
1952	**11** 4,939	**1** 4,963	**0** 131	**1** 2,902	**1** 2,933	**0** 2,400	**4** 1,385	**0** 207	16	2	28	12
1953	**11** 5,828	**2** 6,763	**0** 103	**1** 3,911	**1** 2,946	**1** 2,296	**3** 1,548	**0** 252				
1954	**11** 3,953	**12** 6,265	**1** 1,657	**6** 3,317	**0** 3,104	**1** 2,556	**7** 1,665	**0** 88				
TOTALS	**88** 58,282 XX	**42** 54,982 XVIII	**4** 2,763 II	**19** 27,469 VII	**8** 22,339 IV	**5** 16,756 I	**30** 5,730 II	**2** 3,145 II	24	5	55	43

Roman numerals indicate anesthesia deaths.

Boldface figures indicate deaths with agents listed.

TABLE 46. ANESTHESIA DEATHS—PRIMARY AND CONTRIBUTORY

	TOTAL NUMBER OF CASES	NUMBER OF DEATHS	RATE: 1 DEATH IN:
Ten American University Hospitals (Beecher and Todd Report) 1948–1952	697,600	384	1,560
University Hospitals of Cleveland, Ohio 1945–1954........	136,043	59	2,306

TABLE 47. STUDY OF ALL DEATHS IN WHICH PATIENT HAD CURARE

	NUMBER OF CASES	NUMBER OF DEATHS	RATE: 1 DEATH IN:
Ten American University Hospitals (Beecher and Todd Report) 1948 through 1952......	44,100	118	370
University Hospitals of Cleveland, Ohio 1945 through 1954	5,730	30	192

which the patient's pre-existing disease or injury caused death after the patient was returned to the division are excluded, but those patients who died as a result of disease during their treatment in the operating room are included.

As seen in Table 45, all patients who died were classified as follows: (1) anesthesia sole factor; (2) surgery or disease sole factor; (3) anesthesia major factor, surgery or disease minor factor; (4) anesthesia minor factor, surgery or disease major factor; and (5) indeterminate. These conclusions were reached after documenting the autopsy findings in 97 of the 127 cases and the clinical impressions of the surgical mortality conference composed of 20 or more surgeons and, since 1951, of anesthesiologists or from the obstetric mortality conference. Obviously, all deaths resulting from surgical and anesthesia technic or errors in judgment were preventable.

In view of the widespread interest in the 5-year survey of 10 American university hospitals in the Beecher and Todd report on 697,680 administrations of anesthesia, we have compared our summarized comparable data in Table 45.

Especially because of the implications arising from the use of the muscle relaxants, we have compared our data in Tables 47, 48 and 49. Table 50 is a summary of the mechanism of death in our cases. Table 51 is an inquiry into the incidence of death with multiple agents. No attempt was made to study

TABLE 48. ANESTHESIA DEATHS IN CURARE USES

	TOTAL NUMBER ANESTHESIAS	TOTAL PRIMARY ANESTHESIA DEATHS	RATE: 1 DEATH IN:	MAJOR SURGERY RATE: 1 DEATH IN:	NUMBER CASES OF CURARE	CASES WITH CURARE, RATE: 1 USE IN:
Ten American University Hospitals (Beecher and Todd Report) 1948 through 1952................	697,600	224	2,680	192	44,100	14
University Hospitals of Cleveland 1945 through 1954................	136,043	41	3,318	191	5,730	24

TABLE 49. CURARE STUDY

	University Hospitals of Cleveland, Ohio 1945–1954			Ten American University Hospitals (Beecher and Todd Report) 1948–1952
	Number of Cases	Deaths	Rate: 1 Death In:	Rate: 1 Death In:
Curare in all cases	5,730	30	191	(Major surgery, 192)
Intrathoracic surgery, with curare	1,476	22	67	
General surgery, with curare (all cases)	4,254	8	532	Major and Minor 370
General surgery, with curare (anesthesia sole factor, major or minor)	4,254	3	1,418	
General surgery, with curare (anesthesia primary factor, sole or major)	4,254	2	2,127	(Minor surgery, 2,134)

TABLE 50. MECHANISM OF OPERATING-ROOM DEATH (1945-1954)

ost Frequent Cause	Number	Percentage
Cardiac arrest	32	25.2
Aspiration: Vomit	10	7.0
Blood	2	1.
Uncontrollable hemorrhage	10	7.
Respiratory arrest (includes 4 high spinal blocks and one pneumoencephalogram with 100 per cent oxygen and one Rubin's test with air)	9	7.
Vascular occlusion during surgery with intra-auricular thrombus or coronary thrombosis	9	7.
Toxic or traumatic shock without major hemorrhage	9	7.
Intra-cranial hemorrhage or death during drainage of hydrocephalus	8	6.
Asphyxia and airway obstruction: mucus, kinked intratracheal tube or tube slipping out during surgery	8	6.
Unclassified and miscellaneous (in this group rare and indeterminate causes of death)	30	26.8
Total operating room related deaths in 136,043 anesthesias	127	
AUTOPSIES	97	76.4
NO AUTOPSIES	30	23.6

incidence of operating-room mortality with anesthesia managed solely by nurse anesthetists and surgeons from 1945 through 1950 and by the reorganized department that has seen the use of increasing numbers of physician anesthesiologists and residents in anesthesia since July, 1951. The policy of the departments has been the use of the best available surgical-obstetric anesthesia team for the job at hand.

Table 52 records the incidence of deaths from all causes in general surgery, intrathoracic surgery and obstetrics.

TABLE 51. INCIDENCE OF USE OF MULTIPLE ANESTHETIC AGENTS RELATED TO PRIMARY ANESTHESIA DEATHS IN CONSECUTIVE CASES

	Anesthetic Combinations*					
	One	Two	Three	Four	Five	Total
Total deaths	44	38	13	3	1	99
Anesthetic deaths	14	7	3	2	0	26

* Agents studied: ether, gases, intravenous barbiturates, curare, spinal and local.

TABLE 52. COMPARISON OF DEATH RATE IN GENERAL SURGERY AND OBSTETRICS WITH INTRATHORACIC SURGERY: ALL CAUSES

TYPE OF OPERATION	NUMBER OF CASES	DEATHS	RATE: 1 DEATH IN:
General surgery......	93,234	67	1,391
Intrathoracic surgery..	1,476	49	30
Obstetrics..........	42,789	11	3,890

TABLE 53. COMPARISON OF DEATH RATE IN GENERAL SURGERY, OBSTETRICS AND INTRATHORACIC SURGERY, IN WHICH ANESTHESIA WAS DETERMINED TO BE THE SOLE OR MAJOR FACTOR

TYPE OF OPERATION	NUMBER OF CASES	ANESTHETIC DEATHS	RATE: 1 DEATH IN:
General surgery......	93,234	31	3,007
Obstetrics..........	42,789	6	7,131
Intrathoracic surgery..	1,476	5	295

Table 53 records the incidence of anesthetic deaths, or deaths in which anesthesia was a sole or a major contributing factor. In both these tables it is obvious that the high incidence of deaths associated with intrathoracic surgery makes it imperative to make separate analyses of results in these three major categories in order to determine the specific incidence of mortality in each. Even though the incidence of death in intrathoracic surgery in this series is relatively high, the mortality still is below 4 per cent in this group of critically ill patients; and in both surgery and obstetrics, the incidence of anesthetic mortality is less than $3/10$ of 1 per cent in the former, and a little more than $1/10$ of 1 per cent in the latter.

From Table 54 we can see that no single agent is the cause or is immune to the production of all this mortality. More frequently, the major cause of anesthetic mortality is related directly to the improper administration of the agents; to faulty technic; to inadequate equipment and resuscitative measures; to the policy of "too little and too late" blood replacement; and to improper management of the postoperative period, in which obstructed airway and/or hypoxia are related to depressed ventilation leading to death. In the analysis of 331 maternal mortalities reported by Hellman and Hingson in *Anesthesiology* in 1951, they found that the most common cause of death was aspiration of vomitus (in 161 instances). In most of these cases, patients without proper premedication or determination of their cardiovascular-respiratory status were anesthetized too soon after having eaten a meal.

Macintosh, of England, feels that the most common cause of anesthetic deaths in that country is the nursing of the unconscious patient in a faulty position, permitting hypoventilation and airway obstruction. He points out also the unnecessary high number of anesthetic fatalities resulting from the administration

TABLE 54. INCIDENCE OF SPECIFIC USE OF AGENT IN PRIMARY ANESTHESIA DEATHS

AGENT	NUMBER OF USES OF AGENT WHEN ANESTHESIA DESIGNATED AS PRIMARY (SOLE OR MAJOR) CAUSE OF DEATH	TOTAL USES	RATE: 1 DEATH IN:
Ether........	20	58,282	2,907
Gas..........	13	54,982	4,229
Intravenous barbiturates.	7	27,469	3,924
Curare.......	2	5,730	2,865
Spinal........	4	22,339	5,584
Local........	1	16,756	16,756

of the wrong drug, from a miscalculation of the proper dosage of standard drugs or from the substitution of a gas for oxygen from incorrectly connected cylinders.

In a city in the United States with a population of about 1 million, one of the authors served on a coroner's committee with an anesthesia mortality commission that reviewed 77 anesthetic fatalities in a single year (1950). In 3 of these cases, nitrous oxide was placed mistakenly in the position of the oxygen cylinder. Happily, the anesthetic gas manufacturing companies and machine companies now have developed the safety-pin index system, which should prevent this unfortunate experience.

Great progress also has been made in prevention of explosions—but more is needed.

MATERNAL ANESTHETIC MORTALITY*

Noteworthy progress has been made since Sir James Simpson first administered anesthesia in obstetrics 104 years ago. However, most of the progress in obstetric anesthesia has been made in the last two decades. Unquestionably, better anesthetic technic and agents have been responsible for reducing both maternal and infant mortality. Nevertheless, maternal mortality resulting from the complications of anesthesia used improperly is assuming relatively greater significance as the antibiotics have so greatly reduced maternal death from puerperal and secondary infections; as better prenatal care and diet therapy have reduced mortality from toxemia; and as blood banks, fluid replacement therapy and better understanding of the oxytocics have reduced maternal mortality resulting from hemorrhage. At the present time it is our opinion that maternal deaths resulting from or related to anesthesia are in fifth place after heart disease as a contributor to mortality.

* Hingson, R. A., and Hellman, L. M.: Organization of obstetric anesthesia on a 24-hour basis in a large and a small hospital, Anesthesiology **12**:745-752, 1951.

TABLE 55. STATISTICS COLLECTED FROM 192 HOSPITALS WITH 2,000 DELIVERIES OR OVER PER YEAR

	CASES	PERCENTAGE
Total number of deliveries in survey	2,577,149	
Total number of deaths in survey	66	.0025
Immediate deaths—total	30	44.0
Delayed deaths—total	36	56.0
Number of autopsies—total	34	53.0

From our own files and from the British literature we have collected 331 maternal mortalities resulting from anesthesia. The large majority of these deaths occurred within the last decade.

An analysis has been made of 66 maternal deaths and 8 fetal deaths resulting from aspiration of vomitus during obstetric anesthesia in the years 1945 to 1949, inclusive. Questionnaires were sent to 219 United States hospitals with 2,000 or more deliveries per year. A significant number—192 hospitals—returned the completed questionnaire, reporting a total of 2,577,149 births in that period. The incidence of death from aspiration of vomitus was 0.0025 per cent, or 1 maternal death in each 39,048 deliveries.

Of the 66 maternal deaths, in 35 (53%) the diagnosis of aspiration of vomitus as cause of death was proved by autopsy. Twenty-nine (44%) patients died during induction or during emergence from anesthesia on the delivery table. Thirty-seven (56%) patients died after delivery varying from 2½ hours to 8 days. Five of these deaths occurred during cesarean section.

Ten different types of anesthesia were used in this series. Open-drop ether and

TABLE 56. TYPE OF ANESTHESIA USED

	CASES	PER-CENTAGE
Nitrous oxide, oxygen and ether	24	36.4
Ether—open drop	17	25.8
Cyclopropane	9	13.8
Nitrous oxide and oxygen	4	6.0
Ethylene	3	4.5
Spinal anesthesia	1	1.5
Sodium pentothal	1	1.5
Sodium pentothal, nitrous oxide and ether	1	1.5
Delvinal sodium	1	1.5
Ethylene and ether	1	1.5
Unnamed	4	6.0

TABLE 57. TREATMENT USED IN REPORTED CASES OF DEATHS FROM ASPIRATION OF VOMITUS, 1945-49

	CASES	PER-CENTAGE
Oxygen by mask, intranasally or otherwise	55	83.0
Suction, oral, pharyngeal or/and nasal	50	75.0
Intratracheal suction	30	45.0
Bronchoscopy with suction	17	25.0
Tracheotomy	0	—

nitrous oxide, oxygen and ether produced the majority of the deaths, but death under spinal anesthesia indicates that morbidity and mortality from aspiration of vomitus can occur also under conduction anesthesia. No death resulted from aspiration in deliveries without anesthesia, with local or caudal anesthesia, or with chloroform.

Nineteen of the 192 hospitals volunteered information about nonfatal cases with aspiration pneumonia. Fourteen of the 19 hospitals reported their actual number of cases of aspiration pneumonitis in the 5-year period. There were 75 cases of aspiration pneumonitis in 192,080 deliveries, an incidence of 1 case of aspiration morbidity in every 2560.0 deliveries (0.039%). Prompt and effective treatment of this complication by the anesthetist saved many mothers and babies. In the information given it was noted that hospitals using prompt bronchoscopy with suction of the bronchial tree obtained excellent results in the degree and the duration of the morbidity. A summary of the treatment used is shown in Table 57.

The time of vomiting in relation to birth of the baby indicated that 29 cases occurred before birth, 20 after birth, with 17 cases not reported. There were 8 associated fetal deaths (Table 58).

Since 66 maternal deaths occurred in this collected series of 2,577,149 deliveries in major hospitals, it seems logical to assume that at least 100 maternal deaths per year result from this cause in our nation's approximately 3½ million deliveries.

There were between 5,600 and 4,100 maternal deaths in the United States each year from 1945 to 1948. Thus, 100 maternal deaths per year by this conservative estimate would represent between 1.5 and 2.5 per cent of total maternal mortality. Therefore, we believe that it is significant to call attention to the fact that approximately 2 out of every 100 maternal deaths in the United States are due to aspiration of vomitus.

Analysis by states of the incidence of deaths from aspiration of vomitus reveals the fact that in a Midwestern state in which there were 186,000 live births in 1948, or 5.2 per cent of the nation's

TABLE 58. TIME OF VOMITING IN RELATIONSHIP TO BIRTH OF BABY

	CASES	PER-CENTAGE
Before birth	29	44.0
After birth	20	30.0
Time not reported	17	25.0
Baby affected (stillborn or death within 48 hours)	8	12.1

3,560,000, there was a disproportionately high number of deaths from this cause. In a total series of 149,292 deliveries, this state reported 18 deaths from aspiration vomitus, or 1 death in each 8,294 deliveries. Ether alone or ether-nitrous oxide was the anesthetic agent administered in all these mortalities. In one small hospital in this state there were 10 aspiration pneumonias in 6,048 deliveries with ether the only anesthetic used.

The most common anesthetic causes of death in the more than 300 mortalities analyzed were:

1. **Aspiration of Vomitus in the Improperly Prepared Patient.** During the last 25 years the world's literature listed 50 maternal deaths from this cause. During the last 5 years, through questionnaire study methods, we have added to the published literature an additional 66 aspiration vomitus maternal mortalities. Seventeen of these occurred in a single state. These mortalities could have been prevented in most instances by:

A. Withholding food in labor;

B. Selecting conduction anesthesia for patients who had eaten recently;

C. Providing obstetric tables capable of developing the Trendelenburg position, adequate suction apparatus and transparent face masks; and

D. Providing a round-the-clock competent staff acquainted with the incidence, the treatment and the prevention of this condition.

The occasional obstetric anesthetist who gives chiefly surgical anesthesia or little anesthesia does not understand the problems involved. Hospitals should be encouraged to assign anesthetists to the department of obstetrics for long tenures in such manner that the anesthetists rotate on 8-hour shifts. Since approximately one third of anesthesias are obstetric, enough revenue could be collected to provide increased compensation for obstetric anesthesia and the night duty involved.

Obstetric patients should be educated through ethical propaganda to understand the necessity of competent obstetric anesthesia. This is well exemplified in the experience of the Baltimore City Maternal Mortality Commission, which, in the period 1944 to 1949, reviewed 110 maternal mortalities. Of these, 14, or 12.7 per cent, were related in whole or in part to obstetric anesthesia.

2. **Overdosage of Spinal Anesthesia.** Of the 335 deaths reviewed, 25 resulted from surgical anesthetic doses administered to obstetric patients. Six of these occurred in a single state. We insist that obstetric anesthetists follow the schedule of doses referred to below.

Frequently, the dosage of anesthesia in obstetrics is less than that in patients of comparable size and weight in surgery. This is particularly true in spinal and saddle-block anesthesia, where the dose may be reduced from one half to one third the usual amount. For this reason we should like to emphasize the safe maximum single-dose spinal or saddle-block anesthesia that can be depended upon for vaginal delivery:

Procaine	30 to 50 mg.
Metycaine	22 to 30 mg.
Pontocaine	2 to 5 mg.
Nupercaine	$2\frac{1}{2}$ to $3\frac{3}{4}$ mg.
Xylocaine	25 to 40 mg.

For cesarean section with continuous spinal anesthesia, these doses should not be repeated more frequently than 30-minute intervals. For single-injection spinal anesthesia in obstetrics, procaine, Metycaine or Xylocaine alone is frequently too short acting for this operation to be completed safely. Pontocaine might be used in doses to 8 mg. and Nupercaine up to 5 mg.

3. **The Administration of Transfusions Following Obstetric Hemorrhage**

Under Anesthesia in the "Too Little and Too Late" Policy. Major obstetric hemorrhage may develop at any time, and emergency quantities of 40 Rh negative blood should be available on every obstetric service. We also recommend having readily available the polysaccharide Dextran as a temporary expedient while awaiting transfusion.

4. **The Use of an Agent or a Method Not Understood by the Anesthetist.** Examples of death from this type include:

A. Too light anesthesia with Pentothal Sodium or cyclopropane and

B. Continuous caudal analgesia to patients improperly watched.

5. **The Administration of Incompatible Drugs, Such as Pituitrin and Cyclopropane, Large Intravenous Doses of Ergotrate and Vasopressors.** The anesthetist should know the major incompatibilities of the vasopressors, the oxytocics and the anesthetics:

A. Pituitrin following cyclopropane can precipitate ventricular fibrillation.

B. The use of intravenous Ergotrate or Ergonovine in 0.1 to 0.2 mg. doses following too closely upon intravenous oxytocics after ephedrine or desoxyephedrine can produce dangerous elevations in blood pressure and result occasionally in cerebral hemorrhage.

C. In obstetric toxemia, fluid replacement therapy should take into consideration the desirability of sodium-free infusions.

D. Tetanic uterine contractions induced by oxytocics or occurring spontaneously can be relaxed by drop ether inhalation, without which fetal life is in jeopardy.

6. **Inadvertent Intravenous Administration of Full Dosage Local Anesthetics.**

SUMMARY

The 335 maternal anesthetic deaths collected in our files and from the British literature present justifiable evidence for the need of organized anesthesia in the larger maternity hospitals. This need can be met by (1) relegating simple and basic anesthesia to nurse anesthetists, medical students and interns under proper supervision; (2) training carefully obstetric residents in standard systemic and conduction anesthesia designed for obstetric delivery and cesarean section; (3) providing standard equipment such as delivery tables capable of Trendelenburg positions, adequate suction appartus in each room, plastic transparent face pieces permitting constant surveillance of airway for obstruction; (4) having readily available therapeutic oxygen with and without positive pressure for resuscitation of infants and mothers; (5) having readily available intravenous fluids and whole blood; and (6) assigning a full-time director of obstetric anesthesia from the general department of anesthesia who will organize available personnel through 8-hour shifts round the clock according to the plan herein submitted.

We re-emphasize that our present situation of emergency with shortages of staff calls for an immediate surveillance of this problem by hospital administrators, anesthesiologists, obstetricians and nurse anesthetists.

TABLE 59. ASPIRATION OF VOMITUS DURING OR IMMEDIATELY AFTER ANESTHESIA

British medical literature, 1924 through 1944	50
Merrill, Hingson survey of major 219 American hospitals	66
North Carolina maternal welfare study—Aug., 1946, through May, 1948	3
Massachusetts maternal welfare study, 1941	1
Brooklyn 1936–47 (Charles Gordon study)	26
Memphis Methodist Hospital case (file report, 1947)	1
Philadelphia Lying-in Hospital (file report, 1940)	1
Chicago Lying-in Hospital (Dieckmann, 1945)	2
Supplementary file—personal communications from American hospitals	13
TOTAL	163

TABLE 60. MATERNAL MORTALITIES FROM SPINAL ANESTHESIA (1935-1951)

OVERWHELMING AND ASSASSINATING DOSES	
North Carolina maternal welfare study, Aug. 1946 through May, 1948 (Pontocaine 14 to 17 mg. and procaine 150 mg.)	6
Jefferson Medical School (200 mg. for cesarean section)	2
Charity Hospital, New Orleans (17 mg. Pontocaine and 150 mg. procaine for cesarean section)	3
Grace Hospital, Detroit (200 mg. procaine for cesarean section)	1
Massachusetts maternal welfare report, 1941	2
Hospitals of Brooklyn (Gordon report supplemented by recent maternal mortality conferences)	8
Loretto Hospital, Chicago, 1950 (7.5 mg. Nupercaine plus 1 mg. Adrenalin)	1
Franklin Square Hospital, Baltimore (file copy) (12 mg. dosage of Pontocaine)	1
TOTAL	24
DRUG IDIOSYNCRASY AND PROFOUND RESPONSE TO STANDARD DOSE	
Philadelphia Lying-in Hospital, 1948 (2.5 mg. Nupercaine with ascending paralysis and apnea)	1
Medical College of Virginia, 1948 (2.5 mg. Nupercaine)	1
Margaret Hague Hospital, 1935	2
Detroit Hospital	1
TOTAL	5
MISUSE OF NUPERCAINE IN HYPOBARIC SOLUTION	
New Orleans hospitals (hyperbaric solution and prolonged Trendelenburg position)	2
Baltimore mortality report	1
Chicago file report	1
North Carolina—meningitis	1
New Orleans (contaminated used glucose)	2
TOTAL	7

PROGRAM FOR REDUCING FATALITIES

From the foregoing it can be seen that anesthesia-related mortality at the present time is unduly high—yet in many instances not unrelated to surgical and obstetric factors of preoperative preparation, diagnosis, technical competence and duration of surgery. Obviously, it would be improper prejudicially to assign the cause of death to any one standard agent or technic, even though a few of them, in the classic remarks of Nosworthy, are "fatally easy to give." These unnecessary anesthetic fatalities can be reduced by:

1. More complete and standard training requirements for anesthetists; more careful selection of qualified applicants.
2. The development of close team work among surgeons, obstetricians and anesthetists, who will review the patients' problems, together before surgery and as frequently during surgery as required, through an interchange of progress reports.
3. The improvement of available lifesaving resuscitative equipment such as:
   A. Mechanical airways and devices for intubation;
   B. Suction apparatus;

TABLE 61. ANESTHETIC MORTALITIES RESULTING FROM CAUDAL AND CONTINUOUS CAUDAL ANESTHESIA

Inadvertent spinals and overwhelming respiratory failure	8
Vasomotor collapse in poor-risk cases	5
Infection: peridural abscesses	3
Drug toxicity	3
Overwhelming motor paralysis from neglected cases, without attendant, in continuous drip technic	2
TOTAL	21

TABLE 62

NITROUS OXIDE, ETHER, ETHYLENE AND CYCLOPROPANE	
Atelectasis and anoxia	19
Cerebral hemorrhage during excitement stage in induction	2
Sudden apnea during early induction (sensitivity)	4
TOTAL	25
SODIUM PENTOTHAL	
Apnea on induction without resuscitation	6
Delayed shock manifested by extreme hypotension 1 hour after anesthesia	1
Deaths due to Evipal (Synopias), reported by Dieckmann	42
TOTAL	49

TABLE 63

DEMEROL	
Sensitivity and profound shock from 100 mg. in normal patient	1
CYCLOPROPANE	
Cyclopropane reaction with Pituitrin ventricular fibrillation	4
Cyclopropane shock	1
CHLOROFORM	
Baltimore (anesthesia for abortion administered in home on bed)	1
Buffalo hospitals in 12,000 cases	3
TRILENE	
Heart failure and profound effect	16
Pulmonary edema from prolonged use	2
Shock and bradycardia and liver poisoning	1
BARBITURATES (overwhelming depression)	
Baltimore (7½ gr. Sodium Amytal in toxemia)	1
Philadelphia Lying-in (4½ gr. intravenous Nembutal)	1
HEART FAILURE UNDER ANESTHESIA	12
TOTAL	43

C. Removal of unnecessary resistance in anesthesia apparatus, especially for small children; and

D. Operating tables maneuverable promptly to Trendelenburg positions.

4. Restorative intravenous fluid and blood infusions prophylactically in operation in almost all cases of major surgery and, most important, the development and the maintenance of sufficient anesthesia staffs available for 24 hours of service on divided shifts in both surgery and obstetrics.

5. Use of properly staffed, equipped and situated postanesthesia recovery rooms.

To augment this program, there must be a careful analysis of anesthesia-related fatalities by a scientific team consisting of anesthesiologists, pathologists, coroners, surgeons and obstetricians, who will document and catalog the accumulating facts to be used in teaching programs, thus permitting the experience and the lessons of the past to provide foundations for improved future practice.

BIBLIOGRAPHY

Beecher, Henry K., and Todd, Donald P.: A study of the deaths associated with anesthesia and surgery: based on a study of 599,548 anesthesias in ten institutions 1948–1952, inclusive, Ann. Surg. **140:**2–34, 1954.

Bishop, H. F.: Operating room deaths, Anesthesiology **7:**651–662, 1946.

Brown, J.: Personal communication.

Committee of Investigation of the Council of the Association of Anaesthetists of Great Britain and Ireland: Deaths associated with anaesthesia, Anaesthesia **7:** 200–205, 1952.

Editorial: Pathology of sudden and unexpected deaths, Anesthesiology **10:**105–148, 1949.

Gandevia, E.: Deaths during anesthesia, M. J. Australia **1:**93–94, 1949.

Gillespie, Noel: Deaths during anaesthesia, Brit. J. Anaesth. **19:**1–16, 1944.

Hingson, Robert A., and Hellman, Louis M.: Organization of obstetric anesthesia on a 24-hour basis in a large and a small hospital, Anesthesiology **12:**745–752, 1951.

Kyrle, P., and Poshakrishna, U.: Report on fatalities during the years 1938–1942, Chirurg. **17:**194–199, 1947.

Lyford, J., Berger, O. L., and Shumaker, H. B.: Analysis of deaths in operating rooms of Johns Hopkins Hospital, with special reference to those occurring under general anesthesia and spinal anesthesia, Bull. Johns Hopkins Hosp. **70:**488–503, 1942.

Macintosh, R. R.: Deaths under anesthesia, Brit. J. Anaesth. **21:**107–136, 1949.

Treat, J. C., and Gaster, E.: Fatalities in 54,128 consecutive cases, Ann. Surg. **119:** 954–958, 1954.

Turingston, H., Light, G., Cole, J., and Engel, P.: Fatalities in intrathoracic surgery, Arch. Surg. **55:**545–556, 1947.

8 Infant Mortality and Morbidity

The use of analgesics during labor and anesthetics for delivery has grown steadily since their introduction. They are of particular importance on the obstetric scene in the United States. No observant obstetrician can gainsay the fact that in normal parturition the infant of a mother receiving no anesthetic or analgesic drugs comes more lustily into the world than one whose mother had received general anesthesia. Based on this observation, there is a widespread belief that anesthetics and certain analgesics administered to mothers before delivery constitute a fetal hazard. Opposed to this is the concept that the relief of pain during labor allows for more timely, gentler and slower delivery and, consequently, should yield better, not worse, infant salvage. Furthermore, it has been suggested that in the case of especially jeopardized infants, the proper selection of anesthesia and analgesia might save additional lives.

It is almost impossible to prove these points statistically. By and large, anesthetic and analgesic drugs play no role in the causation of stillbirths, but they may be related to neonatal deaths. The overall neonatal death rates are extremely small, and, as will be shown later, the effect of pain-relieving drugs is of minor importance when compared with the various complications of pregnancy. Consequently, most investigations of the relationship of pain relief to fetal death have failed to yield conclusive answers.

The effect of analgesic and anesthetic drugs on infant survival is not subject to human experimentation. Human beings cannot be divided arbitrarily into experimental groups as one would animals. For example, one hardly could justify the administration of anesthetic drugs that would freely cross the placenta in very premature births just to note their effect. Even if such an experiment could be carried out, the neonatal loss rates are again so small that impossibly large numbers of cases would be needed to determine the issue.

While the issue probably cannot be solved on a statistical basis, some information might be obtained through a carefully documented study of a number of neonatal deaths. However, in such a study, one must be absolutely certain that anesthesia really has played a significant role in the death. It is always possible, and even probable, that one of the complications of pregnancy will have been the more important factor and anesthesia and analgesia merely coincidental.

INFANT MORTALITY

There are at least three feasible approaches to this problem. One is to examine the causes of large numbers of infant deaths in order to determine whether anesthesia and analgesia could possibly have played a significant role. In a study conducted by the Chicago Health Department, the causes of neonatal mortality are given for 8,905 infants. These are listed with their relative importance in Table 64.

It is conceivable that anesthetic and analgesic drugs may have played a role in the first, the fourth and the sixth

TABLE 64

CAUSE OF DEATH	PER CENT
Abnormal pulmonary ventilation	43.7
Injuries at birth	16.6
Malformations	15.8
Infections	13.4
Blood dyscrasias	5.3
Anoxia	3.8
Miscellaneous	1.4

category, namely, abnormal pulmonary ventilation, infection and anoxia.

The first cause of death in this series was abnormal pulmonary ventilation, responsible for 43.7 per cent of the loss. This category included all infants with no specific lesions outside the lungs whose deaths could be accounted for only on the basis of inadequate functioning of the lungs. In some instances, this inadequate functioning was due to depression of the respiratory center, while in others there was immaturity of the lungs. Seventy-five per cent of the deaths were in premature or previable infants. It is quite possible that where general anesthesia was used, it was indicated by obstetric complications which in themselves caused prematurity. Thus it becomes exceedingly difficult to evaluate the role that anesthesia and analgesia may play in this category.

The second possibly related cause of death in the Chicago study was infection, which was responsible for 13.4 per cent of the deaths. Pneumonia was by far the most common form of infection. Deaths from this cause are more frequent during the fifteenth to the twenty-ninth day of life than they are in the first few days. Infection of this type may be caused by premature rupture of the membranes or dystocia with infection of the amniotic fluid. Also, it may result from aspiration of amniotic fluid and meconium during difficult delivery. It is conceivable that depression of respiration in a newborn infant by anesthetic drugs and the consequent efforts at resuscitation also may induce such infection. Except for the last, it is difficult to understand just what role pain-relieving agents may play in this category.

The last possibly related cause of death is listed as anoxia, responsible for 3.8 per cent. When anoxia causes death of an infant born alive, usually it is because the supply of oxygen to the infant was deficient *in utero* prior to birth. Thus, the infant's tissues and particularly the central nervous system may have been damaged, possibly without noticeable effect on the infant during delivery. The obvious cause of such anoxia would be placental insufficiency due to separation of the placenta, placenta previa or abnormal uterine contraction pattern. It is extremely difficult to evaluate the role of anesthesia and analgesia in this category. Most drugs, unless they so depress the mother and thus add further insult, would have no effect. However, it is possible that certain

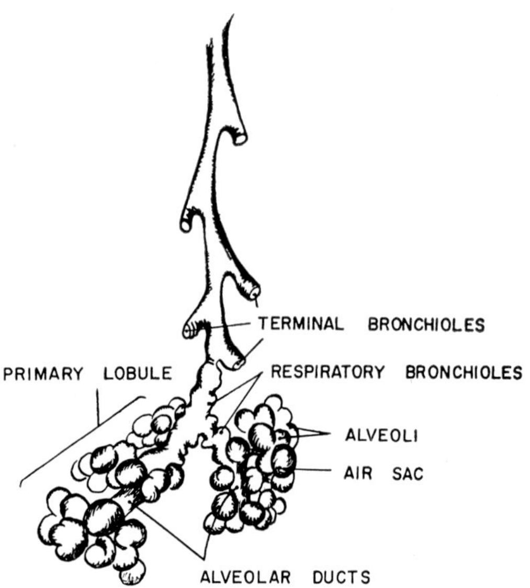

FIG. 104. Diagrammatic sketch of a lung lobule showing the pathway of air to the alveoli. (Bundesen, H. N., *et al.:* Progress in the Prevention of Needless Neonatal Deaths. From the Annual Report of the Chicago Health Department, 1951)

forms of conduction analgesia may produce an increased tone of the uterus, thus endangering, or at least diminishing, the available blood supply to the placenta. This is of theoretic consideration only, and no proof exists that such an effect is present.

INFANT PATHOLOGY

From the standpoint of the pathologist, abnormal pulmonary ventilation includes the following pathologic changes in the lungs:

1. Immaturity
2. Pulmonary hyaline membrane disease and resorption atelectasis
3. Secondary atelectasis
4. Congenital malformations of the lungs and the pulmonary passages

The lungs of a mature infant who has never breathed or been subject to intrauterine anoxia have a characteristic pattern that must be understood clearly in order to understand the pathologic entities referred to above. It is possible to make out the lumens of all portions of the pulmonary tree. The alveolar ducts are irregular in shape and have a "crumpled-sac" appearance. The potential air spaces contain a small amount of fluid. This, along with the elasticity of the parenchyma, gives the spaces a scalloped appearance. These may contain more fluid and be dilated more widely if the infant has made profound respiratory efforts due to intra-uterine anoxia. In these cases, the alveoli may contain squamous debris from the inspired amniotic fluid. They never become roundly and fully distended unless air has been inspired or unless the lungs have been injected with fluids of low surface tension such as benzene.

So long as the fetus is *in utero,* all the lumens of the duct system are filled with fluid. At no time are the walls in apposition in the normal lung. Whether the fluid is a transudate from the alveoli, whether it represents inspired amniotic fluid or whether it is in the alveoli as part of a pathway of flow during exchange of amniotic fluid is unknown. It is well established now that the amniotic fluid is exchanged with the mother at the rate of approximately 300 cc. per hour. That the fetal lungs take some part in this is shown by the fact that radiopaque material injected into the amniotic sac will be concentrated in the alveoli. If this is the normal pathway for exchange, why amniotic fluid debris is not concentrated so heavily there as to interfere with respiration is certainly a question.

In the immature lung, that is, in fetuses weighing less than 1,000 Gm., the spaces of the pulmonary tree are separated widely by connective tissue. Whether expanded by air or fluid, the lining cells are seen clearly to be cuboidal, a sure indication of the immaturity. A small percentage of these fetuses (15%) will survive. Furthermore, a percentage of premature infants (1,000+ Gm.) who succumb will show an immature pattern. In other words, there is no clear demarcation, so far as an intra-uterine existence goes, for lung development in order to support life.

Hyaline membrane disease is a condition known for many years and under many names, such as resorption atelectasis, congestive pulmonary failure, etc. The clinical and the pathologic findings are characteristic. The condition is very rare in term infants. It is present in a higher than expected percentage of infants born by cesarean section. The infants usually breathe spontaneously at birth, and will do so normally for the first hour or two thereafter. There is a gradually increasing difficulty with respiration, with deepening cyanosis and dyspnea. The sternum and the lower ribs show increasing retraction. Death usually takes place within 30 hours. At autopsy,

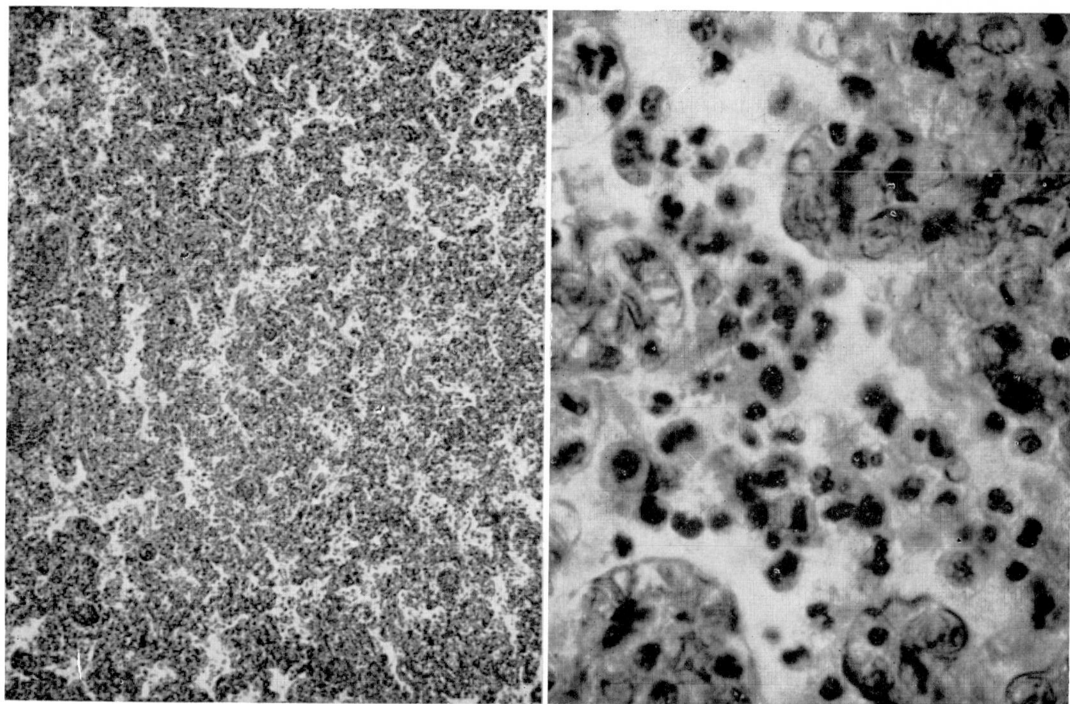

FIG. 105. Intra-uterine pneumonia in stillborn fetus. All potential air spaces are filled uniformly with polymorphonuclear leukocytes. No fibrin present. (*Left*) Low magnification. (*Right*) High magnification. (Potter, Edith L.: Pathology of the Fetus and the Newborn, Chicago, Yr. Bk. Pub.)

the lungs are a deep purple color and of the consistency of liver. Histologically, there is intense engorgement. The most important finding is resorption atelectasis. Most of the alveoli have collapsed, and the walls are approximated. A few of the alveoli and their ducts remain open. Lining the inner surface of some of these is an acidophilic homogeneous material resembling hyaline. The origin of this substance is unknown, but recent evidence suggests that it is fetal. Striking as the hyalinelike material is, the crux of the matter is the atelectasis. The identical clinical picture can occur without the membranes, and in term infants it usually does.

Very rarely does abnormal pulmonary ventilation cause death in term infants. When it does, death may be due to congenital malformations of the major air passages or to the failure of the infant to expand its lungs at birth and before the fluid separating the walls of the lumens of the pulmonary tree is absorbed. Once the fluid is gone, and this occurs quite rapidly, the approximated walls appear to become sticky and difficult to separate. The picture is one of secondary atelectasis. Frequently this is associated with small subplural and intra-alveolar hemorrhages. Very frequently the primary lesion is not in the lungs but in the central nervous system, where either gross damage or severe depression may have occurred.

Pneumonia in the newborn is of two types—that originating *in utero* due to infection of the amniotic fluid and that with onset after birth. In the former, the potential air spaces are filled with leukocytes and amniotic fluid debris.

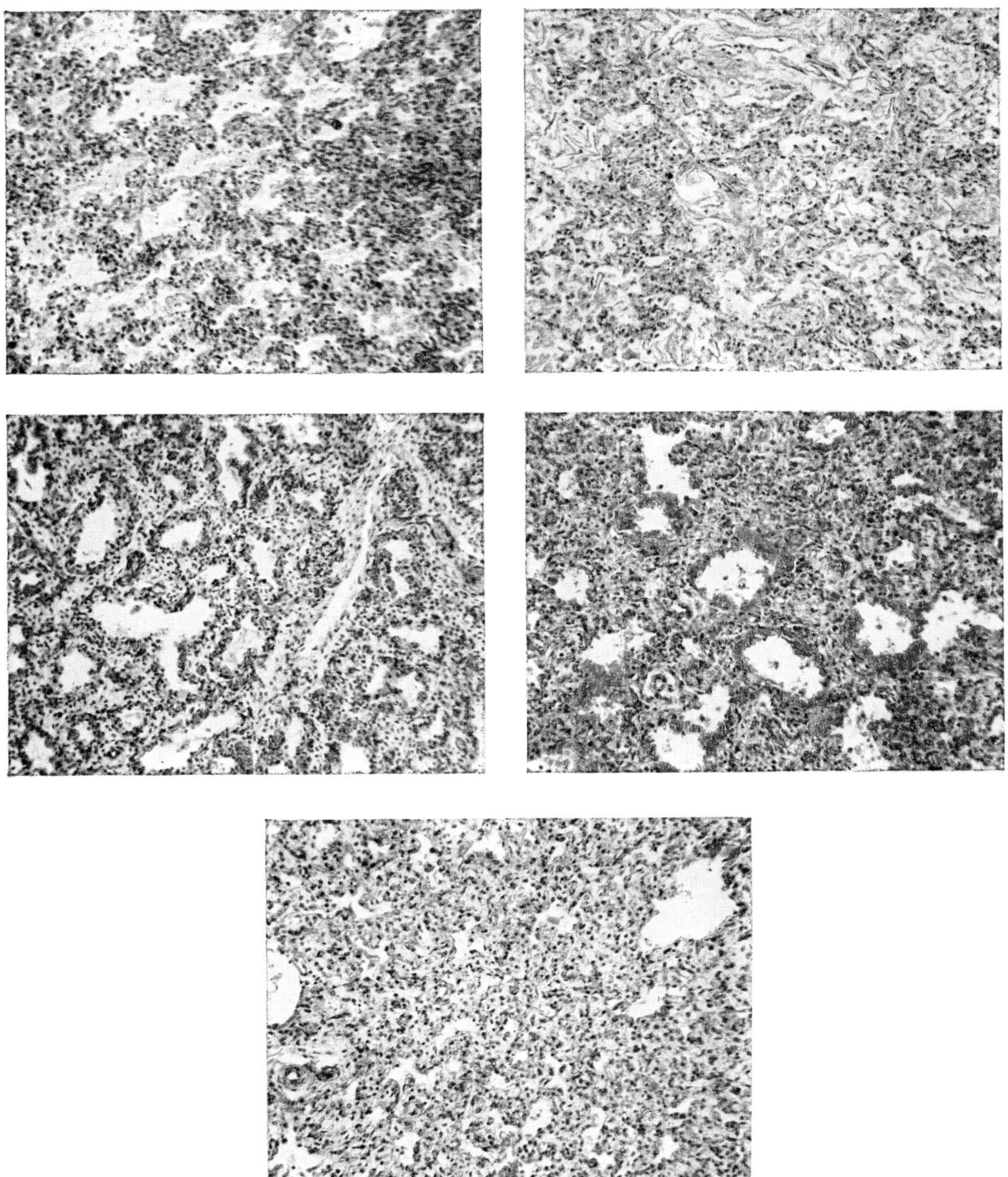

(A) Lung of a mature infant who never breathed. (B) Lung of a term infant who made violent respiratory efforts *in utero*. (C) Lung of an immature fetus. (D) Hyaline membrane disease in a premature infant. (E) Secondary or resorption atelectasis. (See text.)

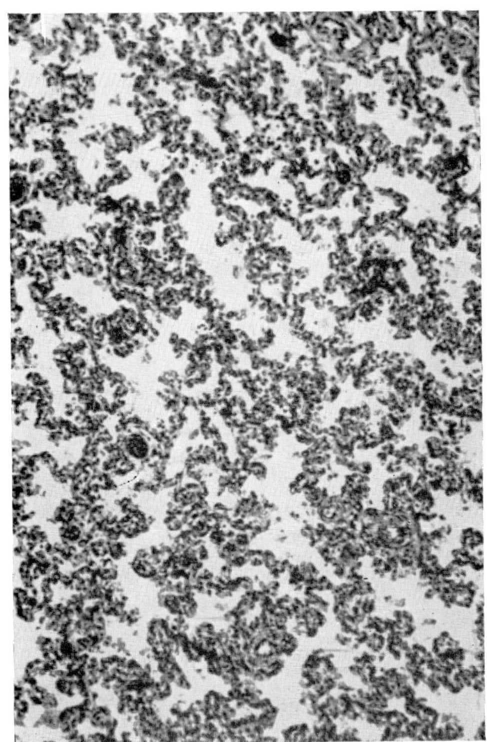

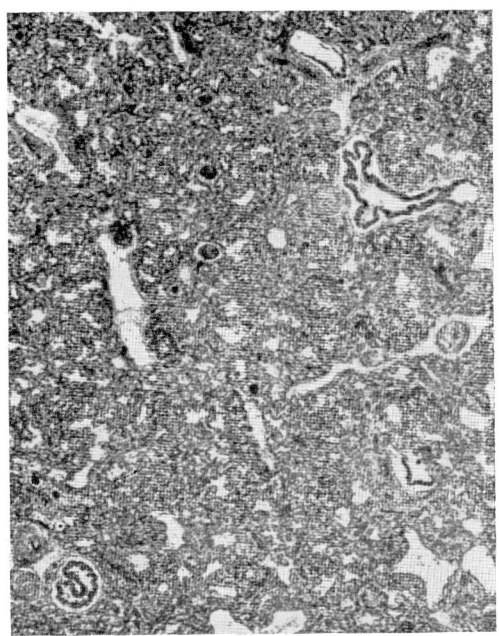

FIG. 106. Lung from stillborn infant and lung from live-born baby, contrasting picture resulting from respiratory efforts made *in utero* and pulmonary expansion after birth. (Potter, Edith L.: Pathology of the Fetus and the Newborn, Chicago, Yr. Bk. Pub.)

Characteristically, there is no fibrin, and this serves to differentiate the intra-uterine from the postnatally acquired pneumonias. Bacteria are present, these being similar to those invading the amniotic fluid, namely, staphylococci and colon bacilli.

The lungs of infants dying from anoxia prior to birth show the potential air spaces widely dilated with fluid and amniotic debris. If the infant is born alive and central nervous system damage has been severe enough, resorption atelectasis will be present.

So far as the other listed causes of death are concerned, anesthesia and analgesia probably play no role.

Two tables are reproduced here from the Chicago study; the first gives the estimated mortality rates by type of anesthetic, and the second indicates the mortality in the various categories of neonatal deaths by type of anesthetic.

In the first of these tables it would appear from a superficial glance that the death rate was lowest (21.46), where "no anesthesia" or regional and local anesthesia was used, and highest with cyclopropane (151.36). However, it must be remembered in examining such tables that in most instances local, regional and "no anesthesia" are administered to patients having simple delivery without complications. Furthermore, anesthesia is omitted frequently for normal multipara experiencing rapid birth, where the mortality normally would be extremely low. On the other hand, cyclopropane is employed frequently in those cases complicated by hemorrhage, dystocia, etc.,

TABLE 65. INFANT DEATHS BY CAUSE AND TYPE OF ANESTHESIA*

TYPE OF ANESTHESIA	CAUSE OF DEATH				
	Infections	*Injuries at Birth*	*Anoxia*	*Abnormal Pulmonary Ventilation*	*All Causes*
None	37.8	31.6	28.3	40.4	34.5
Inhalation	52.9	60.4	64.1	50.8	57.2
Local	6.5	5.1	5.2	5.4	5.7
Analgesics	2.8	2.9	2.4	3.4	2.5
TOTAL	100.0	100.0	100.0	100.0	100.0

TABLE 66. LIVE BIRTHS AND DEATHS, 1936-1949, BY TYPE OF ANESTHESIA ADMINISTERED TO MOTHERS IN FIRST AND SECOND STAGES OF LABOR*

	LIVE BIRTHS 1938		LIVE BIRTHS 1936–1949	ESTIMATED DEATHS 1936–1949	ESTIMATED MORTALITY RATES *per 1,000 Live Births*
	Number	*Percentage*			
Total	48,217	100.0	873,310	18,741	21.46
No anesthesia	20,049	41.59	363,209	6,281	17.29
Local and regional	2,065	4.28	37,378	979	26.19
Barbiturate	136	0.28	2,445	76	31.08
Opiate	275	0.57	4,978	284	57.05
Ether	13,389	27.77	242,518	4,733	19.52
Ethylene and nitrous oxide	6,217	12.89	112,570	3,792	33.69
Nitrous oxide	2,111	4.38	38,251	1,176	30.74
Cyclopropane	239	0.50	4,367	661	151.36
Chloroform	180	0.37	3,231	27	8.36
Other and unknown	3,556	7.37	64,363	732	11.37

* Bundesen, H. N., *et al.*: Progress in the Prevention of Needless Neonatal Deaths. (From the Annual Report of the Chicago Health Department, 1951)

where one might expect a high infant mortality from the complications themselves.

In the second table "no anesthesia" and inhalation give the highest mortality due to abnormal pulmonary ventilation to infection and anoxia. It is hardly conceivable that, on one hand, inhalation anesthesia is the guilty party while, on the other, lack of anesthesia is a major cause of infant deaths in these three categories. It is obvious that neither of these two paradoxical statements is entirely true, and that, on careful study of these cases, it is probable that the complications of delivery—on one hand requiring a deep anesthesia and on the other hand contraindicating its use—carry more weight than do the anesthetics or the lack of anesthetics themselves. Furthermore, it is hard to explain the high rates associated with "no anesthesia" and inhalation anesthesia where birth injuries are the cause of death, on the basis of pain relief or lack of pain relief.

The Chicago study has been cited in some detail to indicate the pitfalls encountered in trying to implicate anesthesia or the lack of anesthesia as a causative factor in infant mortality.

There is another approach to this

problem—one employed by Irving and his colleagues a number of years ago and illustrated in Figure 107.

Dr. Irving's philosophy was that the prevention of pain during labor should enable the doctor to await a more opportune time for delivery and perform delivery in an easier and a gentler manner. If this were so, the number of stillbirths should be reduced, because a number of serious birth injuries would be obviated. Fortunately, Dr. Irving lived in the era in which little pain relief was available to the patients of the Boston Lying-in Hospital. He and his colleagues were of the opinion that the precipitous fall in the stillbirth rate following the initiation of the program was due to the pain relief. Such a conclusion, while possibly true, is not justified by the evidence submitted, for one cannot use as a control a past population that may have differed considerably from the present. Factors other than analgesia may have been influential in causing the reduction in the stillbirth rate.

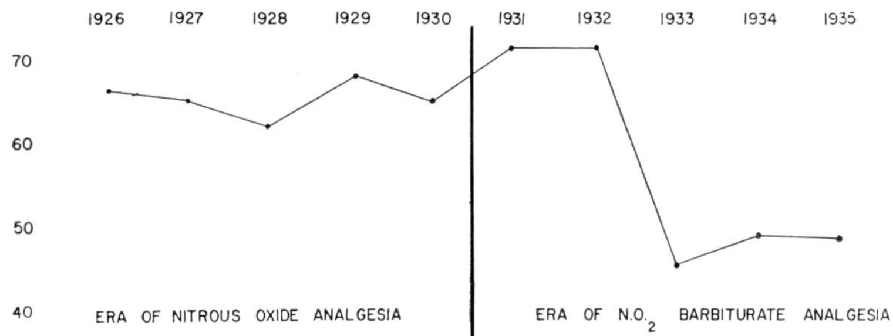

Fig. 107. Stillbirth rate per 1,000 births, including miscarriages and premature nonviable infants. (Clifford & Irving: Surg., Gynec. & Obst. **65**:1)

The authors tried to obtain some answer to this problem from the Baltimore Anesthesia Study. Their approach was somewhat different from that commonly employed, in that they were not concerned with any particular method but divided obstetric anesthesia into two broad systems: the encephalic, in which general anesthesia, either by inhalation or intravenously, was employed; and the anatomic, in which local infiltration and conduction (spinal or caudal) were used. Drugs from the former type cross the placenta freely and in significant amounts; from the latter, only infinitesimally small fractions of drug reach the infant. It is a fairly general clinical impression that the encephalic drugs produce some effect on the infant at birth. In order to test the magnitude of this effect numerically, breathing and crying times were studied for the two classes of anesthesia. If a breathing time of more than 1 minute and a crying time of more than 2 minutes is taken as an indication of poor reaction, then it is quite apparent, as shown in Table 67, that the encephalic approach gives a far greater percentage of poor reactions than does the anatomic.

In the anatomic approach there are certain complications that contribute also to poor infant reaction. Under conduction anesthesia, blood pressure is more labile and far more apt to show a drop. One of us (R. A. H.) has shown that a fall of more than 20 mm. has been observed in 20 per cent of caudal patients. While this drop in blood pressure did not affect the breathing time, it was correlated with a delay in crying time (Fig. 108).

TABLE 67. PERCENTAGE OF INFANTS WITH POOR REACTION ACCORDING TO METHOD OF ADMINISTERING ANESTHESIA

METHOD	NUMBER OF INFANTS				PER CENT	
	Breathing Time		*Crying Time*		*Breathing Time*	*Crying Time*
	Total Known	1 + Minutes	Total Known	2 + Minutes	(1 + Minutes)	(2 + Minutes)
All infants						
Encephalic	3,036	221	3,019	442	7.3	14.6
Anatomic	4,409	153	4,397	407	3.5	9.3
Premature infants						
Encephalic	167	18	164	31	10.8	18.9
Anatomic	414	15	410	45	3.6	10.9

Figure 109 shows only a moderate fall in blood pressure from spinal anesthesia. This patient had been long in labor and had a temperature of 102°. The baby was born at cesarean section with a fetal heart but never breathed. Inasmuch as each degree rise in maternal temperature increases the infant's need for oxygen by 10 per cent, the fall in blood pressure was probably sufficient to reduce the maternal blood flow to the placenta below the critical level. These poor results are rare and can probably be prevented by titrating the patient's blood pressure against an intravenous drip of Neosynephrine (1 cc. in 1,000 cc. dextrose).

From these studies it would appear that certain anesthetic drugs and their coincidental effects upon the mother play a role in the reaction of the infant at birth.

The question of infant survival is not answered by the reaction of the infant at birth, and from clinical impression one may doubt whether one bears any relationship to the other. This is exactly what the Baltimore Anesthesia Study showed. In spite of the fact that general anesthetic drugs of the encephalic type were known to produce more sluggish infants, when death rates were examined for these infants there was no significant difference between the two major categories of anesthesia either in those infants at term or in those in special jeopardy because of prematurity or cesarean section (Figs. 110-112).

These results do not imply that any anesthesia will yield equally good results

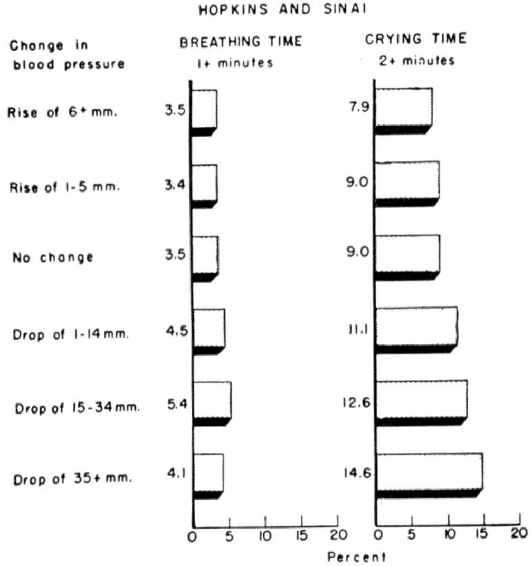

FIG. 108. Relationship between poor infant reaction, as indicated by breathing and crying time and change in blood pressure of mother.

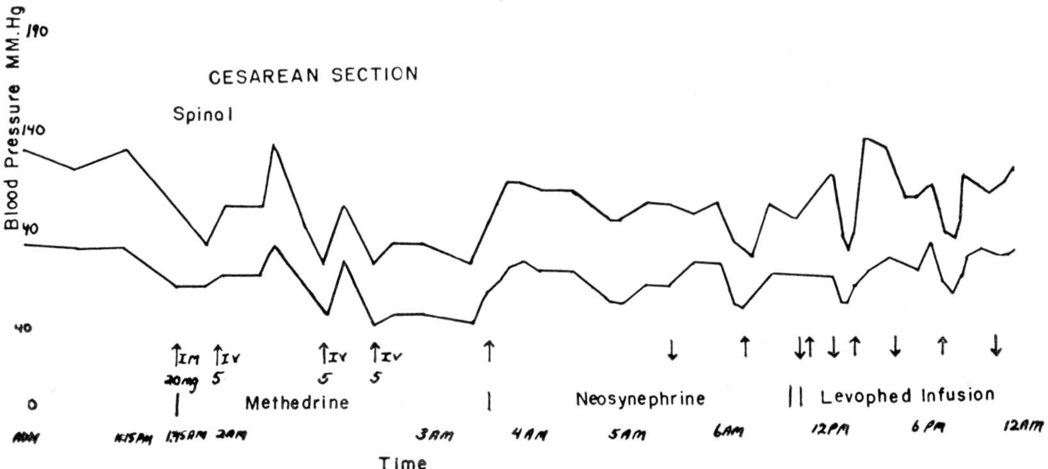

FIGURE 109

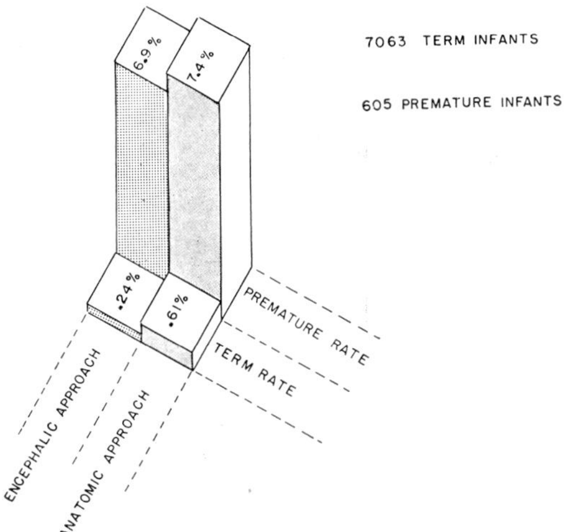

FIG. 110. Total death rate for term and premature infants according to method of administration of anesthesia.

in all situations. They do indicate that when obstetric anesthesia and analgesia are handled round the clock by a corps of well-trained physicians and anesthesiologists aided by a group of alert, specifically trained nurse assistants who follow the patient at the bedside, and when, in addition, drug dosage is kept within reasonable limits, then, and then only, will equally good infant survival be obtained for all methods of anesthesia. More simply stated, there is probably no *best* method of anesthesia and analgesia so far as the infant is concerned. This clarifies the situation somewhat and indicates that it may be more beneficial to select anesthesia and analgesia suitable to the mother's specific situation and complication than to concern one's self unduly with the infant. This, as has been indicated elsewhere in the text, may be of greater significance.

The problem of whether or not "no anesthesia" is better for infants than some maternal pain relief could not be answered from the Baltimore study, nor is a finite solution ever likely to be available to us. In most studies, two groups of patients get "no anesthesia"—

the exceedingly normal and fast-delivering multipara and the patients with such severe complications that they are desperately ill and the infants likely to be dead before birth. In such circumstances, the selection of a satisfactory control is almost impossible. Furthermore, it is impossible in a hospital where the majority of patients have their pains of labor relieved to select arbitrarily a group that will have no pain relief in order to compare infant mortality.

The question is perhaps an academic one anyway. For every shred of evidence seems to indicate that in most situations the infant is primarily unaffected by control of maternal pain. It is only the depression of respiration at the central level that yields the hypoventilating and consequent suboxygenated infant. The main problem that remains with us, and one that should be answered by future investigators, is whether or not the delayed reactions at birth produced by encephalic drugs have any bearing on the mental development of the infant.

INFANT MORBIDITY

Dr. Benjamin Pasamanick, of Baltimore, and Dr. Abraham M. Lilienfeld, of Buffalo, have surveyed *Association of Maternal and Fetal Factors with Development of Mental Deficiency* in *The Journal of the American Medical Association*, Vol. 159, No. 3, September 17, 1955. The infants studied in their report included all of those whose deliveries were managed by the authors of this

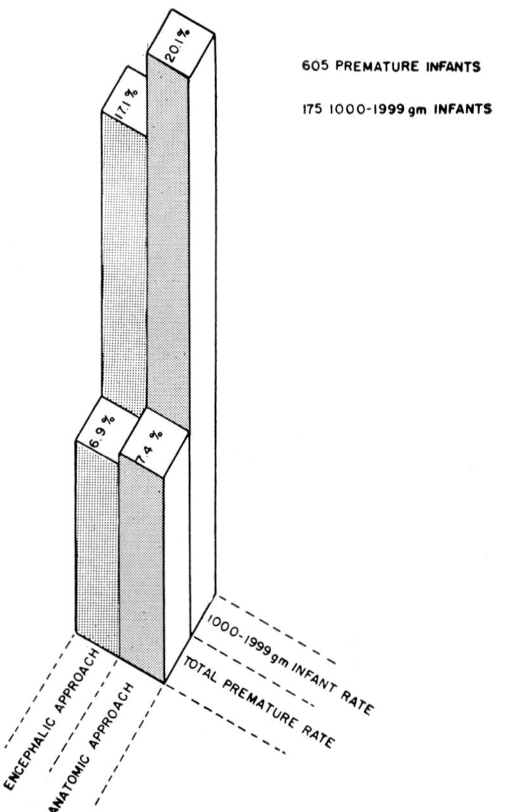

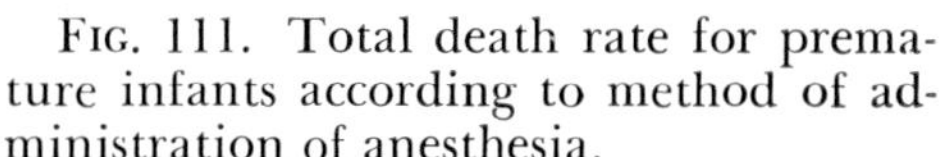
FIG. 111. Total death rate for premature infants according to method of administration of anesthesia.

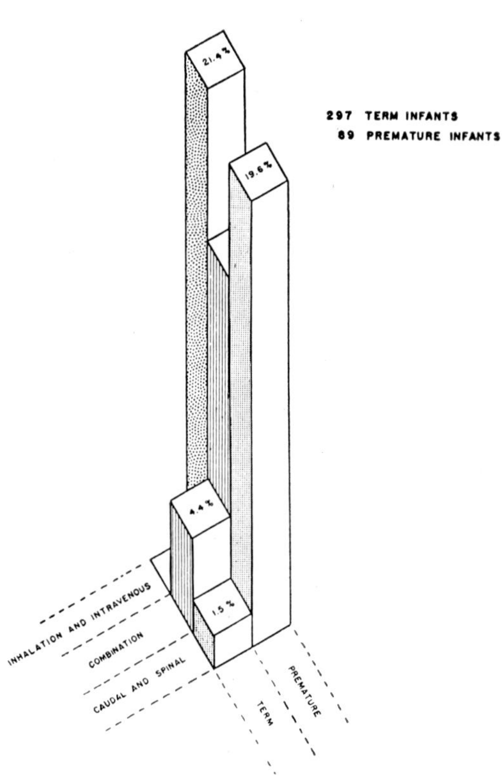

FIG. 112. Total fetal loss in 386 cesarean sections according to method of administration of anesthesia.

book in the Johns Hopkins Hospital during the period June 1, 1948, through July 1, 1951.

They stated:

It has been repeated frequently within recent years that mental deficiency is not in itself a clinical entity but rather a symptom present in a large number of diseases of varying etiology. This symptom, present according to different estimates in from 1 to 2 per cent of the population of the United States, is probably the most serious single public health problem from the point of view of chronicity, cost of care, loss of productive and earning capacity, and tragedy in the family. Within this century, the thinking concerning the etiology of this entity has swung from considering the majority of cases of mental deficiency to be of hereditary or familial origin to the belief that only a small minority of cases falls within this category. As an increasing number of exogenous factors has become causally implicated, the so-called endogenous role of heredity that had previously been applied largely on a *post hoc* basis has accordingly diminished. The familial aggregation of mental retardation is frequently being attributed more to an increased risk of exposure of family members to the same etiologic factors rather than to heredity.

Injury to the brain has long been known to produce sufficient dysfunction to result in mental deficiency, and complications of delivery, such as prolonged and difficult delivery and difficulty in resuscitation of the newborn infant, are often described as major causes of these cerebral injuries. While syphilis had been implicated for many years as an important prenatal factor in the development of mental deficiency, only in the last few decades have we become aware that the period of uterine life is one in which the fetus may be damaged by a number of noxious agents. Among these may be mentioned toxoplasmosis, rubella, and possibly other viral invasions and sensitizations to blood components such as the Rh and other factors. Even dietary inadequacies have been implicated.

A number of studies, such as Windle's, on the effects of anoxia on animals have shown that, with sufficient insult to the brain, it is possible to produce behaviorial malfunction analogous to human mental deficiency. Studies attempting to investigate the relationship of various prenatal or paranatal factors to the development of mental deficiency in children have usually been rather poorly designed. They frequently have been inadequately controlled or based on retrospective information obtained from parents, with all the possibilities of bias this implies. Darke, in a carefully conceived study, found that there was a significant relation between asphyxia neonatorum and low IQ; however, Keith and Norval in a similar study did not find this relationship, although a few individuals were found to be in the defective range. Both studies are open to the serious objection that they eliminated cases with any question of neurologic involvement. It is difficult to conceive of cerebral damage sufficient to cause serious intellectual impairment without even slight neurologic findings. One is led to question the depth of the asphyxia in the cases with completely negative physical findings.

It seemed that a better approach to the question of association of maternal and fetal factors with the development of mental deficiency might be made by selecting a group of retarded children born in a given area and then reviewing the maternal and fetal factors as recorded on birth certificates and hospital obstetric records. Comparison could then be made with an appropriately selected control group. We have used such an approach in a series of similar epidemiologic studies of the association of maternal and fetal factors with the development of the neuropsychiatric disorders, cerebral palsy, epilepsy and behavior disorders of childhood, in which significantly positive associations were found. This is a report of the results of such an investigation with regard to mental deficiency.

Method of Study

The case registers of the Harriet Lane Home, children's psychiatric service of the Johns Hopkins Hospital, and the division of special education of the Baltimore Department of Education were searched for the names and identifying information of patients with diagnosed mental deficiency or intelligence quotients under 80 who were born in Baltimore during the period from 1935 to 1952, inclusive. The registers of 2 institutions for mentally defective persons operated by the State of Maryland Department of Mental Hygiene were likewise searched for institutionalized patients with mental deficiency. The following information concerning each patient was obtained from the clinic or hospital record when available: type of deficiency; presence of associated defects such as epilepsy, cerebral palsy, congenital anomalies, or other defects; and the results of intelligence testing. The records obtained from these different sources were matched to locate duplicates, which were discarded. The birth register maintained by the bureau of vital records of the Baltimore City Health Department was then searched for the birth certificates of these persons. As a control series of births with which the defective patients could be compared, the next birth reported from the same place of birth as the defective patient, matched by race and maternal age group, was selected. The following maternal age groups were used: under 20, 20 to 24, 25 to 29, 30 to 34, 35 and over. If the matched control had died during the neonatal period as determined either from the birth certificate or from the hospital records, this birth was omitted from the control series and the next birth with the characteristics noted above was selected. This was done since there was no chance that mental defect would manifest itself in a child dying during the neonatal period, and this child should not, therefore, be considered as a control whose prenatal and paranatal experiences could be compared with a retarded child who had survived the neonatal period. From the birth certificates the following information was obtained on each defective child and his matched control: place of birth, maternal age, total number of previous pregnancies, number of previous infants born alive and now living, number born alive and now dead, and number born dead.

In those instances in which the retarded child and its matched control were born in a hospital, the following information concerning the pregnancy and delivery was abstracted from the hospital record: total number of previous pregnancies of the mothers, numbers of previous abortions, previous stillbirths, previous premature births, previous neonatal deaths, length of labor, complications of pregnancy and labor, operative procedures, birth weight, and the condition of the child during the neonatal period. The person obtaining this information from the hospital record was not informed whether the birth was of a retarded or of a control child. The hospital records did not contain information concerning the abnormalities studied in a small number of both defective patients and controls. The number differed depending on the specific abnormality, resulting in a slight variation in the totals in the tables presented in this report.

Of the 1,107 retarded children for whom birth

TABLE 68. COMPLICATIONS OF PREGNANCY IN MOTHERS OF PERSONS WITH MENTAL RETARDATION AND CONTROLS BY RACE AND PRESENCE OF ASSOCIATED DEFECTS

Complications	White				Nonwhite		
	No. of Persons with Retardation			No. of Controls	No. of Persons with Retardation		No. of Controls
	Without Associated Defects	With Associated Defects*	Total		Without Associated Defects	Total	
Toxemias of pregnancy	38	2	40	34	50	51	42
Bleeding during pregnancy and labor (cause not specified)	10	2	12	10	7	8	5
Nonpuerperal complications†	35	7	42	25	81	83	83
Breech presentation	10	8	18	13	7	7	2
Dystocia owing to abnormal pelvis	10	2	12	15	29	31	44
Miscellaneous puerperal complications‡	14	4	20	19	11	11	4
Premature separation of placenta	5	1	6	4	1	2	1
Dystocia other than owing to abnormal pelvis	18	5	23	24	..	..	1
Placenta previa	4	3	7	2	2	2	..
Prolapse of cord	2	..	2	..	..	..	1
Malpresentations other than breech	8	1	9	5	11	12	6
No. of hospital records containing information	334	70	404	416	227	235	240

*Associated defects include cerebral palsy, epilepsy, hydrocephalus, mongolism, tuberous sclerosis and craniofacial defects.

†Nonpuerperal complications include diseases associated with, but not related to, pregnancy.

‡Miscellaneous puerperal complications include pyelitis, other genito-urinary diseases and hydramnios.

certificates were located, 430 (or 38.9%) were nonwhite. Sixty-four per cent and 55 per cent, respectively, of the white and the nonwhite births were in hospitals. Thirty-five children, representing 3.2 per cent of the total, were a result of a multiple pregnancy. It is of interest that this percentage of multiple births is higher than in the control group (0.5%) and in the general population (1.2%).

The data developed by Pasamanick and Lilienfeld comparing the implications of the racial factors in this study are not presented in this text, since the authors of the text already have analyzed these in Chapter 1, with the presentation of graphs concerned with these racial factors (Figs. 13 & 14, pp. 29 & 30).

Pasamanick and Lilienfeld surveyed the pattern of factors, such as complications of pregnancy, prematurity and neonatal abnormalities, that appear to be associated with mental defect. They have found these factors to be similar to those previously associated with stillbirths, neonatal deaths, cerebral palsy, epilepsy and childhood behavior disorder. This continuum of reproductive casualty is composed of a lethal component consisting of abortions, stillbirths and neonatal deaths and a sublethal component consisting of cerebral palsy, epilepsy and behavior disorder. The results of this study suggest that this sublethal component should also include mental retardation. It is interesting that approximately one third of persons with cerebral palsy have convulsive seizures, and two thirds have varying degrees of mental retardation, suggesting that cerebral palsy may result from a more severe type of brain damage than epilepsy or mental defect.

The Baltimore study is sufficiently suggestive to warrant further investigation concerning the other possible components of this continuum. Such study, now in the planning stages, has been initiated by the authors of this text with the Child Psychology Division of the Baltimore city schools. It is their plan to compare in

Table 69. Frequency of Complications of Pregnancy in Mothers of Persons with Mental Retardation and Controls by Race and Presence of Associated Defects

	White								Nonwhite					
	No. of Retarded Persons						No. of Controls		No. of Retarded Persons				No. of Controls	
	Without Associated Defects		With Associated Defects		Total				Without Associated Defects		Total			
No. of Complications	No.	%	No.	%	No.	%	No.	%	No.	%	No.	%	No.	%
0	218	65.3	47	67.1	265	65.6	311	74.8	92	40.5	94	40.0	108	45.0
1	96	28.7	17	24.3	113	28.0	78	18.8	85	37.4	89	37.9	90	37.5
2	13	3.9	5	7.1	18	4.5	24	5.8	31	13.7	33	14.0	26	10.8
3	4	1.2	1	1.5	5	1.2	1	0.2	14	6.2	14	6.0	11	4.6
4	3	0.9	..	....	3	0.7	...	....	3	1.3	3	1.2	5	2.0
5	...	....	..	....	...	....	1	0.2	2	0.9	2	0.9	...	....
6	...	....	..	....	...	....	1	0.2	...	....	...	....	...	....
Total	114	100.0	70	100.0	404	100.0	416	100.0	227	100.0	235	100.0	240	100.0
No. having one or more complications	116	34.7	23	32.9	139	34.4	105	25.2	135	59.5	141	60.0	132	55.0
No. having two or more complications	20	6.0	6	8.6	26	6.4	27	6.5	50	22.0	52	22.1	42	17.5

1965 intelligence quotients of suboxygenated children with controls born in the Johns Hopkins and Sinai Hospitals during the period 1948 through 1951. These children, in age groups, with recorded documentation of suboxygenation and hypoventilation for varying intervals of 1 to 10 minutes after birth, will be studied in comparison with undamaged controls born in the same hospitals. By 1965 the children born in 1948 will be near the end of their high school courses, and children born in 1951 will be completing their junior high school courses. Such a study is planned to support the one reported herein and to add further information on the latent and the temporal effects of anoxia in its relationship to mental retardation.

We agree with Pasamanick and Lilienfeld that no longer is one quite justified in speaking of cerebral palsy, epilepsy, mental deficiency and childhood behavior disorder as distinct, separable and indivisible clinical entities; rather, one must think in terms of chronic cerebral injury, with cerebral palsy and/or convulsive seizures, mental retardation and behavior disorder as distinct clinical entities. This focuses attention not only on the need for care in diagnosis but also, since it is now well known that individuals with brain injuries require specific types of management and education, on the fact that a good deal of effort should be exerted to develop precise methods of diagnosis.

Above all, this conceptual framework indicates an area within which lies the possibility of prevention of these neuropsychiatric disorders. It indicates the need for extensive studies of the factors causing or associated with the complications of pregnancy and labor, since these not only influence maternal health and infant loss but appear to have an influence on the surviving infant. Of necessity, any effort toward the prevention of the components of this continuum must be directed at an improvement of conditions associated with maternal health.

We emphasize the conclusions of Pasamanick and Lilienfeld that:

1. The prenatal and the paranatal records of mentally defective children born in Baltimore between 1935 and 1952 showed significantly more complications of pregnancy and delivery, prematurity and abnormal neonatal condition than a similar number of matched controls.

2. The nonmechanical abnormalities such as bleeding during pregnancy and toxemia appear to be important factors of delivery previously described.

3. There is a continuum of reproductive casualty, consisting of brain damage incurred during the prenatal and the paranatal periods as a result of abnormalities during these periods, leading to a gradient of injury extending from fetal and neonatal death through cerebral palsy, epilepsy, behavior disorder and mental retardation.

4. This continuum has implications for further research in the etiology, the diagnosis, the management and the prevention of these neuropsychiatric disorders.

Very probably the problem of reducing neuropsychiatric disorders can be resolved in large measure by initiating promptly and maintaining adequate transalveolar oxygenation.

Dr. Edith Potter, in her paper on *State of the Lungs at Birth* in *The Journal of the American Medical Association,* Vol. 159, No. 14, December 3, 1955, summarized as follows her study of the reasons why the infant does not breathe:

> There are many reasons why an infant does not breathe, but by far the commonest are cytotoxic states of the respiratory center caused by anoxia, by depressant drugs or by other toxic states in the mother. Some of these effects are temporary, and it is to provide oxygen until

such time as that effect shall have passed that resuscitation is undertaken.

The mouth and the pharynx of the infant are usually full of amniotic fluid and mucus at birth, and these are usually inspired without ill-effect with the first breath. Unless an infant has been anoxic for a prolonged period before birth so that its alveoli have been distended by debris from the amniotic fluid, there will be no direct mechanical obstruction to breathing. Even then the effect on the brain of the anoxia that was responsible for excessive intra-uterine activity is more important in failure to breathe than is the direct effect on the lungs. Plugging of a bronchus with mucus sufficient to interfere with establishment of extra-uterine respiration is of almost unknown occurrence. Except in malformations or the more massive intra-uterine pneumonias, a local disturbance in the lungs is almost never responsible for immediate postnatal apnea. All infants who do not breathe are ill; this must never be forgotten when treatment is instituted.

BIBLIOGRAPHY

Bundesen, H. N., Potter, E. L., Fishbein, W. I., Bauer, C. F., and Plotzke, G. V.: Progress in the Prevention of Needless Neonatal Deaths. From the Annual Report of the Chicago Health Department, 1951.

Hellman, I. M., and Hingson, R. A.: Effects of various methods of obstetric pain relief on infant mortality, New York J. Med. **53**: 2767, 1953.

Irving, F. C., Berman, S., and Nelson, H. B.: Barbiturates and other hypnotics in labor, Surg., Gynec. & Obst. **58**:1, 1934.

Potter, E. L.: Pathology of the Fetus and the Newborn, Chicago, Yr. Bk. Pub., 1952.

Tran-Dinh-De, and Anderson, G. W.: Hyaline-like membranes associated with diseases of the newborn lung: a review of the literature, Obst. & Gynec. Surv. **8**:1, 1953.

9 Maternal and Infant Safeguards

VIRGINIA APGAR, M.D.*

The most important maternal complications that demand emergency treatment are:

Hemorrhage
Aspiration of vomitus
Marked hypotension
Convulsions
Marked respiratory depression
Extreme uterine spasm
Severe hypertension
Cardiac arrest

The prophylaxis of these conditions has been discussed elsewhere, but their continued occurrence and mismanaged or neglected treatment still lead to a preventable mortality.

HEMORRHAGE

When the cause of hemorrhage is not immediately obvious or when the rate of blood loss is excessive, a sample of blood should be drawn with a large-bore needle (No. 18) for crossmatching and Rh determination, and a second tube should be drawn with a sample for observation of clot formation. If facilities for quantitative fibrinogen determinations are available, another tube containing dried oxalate is used. These samples should be drawn before the veins become empty and before the blood has been diluted with other fluids. Gross diagnosis of hypofibrinogenemia can be made by observing a tube of clotted blood. Lysis of the clot usually will take place within an hour. The friability of the clot can be tested by agitating it gently with a wooden applicator. A quantitative determination of less than 100 mg. per cent of plasma indicates the need for fibrinogen replacement. Excessive bleeding in cases of placental separation, abruptio placenta and placenta praevia, especially with a dead fetus, should suggest the diagnosis of hypofibrinogenemia. Sometimes it accompanies the rare complication of amniotic fluid embolism. As with blood transfusion, the possibility of viral hepatitis should be kept in mind when giving fibrinogen. The usual dosage is from 10 to 15 Gm. dissolved in dextrose and water.

In all cases of hemorrhage, the large-bore needle is left in place and connected immediately to a bottle of 5 per cent dextrose in water or a plasma expander (dextran, polyvinylpyrrilodone, gelatin, serum albumin). If blood is to be used under pressure, a bottle of normal saline should be interposed between the blood and the patient to prevent agglutination of blood in dextrose and to guard against air embolism.

It is the duty of the physician or the nurse whose task it will be to administer fluids to select at least 2 veins for future use should such an emergency arise. This is especially important in obese individuals. Much time can be lost and a fatality result while search is being made for a satisfactory route for blood administration. The suddenness with which obstetric hemorrhage occurs causes a rapid drop in venous pressure, making venipuncture even more difficult

* Professor of Anesthesiology, Columbia University, and Attending Anesthesiologist, Anesthesia Service, Columbia-Presbyterian Medical Center.

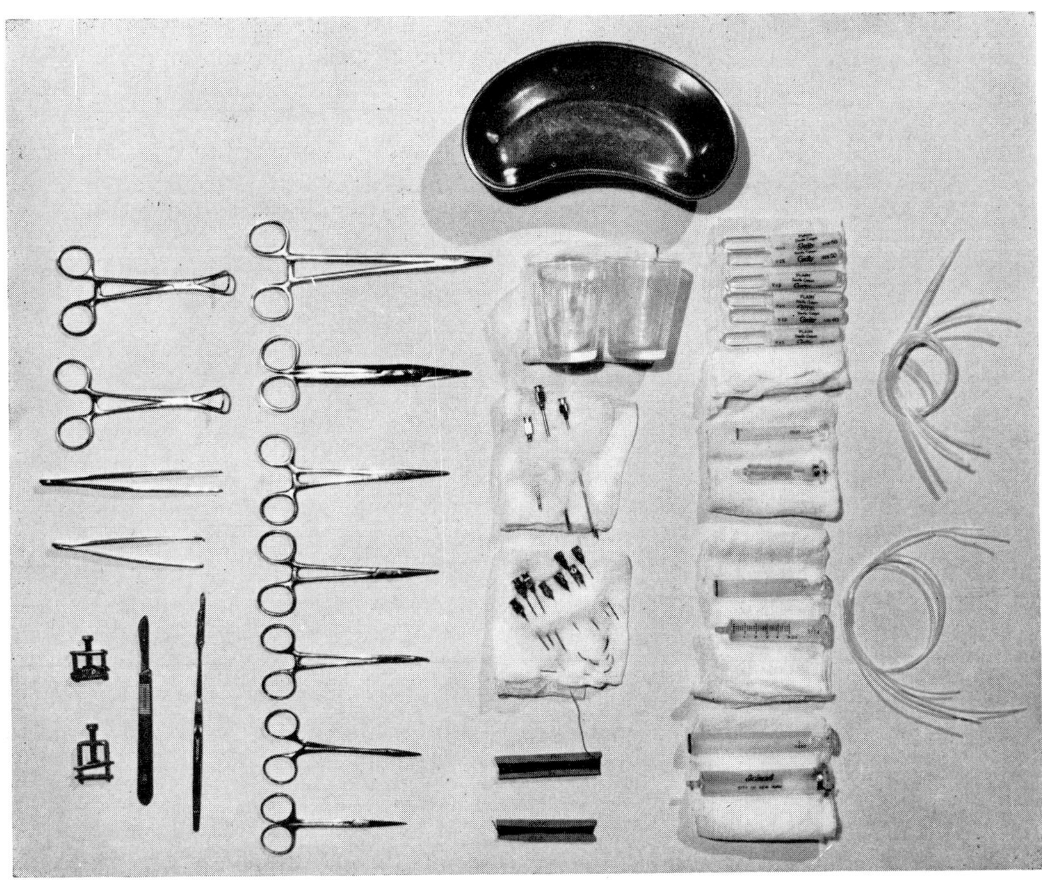

FIG. 113. Cut-down set. (Department of Obstetrics, Kings County Hospital, Brooklyn, N. Y.)

than in the usual type of hemorrhage. With the legs in the lithotomy position, ankle and femoral veins are useless. The hands, the arms and the neck are the only available sites for venipuncture. When a hemorrhagic emergency occurs, a tourniquet should be placed promptly round the upper arm to preserve some blood in the veins to demonstrate their course. If venipuncture is unsuccessful in the upper extremity, the external jugular vein is very useful for blood replacement. To find it quickly, the patient is put in a slight head-down position, and the operator's finger is laid just above and parallel to the clavicle. The broad flat vein can be seen or palpated easily. Venipuncture is easy if the patient is not restless or conscious. Light planes of general anesthesia to produce vasodilatation enough to demonstrate the site of veins are infinitely better than the administration of vasopressors to keep the blood pressure audible. These latter drugs all cause venoconstriction to some degree.

When indirect venipuncture has failed, instruments for cut-down technics should be immediately available (Fig. 113). Recently it was demonstrated that intra-arterial transfusion had no advantage over rapid intravenous blood replacement. Furthermore, this type of transfusion may cause loss of digits through arterial spasm. The occasional absence of anastomosis between the superficial and the deep volar arches in the hand cannot be determined in an emergency, and this anomaly is the probable cause of gangrene. Direct aortic replacement of blood is impossible from the posterior approach because of the supine position necessitated by the obstetric complication. To insert a needle under direct vision in a patient with empty veins, an empty vein, an artery in spasm and a tendon must be differentiated.

The most rapid and simple route in circumstances of decompensated hemorrhage is *marrow transfusion*. The sternum and the iliac crest both are possible sites for transfusion, though use of the former will deliver blood to the coronary arteries more rapidly than will the latter. Sternal puncture carries slightly more hazard of a serious nature than that of the iliac crest, but perforation into the mediastinum, the pleura or the vena cava can be avoided with proper technic. No special equipment is necessary. An 18-gauge needle attached to a 2-cc. syringe makes a convenient instrument for puncture. The manubrium is preferable to the body of the sternum, for there is more space available both laterally and in an anteroposterior direction. The mid-line is identified quickly by palpation of the suprasternal notch. The lower border is at the chondral junction of the manubrium and the body. The lateral limits are noted at the costal border. One centimeter cephalad to the articulation between the body and the manubrium, the outer bony table is thinnest and easiest to penetrate. The needle, held in the right hand, is introduced at a 45° angle; it is advanced with considerable forward pressure but with calculated restraint immediately after the upper table of bone is penetrated. A twisting motion upon introduction of the needle makes perforation of the bone easier. The moment lessened resistance is felt, forward motion is stopped. Withdrawal of the piston with the thumb produces a flow of blood and marrow. Time is not taken to identify fat droplets in marrow. This mixture of blood and marrow can be used for crossmatching if all other attempts to obtain a blood sample have failed. The piston is depressed before the mixture has time to clot, and the appropriate fluid is introduced into the sternum. On 6 obstetric occasions at the Sloane Hospital for Women, sternal transfusion was successful with recoveries in all patients. One obese Negress died of hemorrhage, even though ample blood was available, for all cut-down routes were unsuccessful and sternal puncture was not considered.

The sternal route has been used for fluid administration for as long as 12 hours, but rarely is it necessary for more than a half hour, for hemorrhage either has been stopped or has been fatal. Blood can be introduced as easily under pressure as with the intravenous route; in one case, 500 cc. was administered in 5 minutes. In hemorrhagic emergencies, the mention of the sternal route seems to be a signal for much discussion and wasted time. It is recommended that the sternal needle be placed and blood started before discussion begins.

ASPIRATION OF VOMITUS

Death from this cause is quite unnecessary if there is a plan of action and it is carried out. Obstetricians can be of great assistance if, toward the end of antenatal care, the husband and the wife both are warned about celebrating the onset of the long-awaited contractions by having a big meal preceded by ample alcoholic fluid therapy. Likewise, when in the hospital, if labor actually is present, *no* solid food should be given. It is unlikely that any death from this cause has occurred wholly from aspirated *fluids.* All the usual measures of emptying the tracheobronchial tree are of no avail if much solid food is present. Vision is greatly hampered during laryngoscopy, endotracheal tubes become filled with solid vomitus, and suction equipment is useless.

On a general surgical service it is customary to empty the stomach before anesthesia is induced. Such a plan is equally good on an obstetric service, but it is somewhat more difficult to carry out; in fact, sometimes it is impossible and unwise. If there is no hurry to deliver the infant, and if for some reason regional anesthesia cannot be used, a patient can best be made to empty a stomach full of solid food by stimulating the pharyngeal reflex with a catheter or a stomach tube. It is strongly advised not to introduce extra fluid into the stomach, as is usual with gastric lavage, for the displacement of the stomach by the full-term uterus and its contents may prevent the retrieving of any or all of it and thus increase the problem. Apomorphine is not advised because of its continued action as an emetic.

A frequent situation is the admission of an active multipara who has eaten recently or from whom for reasons of language difficulty such a history cannot be obtained. Delivery is imminent. The safest method of anesthesia is to avoid general anesthetics and to use any regional method, if indeed anesthesia is necessary at all. Local infiltration of the episiotomy site, pudendal block, caudal or spinal anesthesia—all protect the glottic reflex should vomiting occur.

A much more difficult situation is presented by a woman with placenta praevia, an unknown amount of blood loss and fetal distress. Immediate cesarean section is indicated. Local infiltration of the abdominal wall is too time consuming to obtain a live baby. Spinal, caudal or lumbar epidural anesthesia is not wise in the presence of increasing hypovollemia. A quick, skillfully administered general anesthesia produces the best results for both mother and infant. Cyclopropane is an ideal agent to use in this circumstance, but the choice of agent and technic must be left to the anesthesiologist. Some prefer Pentothal Sodium induction, the use of relaxants and rapid intubation with a cuffed endotracheal tube. Nitrous oxide ether sequence is satisfactory but somewhat slower in achieving surgical anesthesia than cyclopropane. In our own experience, the use of relaxants in the presence of a full stomach is associated frequently with silent regurgitation of gastric contents. It is likely that when the technical difficulties of esophageal or gastric blockers are overcome, such a device will find a place on obstetric services.

In spite of the most careful planning and execution of such plans, the grave emergency of flooding the pharynx and the trachea will still occur occasionally. At this time a plan of action is invaluable. If an extra person is available, he is assigned to follow the radial pulse *at all times,* and report any and all changes. A suddenly weak or slow pulse may force the decision for tracheotomy. In the meantime the anesthesiologist discontinues the anesthesia and removes the mask immediately. In the standing position, he inserts his left index finger between the cheek and the jaw until it meets the molar area. With as much force as needed, he pries open the mouth *behind* the last tooth, and with the right hand scoops out as much solid material as fast as he can. Suction is useless, and nasal manipulations, such as suction catheter or nasal airway, only add to the problem by providing explosive bleeding. When there is room in the mouth for a laryngoscope, removal of solid material will be speeded by direct vision. A curved clamp is helpful in reaching the depths of the pharynx. When the pharynx is reasonably clear, the mask is

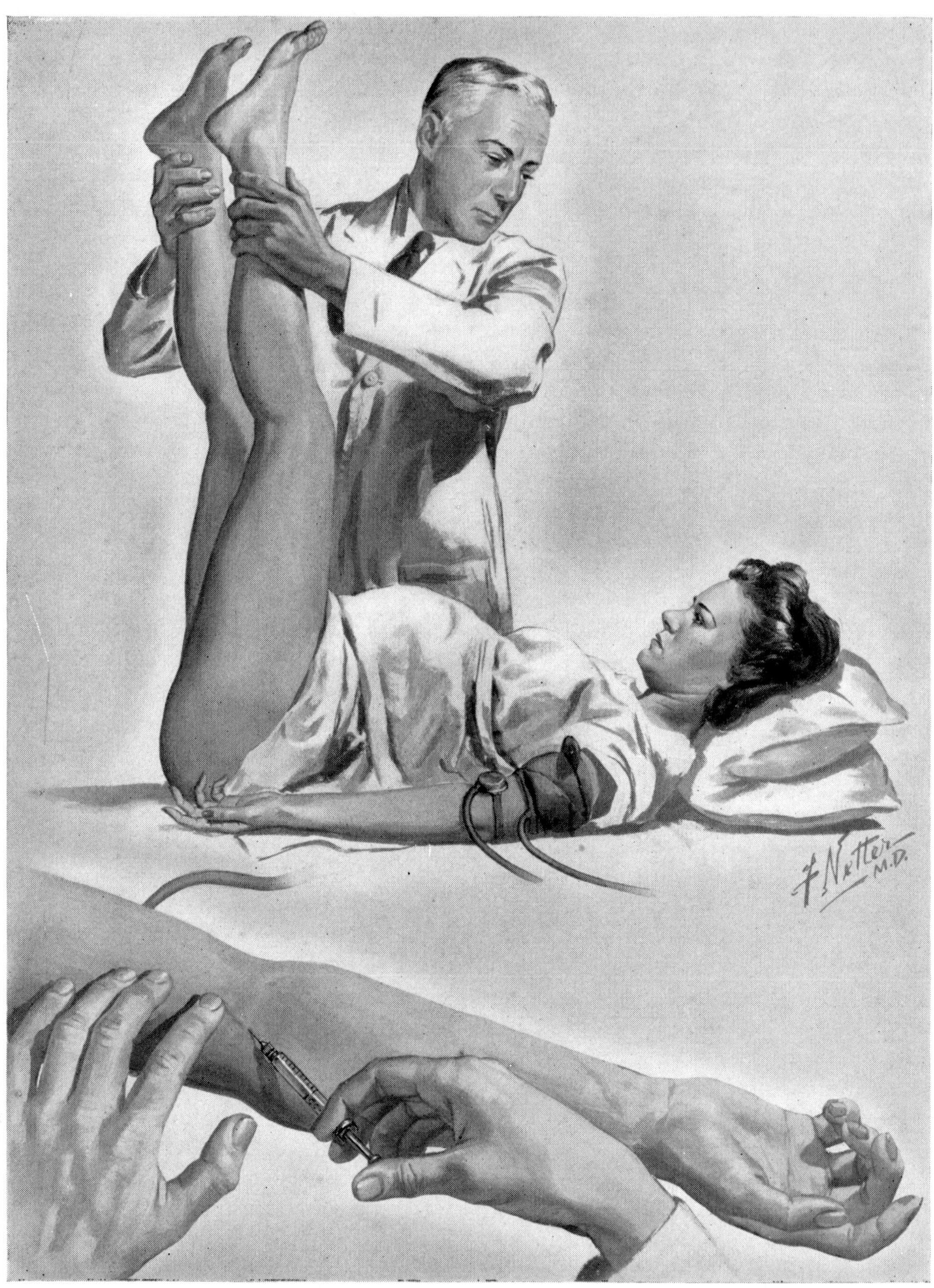

FIG. 114. Steps to combat hypotension. Step 1: Raising the patient's legs vertically provides an "autotransfusion" of 600 to 800 cc. Step 2: Ephedrine or Wyamine 15 to 25 mg. should be injected *intravenously*. (Copyright—Ciba Pharmaceutical Products, Inc.)

reapplied, and oxygen is forced in under pressure through the tight vocal cords. Reports from the pulse-taker or a quick feel of the carotids will dictate further therapy. A stiffened endotracheal tube may be forced through the glottis; or, if this fails, a tracheotomy should be done by the surgeon. This request should not come as a surprise to him, for conversation regarding the impending need, the direction of incision and the palpation of landmarks should have been going on. During this emergency, the surgeon, if possible, has desisted from surgical manipulations except for hemostasis or rapid delivery of the infant. He may assist greatly by palpating directly the uterine, the iliac or the aortic pulsation especially if no pulse-taker is available. Emergency tracheotomy should be done through the cricothyroid membrane, with horizontal incision both through skin and membrane. Oxygen should be administered through the opening and solid material removed with a long clamp or bronchoscopic forceps through a bronchoscope placed in the tracheal opening. Inflation of the lungs is imperative, whether directly by mouth or by blowing into an endotracheal tube placed in the tracheotomy opening or a bronchoscope. Cardiac massage through a thoracotomy wound is of *no* avail unless lung inflation can be obtained.

If this overwhelming emergency should occur during a vaginal delivery, the usual cause of failure is the lack of a *knife* blade for tracheotomy. Episiotomy scissors are poor substitutes, but even they could be used once the decision to perform a tracheotomy was reached. Sterile knife blades should be a part of the emergency equipment of every obstetric service.

If the emergency is circumvented without tracheotomy, it still is the anesthesiologist's duty to aspirate the trachea as soon as feasible. With fluid vomitus it is surprising how much may be inhaled before tight laryngospasm takes place. Postanesthetic orders should include an absolute minimum of opiates, special nursing or a prolonged stay in the recovery room, antibiotics, encouragement to cough, cool humidity, increased oxygen atmosphere if pneumonia is extensive, frequent turning and use of the cough machine if the patient will not, or cannot, co-operate.

In the last 17 years at the Sloane Hospital for Women, the incidence of this complication that caused death is 1:25,000. One death occurred in a conscious patient in 1938 and one in 1949 in a patient anesthetized with nitrous oxide-ether for cesarean section. During this time there were over 51,000 deliveries.

MARKED HYPOTENSION

The treatment for hypovolemic hypotension from hemorrhage was discussed earlier.

Hypotension relating directly to the use of drugs often results from a temporary overdosage of regional anesthetic agents by the infiltration, the pudendal, the caudal or the epidural route. Hypotension following spinal anesthesia usually results from too high a block of sympathetic fibers in the thoracic region. Occasionally this is the explanation of hypotension following caudal and epidural anesthesia, though much more frequently too much drug is given too fast. Rarely is intravenous administration of the drug the real cause. Elevation of the legs usually reverses the hypotensive trend; if it does not, intravenous injection of 15 to 25 mg. ephedrine will correct the hypotension. Oxygen therapy to the mother is indicated, of course.

Hypotension may result also from antepartum administration of Pitocin intravenously for induction of labor. It should be remembered that by *U.S.P.* standards 5 per cent Pitressin may be included in Pitocin, and we personally believe that this amount accounts for the rare case of hypotension following the intravenous use of Pitocin for induction of labor. Again, discontinuance of the oxytocic drug, elevation of the legs and intravenous introduction of a vasopressor drug should correct the complication.

As McRoberts has pointed out, postural hypotension in the full-term obstetric patient is a real entity. We have encountered it twice in 6 years. Turning the patient into a lateral position corrected the hypotension immediately. The explanations of the cause and the cure of such hypotension are far from satisfactory, but clinical evidence strongly suggests that if a patient exhibits undue hypotension when lying supine, it is well to turn her into a lateral position and deliver her in that position.

CONVULSIONS

The management of convulsions resulting from toxemia of pregnancy is discussed in a previous chapter.

Overdosage of regional anesthetic drugs may be a cause of convulsions. The importance of *time* taken for injection of regional drugs has not been stressed enough. Minimal lethal doses of regional drugs in animal experimentation rarely have taken into consideration the *time* taken for the injection of a given dose. If an injection must be done rapidly, as with a precipitate delivery, the *concentration* of the drug should be dropped to an absolute minimum. If the *volume* of drug is necessarily large, as with infiltration technic for cesarean section, concentration of the anesthetic drug again should be minimal. Premedication with depressant drugs, such as barbiturates or opiates, will minimize the chance for convulsions from this cause, but it will not necessarily prevent them. Should convulsions occur, a small dose of soluble barbiturate should be administered intravenously. Apnea should be expected to follow successful treatment of the convulsion, and equipment for endotracheal intubation and assisted ventilation always should be at hand. Fifty milligrams of Pentothal Sodium has been observed to produce apnea in a 200-lb. patient convulsing from an accidental overdosage of Pontocaine caudal anesthesia. Intubation and proper ventilation resulted in complete recovery.

Convulsions during labor are not infrequently related to unsuspected central nervous system disease. In the last 6 months we observed convulsions due to epilepsy, brain tumor and cerebral aneurysm. If fetal distress accompanies the convulsions, extraction of the infant is indicated. Depressant drugs, such as the barbiturates, should be used in small doses, with oxygen therapy and assisted ventilation if convulsions persist.

MARKED RESPIRATORY DEPRESSION

Usually, this condition is associated with attempts to prevent eclampsia. Too frequently, the infant is premature as well. Sedation, whether with chloral, paraldehyde, morphine or barbiturates, not infrequently produces a slow, ineffective ventilation in the mother. Oxygen therapy by a comfortably fitting face mask should be instituted to maintain as nearly normal placental oxygen tensions as possible. Most of these respiratory depressant drugs produce circulatory depression as well, which further indicates oxygen therapy. The high death rate in infants of toxemic mothers may be related in large part to poor antenatal oxygenation.

Respiratory depression related to central nervous system disease, such as myasthenia gravis and multiple sclerosis, needs special treatment. Pain-relieving drugs with central nervous system action should be avoided. Continuous caudal anesthesia is especially satisfactory in cases of myasthenia gravis. Tracheotomy is necessary in an occasional patient with severe neurologic disease, both for suction and for ventilation.

Severe respiratory depression from accidental high spinal or epidural anesthesia should be treated immediately with assisted ventilation, added oxygen and intubation of the trachea if ventilation without it is not satisfactory.

EXCESSIVE UTERINE SPASM

This condition is rare except with misuse of Pitocin inductions of labor, with delivery of the aftercoming head in breech presentations or with delivery of a second twin, whose position demands a version and breech extraction. In our experience, only *one* method is available to relax a uterus, and that is *deep general anesthesia.* The agent is of no importance, though we have found cyclopropane to be the most useful drug. Ether, chloroform, Trilene, Vinethene or ethyl chloride also may be used to produce third-plane anesthesia, but we have found cyclopropane to be by far the most expeditious agent to administer because of its relatively nonirritating qualities. The skeletal relaxants, such as curare and succinylchloride, are of no use in this situation; perineal relaxation may well be obtained, but not uterine muscle relaxation.

SEVERE HYPERTENSION

This complication is much less frequent than hypotension, but still it may be a cause of maternal death. By U.S.P. regulations Pitocin may contain as much as 5 per cent Pitressin, which in some patients results in hypertension, but in others in hypotension. Assiduous attention to the blood pressure is the only way to distinguish the difference in reaction to the drug. Ergotrate in its many commercial forms almost always causes hypertension. Overdosage of vasopressor drugs in spinal anesthesia will result in maternal hypertension. The main form of treatment is to discontinue the hypertensive-producing drug. Other suggestions are the production of general anesthesia, the use of vasodepressants, such as Arfonad or hexamethonium, though clinical success is far from established.

Whenever unexpected hypertension occurs, the possibility of pheochromocytoma exists. The use of true sympathetic blocking agents is definitely indicated in suspicious cases; Regitine, 5 to 10 mg., or benzodioxane, 15 to 20 mg., intravenously will control the immediate situation.

The following equipment is considered to be minimal to prevent maternal mortality. However, equipment never can supplant an intelligent obstetrician, anesthesiologist or obstetric nurse.

1. Oxygen. Piped-in system preferable because of minimal human failure; otherwise, "d" tanks, fitted with yokes, wrench and delivery tube.
2. Mask for patient who is breathing (Oxygen Equipment Manufacturing Company or Boothby, Lovelace & Bulbulian). The former type is fitted with a device for expiratory positive pressure in cases of cardiac failure with pulmonary failure.
3. Mask, headstrap and bag for patient who is *not* breathing. Bellows type hand resuscitators also are useful. Mouth-to-mouth (or nose) respiration always available without equipment.
4. Pharyngeal airways, plastic or metal, Sizes 3, 4 or 5; nasopharyngeal airways, small and medium sizes.
5. Endotracheal tubes, Sizes 32, 34 and 36, with metal stylets in each.

6. Laryngoscope in functioning condition. Macintosh blade the most useful.

7. Tracheotomy tubes, Size 5 or 6, with appropriate instruments for insertion; forceps, clamps, retractors, *knife* blade and handle.

8. Knife blade for tracheotomy or cardiac massage; No. 11, Bard Parker.

9. Suction machine; any type that works; proper adapters to fit all electrical outlets in delivery and labor rooms.

10. Stomach tube, large bore; occasionally useful as stimulus for vomiting.

11. Sterile syringes, 2, 10 and 50 cc.

12. Sterile needles; Lindemann type; 18 and 22 gauge, 2 in.; 20 gauge, 3 in., for regional injection.

13. "U" sterile tubes for blood collection; grouping, crossmatching, Rh and fibrinogen determinations.

14. Plasma expanders; dextran; polyomylpyrollidone; gelatin, serum albumin.

15. Vasopressor drugs; in solution; 5 per cent ephedrine sulphate; 0.2 per cent neosynephrine (20 mg. in 1,000 cc. solvent) with attached tubing; Regitine 10-mg. ampuls; benzodioxane 20-mg. ampul.

16. Barbiturate in solution; Nembutal 5 per cent, Seconal 5 per cent, Pentothal Sodium 2 per cent.

17. Local anesthetic in solution; procaine 1 per cent or Xylocaine 1 per cent.

18. *Beds* in labor rooms and *tables* in delivery rooms that can be put in head-down position.

CARDIAC ARREST AND RESUSCITATION*

While it might be possible to carry out successful resuscitation of patients who died elsewhere in the hospital, the major problem concerns the resuscitation of patients who die in the operating room or the delivery room. The necessary apparatus is available in both. If it is not available, it should be. Methods for successful resuscitation have been in existence for a good many years.[1] We surgeons and anesthetists have been slow in applying these methods. Every surgeon who operates should be familiar with these methods. We owe this to society. Indeed, it can be stated that any patient with a good heart and with good lungs who dies in the operating room or the delivery room can be resuscitated successfully. It is tragic loss of life if the surgeon is not prepared to take care of one of these emergencies when the crisis occurs. We have been giving a course in resuscitation to surgeons and anesthetists for the past six years under the direction of the Cleveland Area Heart Society. In the first 18 months we know of some 20 or more patients whose lives were saved by surgeons and anesthetists who had taken this course. The number of lives salvaged by these trained men now is more than 70.

The resuscitation procedure should be divided into two parts. Part 1 concerns the restoration of the oxygen system, and Part 2 concerns the restoration of the co-ordinated heart beat. These 2 parts of the resuscitation procedure should be regarded as separate and independent steps in the procedure.

Part 1

Restoration of the Oxygen System

This is the emergency part of the resuscitation procedure. In order to maintain life, a constant supply of oxygen to the brain is necessary. Brain cells disintegrate in a few minutes from lack of oxygen. (Probably damage demonstrable clinically begins in 3 minutes; and total brain death is complete in 11 minutes at normal body temperature.) Lack of oxygen to the brain is responsible for a good many of the children with cerebral palsy. The child at birth may not be breathing adequately, the airway may be obstructed, and the newborn baby may need mechanical respiration. If proper steps are not taken at the time of birth, the child may become one of this large group of children classified under cerebral palsy. In the operating room, if the patient stops breathing or if the heart stops beating, the brain immediately begins to undergo degenerative changes. If the anoxia continues for 5 minutes or so, these degenerative changes become irreversible. Usually it is a simple matter to restore the heart beat. If the resuscitation procedure is not carried out properly, the heart beat may be restored to a patient who has entered a vegetative condition. The period of an-

* This section, by Dr. Claude S. Beck, Professor of Cardiac Surgery, Western Reserve University, was read before a General Session of The Medical Society of the State of Pennsylvania in Pittsburgh, September 23, 1953, and published in *The Pennsylvania Medical Journal,* vol. 56, pp. 969-974.

oxia that can be tolerated by the brain cells without damage is influenced by temperature. The oxygen requirements are greater in high temperatures and reduced by low temperatures. Individuals have been taken out of a cold lake after having been submerged for a period of 10 minutes and complete recovery was obtained. For our purpose we can assume that there is a period of 3 to 5 minutes which can be taken to restore the oxygen system after it has once broken down.

The oxygen system can be restored by doing 2 things: (1) delivering oxygen into the lungs by intermittent positive pressure, and (2) circulating the oxygen by squeezing the heart. In order to do these 2 things, an intratracheal tube is necessary. A laryngoscope also is necessary, and someone must be available to introduce an endotracheal tube of proper size into the trachea. If an intratracheal tube cannot be introduced, then tracheotomy should be done. A rubber bag filled with oxygen also is necessary, and someone must squeeze the bag intermittently to deliver the oxygen into the lungs. In order to do these various simple steps within the time limitation we must be prepared. We are not doing the best for our patient if someone has to get an intratracheal tube and if someone else has to run off for oxygen and a rubber bag. These things should be available at the head end of every patient who has any surgical procedure done on him, whether it is done under general anesthesia or local anesthesia. Every hospital should make it a rule that these items are immediately available for every patient.

After the oxygen has been delivered to the lungs, it must be circulated so that the brain can pick it up. This can be done only by squeezing the heart. In order to do this, one must slit open the chest immediately and get the hand on the heart. Time is not taken to count the ribs for the incision, to put on gloves and gown, or to cleanse the skin. One knows approximately where to make the incision. It is made from the sternum out to the left axilla and is carried through the intercostal tissues; the cartilage above and below is cut across with a knife and a retractor is inserted into the wound so that the wrist of the person who is going to squeeze the heart will not become strangulated by the pressure of the ribs on the wrist. Someone can pull the ribs apart while a self-retaining retractor is obtained. The heart then is grasped by the hand, and it is emptied of blood. The rate of squeezing the heart is limited by the rapidity of the filling of the heart. It does not fill fast enough as a rule for it to be squeezed more than about 60 times per minute.

There are several methods by which the heart can be squeezed. One can put the right hand beneath the heart and squeeze it against the sternum. In children, the thumb can be placed over the right ventricle and the fingers over the left ventricle, and in this way the heart can be emptied satisfactorily. A third method is to use the fingers of the right hand over the left ventricle and 2 fingers of the left hand over the right ventricle. With experience one can make a blood pressure of 80 mm. of mercury, or even higher. However, there are precautions concerning this maneuver. The heart should not be squeezed so hard that the heart muscle is ruptured or bruised. It has happened more than once that a student in our resuscitation course actually stuck his finger into the left ventricle. Another point in the technic is to reduce all pressure on the heart during the phase of filling. The pressure that brings about cardiac filling is very slight, and the heart must be free to receive blood. Some years ago Mr. James Rand made suction cups that we could apply to the heart. These suction cups were used to pull the heart apart, so to speak, and in this way blood filled the heart more rapidly than was possible without them. With this more rapid filling the heart could be squeezed more times per minute, and in this way a larger volume of blood could be moved.[2]

It is not always necessary to split open the pericardium from base to apex, and I would not take the time to do this as soon as the chest is opened. I would squeeze the heart immediately and create some circulation, and later, if the heart cannot be grasped satisfactorily, the pericardium should be opened and the heart examined. As a rule, the pericardium is opened. The lungs should be well inflated and well deflated. The lungs should come up and go down nicely in repeated cycles about 20 times per minute. Lack of proper inflation and deflation of the lungs may be the cause of failure. The surgeon may be so intent on squeezing the heart that he does not notice the movement of the lungs. The lungs should not be distended constantly. They should come up and go down nicely in each cycle. A breathing machine is helpful if the procedure extends over a long period of time. In most instances, however, success is achieved in 10 or 15 minutes, and the bag of oxygen can be squeezed satisfactorily by the anesthetist for that period of time. Once the oxygen system is established, the crisis is over. The surgeon then can take time to take a few breaths for himself and reduce his own tension. Things are under control after these various steps have been taken properly. One can take an hour or several hours before the second part of the resuscitation procedure is carried out.

Are these the only effective steps in order to restore the oxygen system? In my opinion, these are the most effective steps that can be taken. If the necessary equipment is not available, then the surgeon considers alternative steps, such as trying to inflate the lungs by blowing into the patient's mouth or by squeezing the chest. Precious time may be taken by injection of Adrenalin into the heart through the chest wall. Someone might even try to give an intra-arterial transfusion of blood. Someone else might get an electrocardiogram to see for sure whether the patient is dead. Can the heart by emptied by squeezing it from beneath the diaphragm? The heart has been started by this maneuver, and it is probable that touching it or squeezing it started it to beat. My experience is that a satisfactory blood pressure cannot be produced by trying to squeeze it from below the diaphragm. An electric shock to defibrillate the ventricles cannot be applied effectively from below the diaphragm. If the abdomen is open when the heart stops beating, the surgeon can try this manipulation, but I would not waste opportunity if the heart does not start to beat immediately. I would be in favor of opening the chest and working on the heart under direct vision. If a tube cannot be inserted into the trachea, I would be in favor of doing a tracheotomy. We cannot accept failure because of inability to introduce a tube into the trachea.

The position of the patient is flat on the back. The table might be tilted so that the head is on a lower level than the feet by about 6 to 12 inches. This allows blood to drain from the legs and the abdomen into the heart, but at the same time the veins in the arms and the head do not empty as well as if the patient were horizontal.

Part 2

Restoration of the Heart Beat

When the heart stops beating it shows one of two conditions: either the heart is in ventricular asystole or it is in ventricular fibrillation. It is usually possible to differentiate these two conditions by examination of the heart. When the heart is in standstill, there is no motion of the ventricular musculature. When it is in ventricular fibrillation, one can see fine or coarse contraction waves that pass over the musculature. Sometimes these waves, like ripples on a quiet pond, begin in one small area on the heart and move out from this area to the entire musculature. Sometimes the fibrillation is so fine that an electrocardiogram is necessary for its recognition. In any event, an electrocardiogram is valuable as proof that the ventricles are fibrillating. Methods of handling standstill and fibrillation are quite different.

For Cardiac Standstill. Squeezing the ventricles often is sufficient to start a co-ordinated heart beat. Often the heart will start beating after the ventricles have been squeezed a few times. In these instances, restoration of the heart beat is no problem. I had 1 patient whose heart started beating without the pericardium's being opened. The individual who is squeezing the heart notes the tone of the ventricles. He knows whether the ventricles are flabby and soft or whether the myocardium is firm. If it is firm, a co-ordinated beat can be restored quickly. If it is flabby, then the tone of the heart must be improved by the use of Adrenalin. A small amount of Adrenalin is injected into the cavity of the right ventricle. This Adrenalin is moved through the lungs by squeezing the heart. It comes back to the left ventricle, and then small traces of the drug enter the coronary arteries and reach the myocardium. It is possible to feel the tone restored to the heart, and when one feels this, he can be assured that the heart is going to start beating. A normal heart wants to beat, provided the conditions are proper for it to do so.

For Ventricular Fibrillation. In the human heart ventricular fibrillation rarely stops spontaneously. As a rule, it is necessary to shock the heart out of fibrillation. This is done by using special apparatus, which should be available in every operating room. It is dereliction of responsibility for any hospital not to be provided with a defibrillating instrument. This defibrillating device can be made by an electrician, or it can be purchased from the Rand Foundation of Cleveland, which makes them without profit. A current of 110 volts is used. Resistors are placed in the apparatus to reduce the amperage to about 1½ amperes. The amperage can be increased or reduced. The electrodes are large, approximately 6 cm. in diameter. If they are small, they may burn the heart. The surgeon must protect himself against the current. The handles of the electrodes are insulated. In our operating rooms these electrodes are kept in a sterile package. The current is turned on for about a second or two. Sufficient time must be given for the current to go through the myocardium. A circuit is made and broken as the current is applied to the heart. The skeletal muscles will contract, and a jerk of the patient can be expected. The passage of the current through the myocardium causes all the muscle fibers to contract at one time while the current is applied. Then, when the current is broken, it is to be expected that the muscle fibers will relax uniformly without some of them going back into fibrillation. If the fibrillation ceases with the shock, one then has simplified the problem to that of standstill, and the same procedure as outlined in the discussion under "Standstill" is carried out. Sometimes the heart will go back into fibrillation, and, when this occurs, the shock must be reapplied. It may be necessary to use a drug to reduce the irritability of the heart so that it will remain in standstill. We discovered that procaine was effective in reducing the irritability of the heart so that it would remain in standstill after the electrodes were removed.[2]

Drugs and Their Application

In general, only 2 drugs are necessary for successful resuscitation. These drugs are Adrenalin and procaine. We advocate the use of small quantities of these drugs. The drug effect is obtained by way of the capillary circulation rather than injection into the myocardium. If a drug is injected locally into the myocardium, only a localized effect is obtained. If it is injected into the blood stream so that it reaches the capillary bed, then a generalized effect is obtained. We found that perhaps the most satisfactory way to administer drugs was to inject them into the cavity of the right ventricle. Two 10-cc. syringes should be available, and an 18-gauge needle is about the proper size. Adrenalin solution 1: 1000 is diluted 10 times with normal saline. From 3 to 5 cc. of this diluted solution is the usual dose of Adrenalin. The needle should be inserted at an acute angle through the myocardium rather than inserted perpendicularly to the surface of the heart. If the puncture wound is at an angle, there is less likelihood of bleeding after the needle is withdrawn. The surgeon should be careful not to stick the needle into a coronary vein or artery. Procaine is used in either a 1 or a 2 per cent solution, and the usual dosage is 5 cc.

Another drug that we have found to be of value is digitalis. We made this discovery in our course in resuscitation. Dogs that have been given Cedilanid (intravenous digitalis preparation) showed remarkable tendencies toward defibrillation. The hearts that were digitalized could be thrown into and out of fibrillation almost as many times as one desired. If we are having difficulty in restoring the heart beat in the human patient, I suggest that an intravenous digitalis preparation be administered. Other drugs have been advocated for the resuscitation procedure. Calcium gluconate will increase the tone of the heart, but I do not think that it is as effective as Adrenalin.

Closure of the Chest

The surgeon should observe the heart beat for a sufficiently long period of time so that he can be reasonably certain the heart is going to keep on beating after he closes the chest. It is unnecessary to suture the pericardium. If the pericardium is not closed, the opening in it should be large enough to prevent herniation. In other words, the pericardium should either be widely open or closed, allowing only for drainage of fluid. One should be careful about the internal mammary vessels, because these vessels might be cut when the incision is made, and because there is no blood pressure there will be no hemorrhage. These vessels might begin to bleed if cut and not ligated. Intercostal vessels also should be clamped and ligated. The incision in the chest then is closed as any thoracotomy is closed. It is advisable to put in a drainage tube and also to introduce antibiotics into the chest cavity and to administer these for several days thereafter. The patient may require oxygen or even mechanical respiration after the heart beat has been restored. In some instances, intravenous fluid should be given, and, if the heart beat is weak, Adrenalin should be added to the intravenous fluid so that a small amount of this drug goes in with the glucose or saline.

Causes of Failure

1. Too slow to get started. This is one of the most common causes of failure. The anesthetist may not recognize that the heart beat has stopped. The surgeon also may not recognize that death has occurred. One may feel for the pulse or listen for the heart beat for too long a period of time. In some instances, time is even taken to get an electrocardiogram during these moments of crisis. In one instance of which I know, the surgeon called in the Baltimore Fire Department to bring a pulmotor to the Johns Hopkins Hospital. Some surgeons have exposed an artery and given an intravenous transfusion during these first few minutes of crisis. In other instances the surgeon was so confused that he did not know what to do. Every surgeon who operates and every anesthetist who gives anesthetics should know what to do without thinking about the problem. The steps to be taken should be established by reflex mechanism brought about by training for the emergency. Hospitals should have a "fire drill" on resuscitation in which a dog's heart is fibrillated and defibrillated, and everyone on the staff should be familiar with the procedure. Such an exercise should be done once every year so that surgeons and anesthetists will be constantly prepared. As soon as the heart stops beating there is no alter-

native to the immediate establishment of the oxygen system.

2. Inadequate oxygenation of the lungs. As already stated, the lungs must come up nicely on inspiration and then go down nicely on expiration. The lungs should not be kept in a state of continued distention. I feel that I cannot overemphasize this point. A properly fitting intratracheal tube with inflatable cuff is essential. If a good fit is not obtained, the lungs cannot be inflated properly.

3. Inadequate circulation. The brain will be damaged if adequate circulation is not maintained. At no time can the oxygen system be stopped for more than a few moments in order to observe the heart or to apply electric shock. At all other times oxygen must be circulated by proper squeezing of the heart. This part of the procedure may have to be maintained for 1, 2 or 3 hours. Adequate exposure of the heart is necessary to empty the heart. Both ventricles must be emptied, and not just the left.

4. If the procedure is applied for a period of several hours and if a closed gas system is used, it may be necessary to change the soda lime for absorption of carbon dioxide. Failure to absorb carbon dioxide can interfere with the restoration of the heart beat.

5. Intrinsic heart disease. Anatomic conditions may be present in the heart which preclude successful resuscitation. In my experience these conditions have been glycogen storage disease, or von Gierke's disease, coronary artery disease, congenital defects of the heart such as interventricular septal lesions, pulmonic stenosis, and mitral stenosis. In one of my patients undergoing operation for mitral stenosis whose heart stopped beating before the valve was opened, the mitral valve was opened in about 10 seconds, and a co-ordinated heart beat was restored in 12 minutes. The oxygen system was maintained during this period so that there was no brain damage. In this instance mitral valvulotomy became a prerequisite to successful resuscitation. One of my patients with severe coronary artery disease was resuscitated successfully, but I have also had a number of patients with severe coronary disease who could not be resuscitated after working on them for several hours.

Conclusions

Any patient with normal heart and normal lungs can be resuscitated successfully if the proper steps are taken. Every surgeon and anesthetist should be familiar with the resuscitation procedure. Every hospital administrator should be obligated to provide a defibrillating device for use in the operating room. An exercise such as the "fire drill" should be carried out once a year in every hospital so that the staff always will be alerted to the requirements of the procedure.

Bibliography

1. Beck, Claude S., and Mautz, Frederick R.: The control of the heart beat by the surgeon with special reference to ventricular fibrillation occurring during operation, Ann. Surg. **106**:525, 1937.
2. Beck, Claude S., and Rand III, H. J.: Cardiac arrest during anesthesia and surgery, J.A.M.A. **141**:1230-1232, 1949.

Table 70. The Evaluation of the Newborn Infant (Method of Scoring)

Sign	Score 0	Score 1	Score 2
Heart rate	Absent	Slow (below 100)	Over 100
Respiratory effort	Absent	Slow; irregular	Good; crying
Muscle tone	Limp	Some flexion of extremities	Active motion
Response to catheter in nostril (tested after oropharynx is clear)	No response	Grimace	Cough or sneeze
Color	Pale blue	Body pink; extremities blue	Completely pink

Sixty seconds after the *complete* birth of the infant (disregarding the cord and the placenta), the 5 objective signs are evaluated, and each is given a score of 0, 1 or 2. A total score of 10 indicates an infant in the best possible condition.

INFANT SAFEGUARDS

It is not possible to define which individual should be taught the principles of infant resuscitation. It may well be that the obstetrician, the pediatrician, the anesthesiologist and the obstetric nurse all should be taught to take care of a depressed newborn infant, for each is free at different times. All should be well acquainted with the principles and the practices thereof.

Perinatal mortality taken from onset of labor until 48 hours of life has been reduced little in the last 30 years. The lack of good records at the time of birth is appalling; maternal delivery room records do not appear on the infant's chart. Furthermore, lack of neonatal "recovery

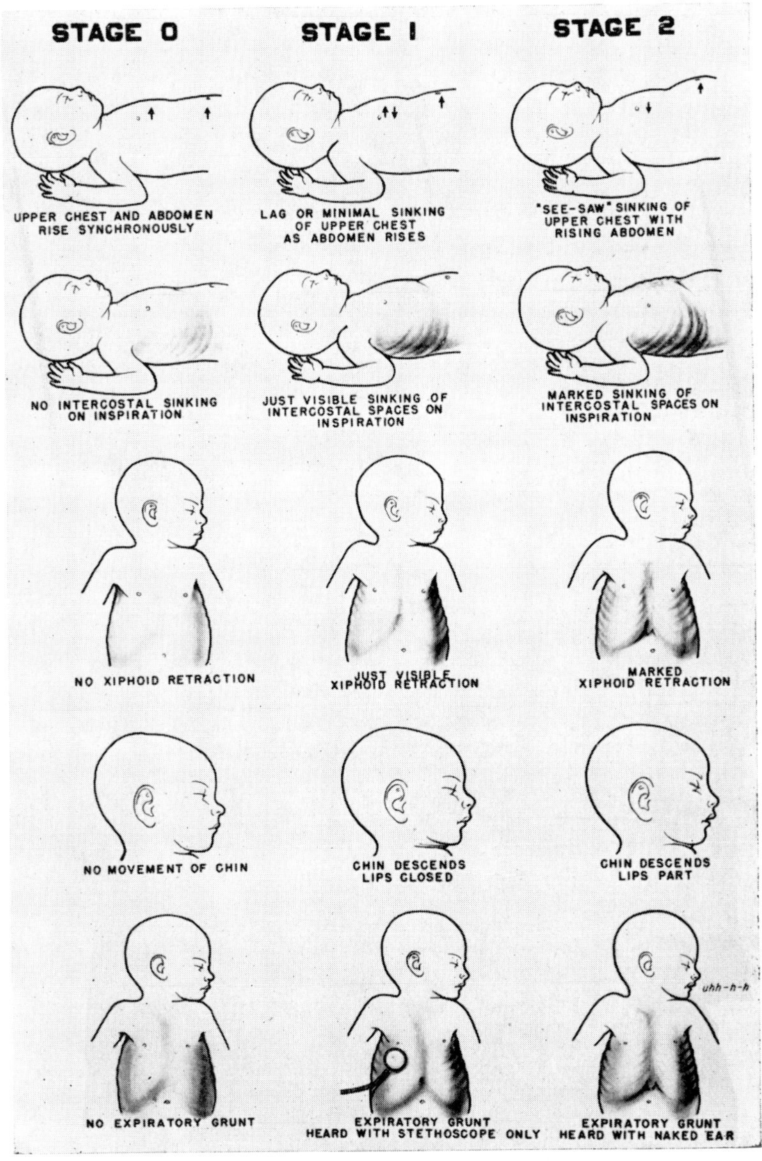

Fig. 115. Retraction score for premature infants.

rooms" has prevented much important recording of respiratory distress in the first 24 hours. Improvement as a result of better records can be hoped for, not without optimism.

As a beginning, for observation at birth a scoring system has been devised to be applied 60 seconds after birth by whatever route birth occurs (Table 70). Aside from focusing the attention of the obstetrician on the condition of the child, the pediatric nurse receiving the infant also notes the "score" and gives better attention to those infants with lower score. The initial score is definitely related to mortality (Table 71).

TABLE 71. RELATIONSHIP OF INFANT SCORING SYSTEM TO DEATHS (SLOANE HOSPITAL FOR WOMEN, 1953)

Score	Number Cases Scored	Percentage of Total Cases Scored	Percentage of Deaths
0-1-2	186	5.85	12.5
3-4-5-6-7	764	23.83	1.5
8-9-10	2,256	70.32	0.35

A different "retraction" score has been devised (Fig. 115), especially for premature infants. Quantitative estimation of respiratory distress by the "retraction" score checks closely with mortality rates in different age groups.

In general, we feel that no anesthetic agent or technic influences infant mortality, provided that maternal circulatory and respiratory depression is avoided. Also, a declining infant mortality rate is related directly to the presence of trained personnel who can immediately ventilate depressed infants or intubate them if necessary.

There are no reliable signs of fetal distress. Half the fetal hearts that are inaudible just before birth result in infants born in good condition; the remainder are stillbirths. Electrical amplification of fetal heart sounds will focus attention on cardiac irregularities, but it is of no use when sounds are absent. The presence of meconium in amniotic fluid before delivery may lead to difficulty through intra-uterine aspiration of meconium, the development of obstructive emphysema, which may proceed to spontaneous pneumothorax and prove fatal if it is unrecognized and untreated. If an infant survives aspiration of meconium, there is no evidence that breathing time or crying time is prolonged, that oxygenation at birth is unusually deficient, or that later intellectual development is delayed. Likewise, bradycardia or tachycardia of over 160 beats per minute in the antenatal period presages no future trouble if the infant survives the period of fetal distress. Fetal electrocardiographic methods need further development, for their accuracy surpasses that of auscultatory methods, but many technical problems remain to be solved. As yet, no device yielding good fetal cardiographs is available commercially.

The importance of a free airway in the infant cannot be overrated. Gibberd recently stressed this point. The infant can well be drowned by his first breath. The head-down position during and immediately following delivery is imperative. Prompt suctioning of visible pharyngeal fluids is indicated by either a bulb syringe or a suction catheter. A bulb has the advantage of being short enough to avoid touching the vocal cords, while a suction catheter with glass trap has the advantage of making visible the material aspirated and reaching deeper into the pharynx. If nothing is obtained by suctioning, it should not be continued, for vagal stimulation with accompanying bradycardia is frequent, and both oxygen and carbon dioxide are

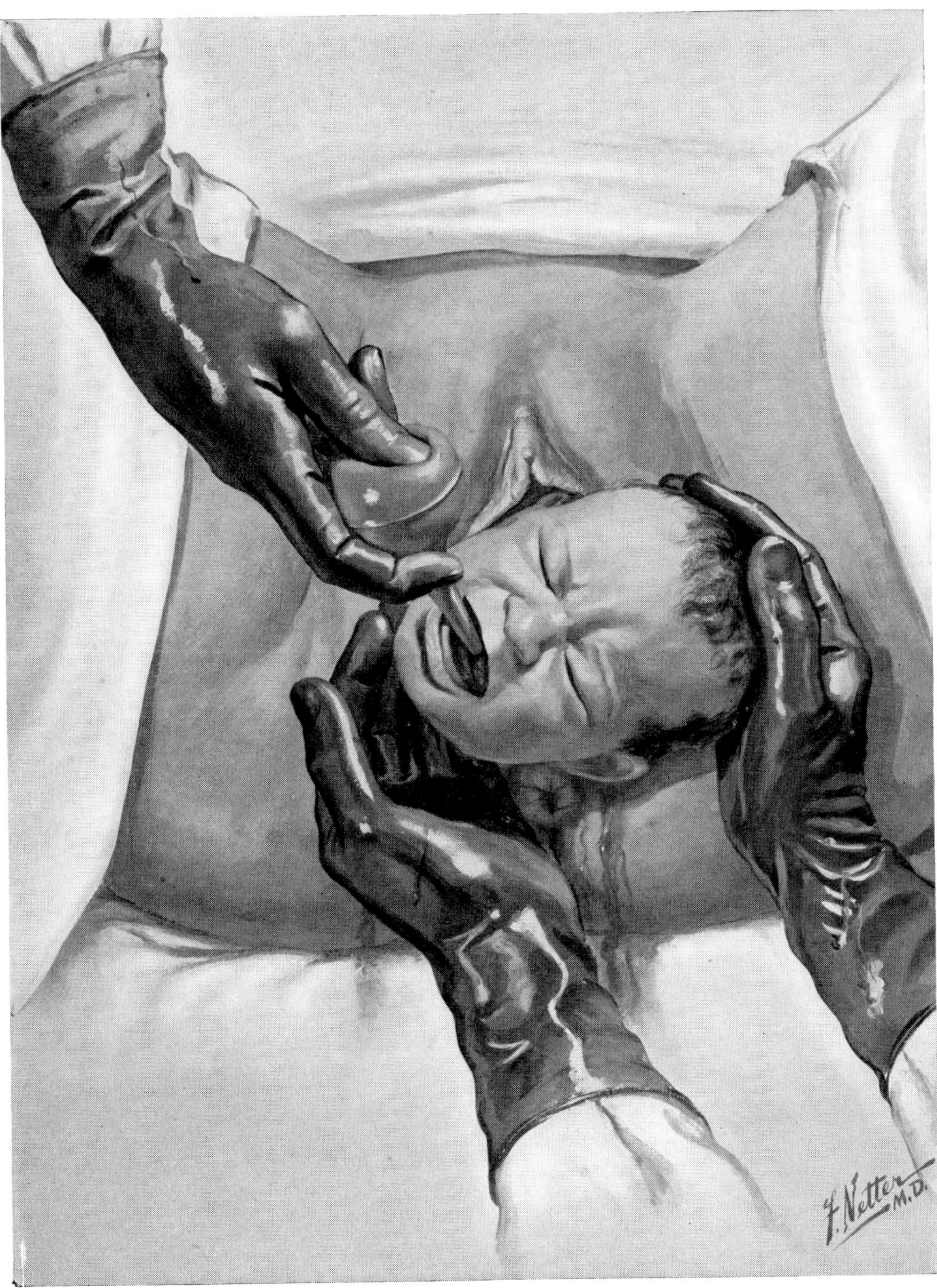

FIG. 116. Aspiration of mucus before complete delivery. Babies born under conduction anesthesia usually cry immediately. Mucus should be aspirated before delivery is completed. (Copyright—Ciba Pharmaceutical Products, Inc.)

removed from the pharynx. Direct laryngoscopy is a simple and a sure way to ascertain a free airway should resuscitative efforts be unavailing. If an infant is flaccid enough to "need" inflation on his lungs with oxygen, he also needs a pharyngeal airway to lift his tongue up from the posterior pharyngeal wall or palate. An infant plastic airway has proven to be satisfactory. If administration of oxygen is ineffective with a pharyngeal airway in place, endotracheal intubation is indicated. This is much quicker and more accurate with direct laryngoscopy than tactile intubation. A "premature" blade attached to a pencil handle is simple to use. All delivery room personnel should be familiar with its use, practice being obtained on stillbirths and recent neonatal deaths.

Circulatory adjustments at birth and their importance are far from settled.

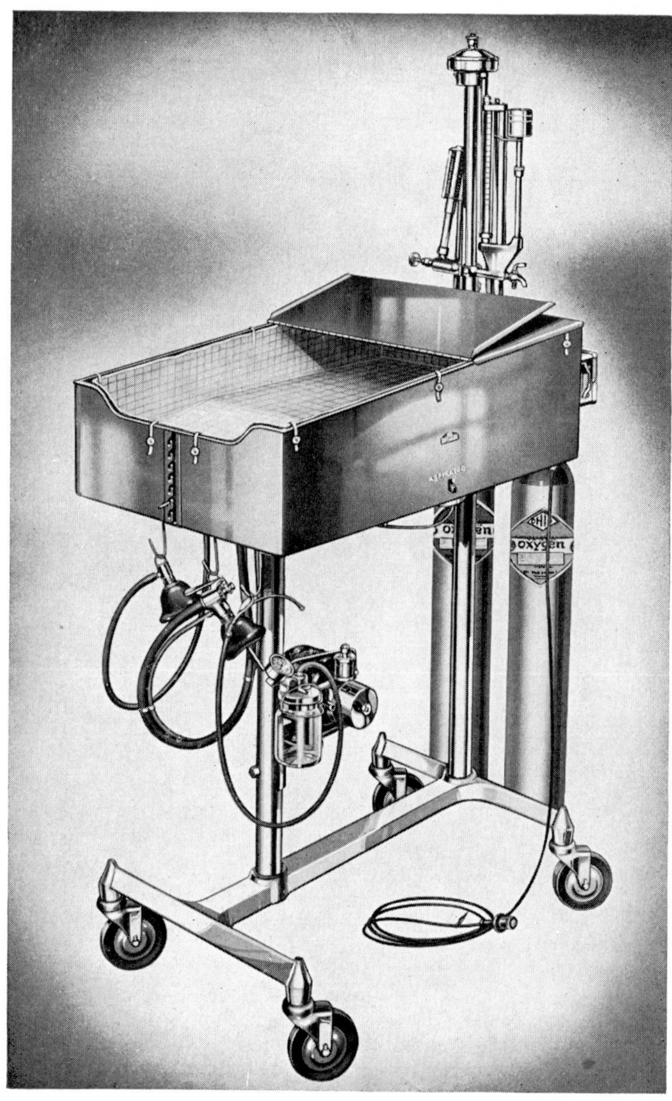

Fig. 117. Kreiselman infant resuscitator. (Ohio Chemical Company)

Marked changes occur in the first few minutes after birth. Heel blood samples taken during this period are not related in any way to cord blood taken just after birth. Reynolds has demonstrated a drop in blood pressure in new born lambs with the first breath; Everett has measured the 130 per cent increase in pulmonary blood in the first 24 hours in guinea pigs. It is an accepted fact that fetal blood can be shunted into the newborn infant or the placenta merely by holding the infant higher or lower than the placenta. Proponents of "holding the infant lower than the placenta before the cord is clamped" theory mention the increased iron thus obtained that tides the infant over the preliminary nursing period; on the other hand, the hypervolemia of viscous, high hematocrit blood thus produced may be a factor in etiology of "hyaline membrane" syndrome in premature infants. Holding the infant higher than the placenta may well be utilized in Rh-sensitized infants who will receive exchange transfusions. It is safer to have such an infant hypovolemic, so that overloading of the circulation with exchange transfusion will be less apt to occur.

No real evidence exists as to whether or not ventilation needs to be assisted, and if it does, when. Higgins questions the advisability of any resuscitative efforts. There is real need for random selection of resuscitation methods in depressed infants to prove or to disprove this idea.

As yet there is no satisfactory method of ventilating newborn lungs artificially. Aside from the question of whether or not such ventilation should be attempted at all, the methods already developed are open to serious question, not only as to their efficacy, but also as to what is expected of them. Proponents of low pressure methods (Fig. 117) probably expect safety with assisted respiration through absorption of oxygen in the smaller bronchioles. Pressures below 12 cm. of water probably cannot expand collapsed alveoli, particularly those with absorption atelectasis. It has been shown by Day and his co-workers that such collapsed lungs, at least in rats, can be expanded safely by sudden short high pressure resuscitation. At present, this can be accomplished in the human being by one of two methods: mouth-to-endotracheal tube inflation with added oxygen to the operator's mouth; or the GBL inflator (Fig. 118), which allows pressures as high as 60 cm. of water. The time of such high pressure inflation always should be kept as short as possible. There always is danger of alveolar rupture, particularly in the mouth-to-mouth or mouth-to-endotracheal tube method.

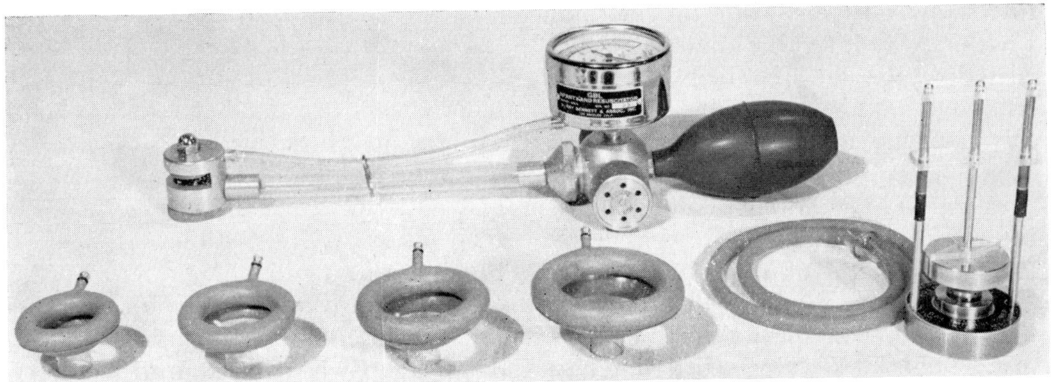

FIG. 118. GBL infant hand resuscitator.

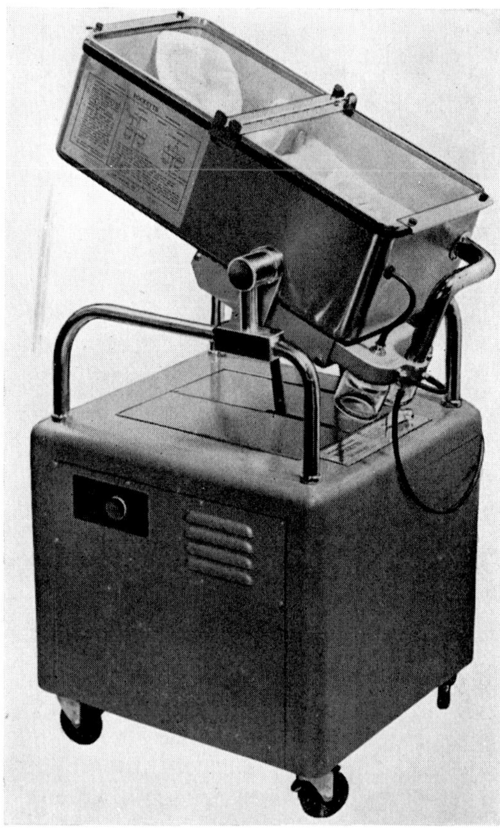

FIG. 119. The Rockette Millen-Davis rocker.

If the latter has been used, antibiotics should be given routinely. The efficacy of these high pressure methods in the human being is unknown, but it is our feeling that these may be more effective than anything hitherto tried. If the infant already is breathing but is somewhat depressed, respiration may be stimulated with a rocking bed (Fig. 119). Although recent studies have shown that this machine affected respiration profoundly, its real merit has yet to be affirmed. The essential point is that so little is known about the initiation and the maintenance of respiration in the first few minutes of life that only the crudest and perhaps totally ineffective instruments for assisting ventilation have yet been developed.

We feel strongly that a "newborn recovery room" should be established in clinics with over 2,000 births. The many advantages gained from a postoperative, or postanesthetic, room are overwhelming as to patient care observation of the newborn infant, regardless of color and economic status, for 24 hours cannot help but bring benefit to both infant and nursing and medical personnel. Visiting hours for fathers and grandparents can be arranged easily. The scoring of retraction of respiration, as well as the results of treatment, can be undertaken easily; equipment for resuscitation can be centered in such a nursery rather than in 6 or 7 places in larger hospitals. The best nursing care can be congregated in such a nursery.

Before the infant leaves the delivery room, but after good respirations have been established, we feel that gastric aspiration is indicated in all infants when there is any reason to suspect tracheo-esophageal fistula with atresia of the esophagus. At present we have no reason to feel that emptying the stomach will prevent respiratory complications. However, with a maternal history of polyhydramnios, a large amount of stomach contents indicates duodenal atresia or volvulus. In 2 recent cases, 50 and 120 cc. were present, with duodenal atresia in one case and volvulus in the other. Immediate operation should result in complete cure.

Diaphragmatic hernia not infrequently causes respiratory difficulty. Almost always it is fatal if it is not diagnosed shortly after birth. If it has developed *during* intra-uterine life, the mother may have polyhydramnios because of the fetal intestinal obstruction. However, if the defect in the diaphragm does not become apparent until the infant cries and forces abdominal viscera into the chest, diagnosis may be delayed until the infant cries. Then auscultation will reveal *no* breath sounds on one side and a marked displacement of the heart to the left or the right. Such infants sometimes become quite pink in the first few minutes but cyanosis returns and deepens as the viscera are pushed higher in the chest by crying. Displacement of the heart, which originally was placed centrally, and absent breath sounds suggest the diagnosis. Spontaneous or mechanically produced pneumothorax offers the only other possibility. Percussion and a roentgenogram enable the proper diagnosis to be made.

In 20 to 30 per cent of cases, maternal polyhydramnios is associated with fetal abnormalities. Why this should be so is unknown, but it may be that, in some way yet to be discovered, the anomaly interferes with the role of the fetus in the dynamics of amniotic fluid exchange. The conditions in the infant that we have observed in the past few years to be associated with polyhydramnios were anencephalia, only if the medulla itself was involved; 75 per cent of the tracheo-esophageal atresias and fistulas in those in whom the opening of the fistulous tract was too stenotic to accommodate such a transfer of amniotic fluid from the lungs to the stomach; diaphragmatic hernia; certain undetermined types of congenital heart disease; acute volvulus with gangrene of the small intestines and duodenal to mid-jejunal atresias.

Immediate emergency operation is urged in any anomaly amenable to the surgical approach. The newborn infant is much more resistant to the insult of anesthesia and surgery the first day than 2 to 7 days later. Whether this is due to his inherent ability to carry on some of his metabolism anaerobically, or whether there has not yet been time to upset his fluid and electrolyte balance, is not known. Both factors probably play a part. In demonstrating atresia of the esophagus, the radiologist should refrain from using barium, bismuth or Lipiodal in making the diagnosis, for aspiration of these materials may cause severe anoxia.

Of the anomalies mentioned so far, tracheo-esophageal fistula, diaphragmatic hernia, perforation of the stomach, duodenal atresia and volvulus should be corrected a few hours after birth. Other anomalies not associated with polyhydramnios in which immediate operation is indicated are omphalocele, imperforate anus and meconium ileus. When diagnostic methods for congenital cardiac lesions in the *newborn* infant are perfected, some of these also will be treated surgically. Ligature of a large ductus arteriosus should not be difficult. Intracardiac surgery depends not only on perfecting diagnostic methods but on increasing the safety of hypothermic technics and extracorporeal circulation technics.

The behavior of the infant's temperature at different environmental temperatures and at different ages has not been studied well. It seems illogical, though firmly established by centuries of practice, to attempt to increase the body temperature of infants who are having difficulty with oxygenation. Drawing a parallel from cardiac surgery in young children, it is more logical to cool off such an infant. All warmed living tissues have a higher oxygen consumption than when cooled. A hypoventilating infant has difficulty in maintaining sufficient *tissue* oxygenation. This situation should be assisted by cooling rather than by warming the infant.

In a series selected at random and controlled completely, there is no evidence that excessive humidity or the use of wetting agents, such as "Alevaire," is of any benefit to an infant with respiratory distress.

There is much evidence that high concentrations of oxygen should be avoided, especially in the premature infant. Retrolenticular fibroplasia is related definitely to high concentrations of oxygen, time of exposure and age of infant; the toxic effects of high oxygen on an infant's lung are less well known. A suggested relationship of pulmonary hemorrhage to excessive oxygen in small laboratory animals is possible. The rapid occurrence of atelectasis in lungs that contain high oxygen and then are subjected to tracheal obstruction is common knowledge. For these 3 reasons, all delivery and nursery room oxygen outlets should be fitted with a valve that reduces the inflow from an oxygen source to about 40 per cent or less. This is harder to achieve in equipment designed to give positive pressure to the face or the lungs, but at present 50 per cent can be achieved.

There is room for great improvement in the keeping of records of the perinatal period. Several hospitals have introduced improved forms and methods of collecting data, but their value lies mainly in interested, conscientious personnel. No record keeps itself. At present we feel that before the infant *leaves* the delivery room, the following data should be entered upon the mother's anesthesia chart, preferably in triplicate, by the anesthesiologist: signs of fetal distress (meconium before delivery; fetal heart under 100 or over 160); amount of fundal pressure + to ++++ (hidden placental separation may cause severe unrecognized intra-uterine anoxia); the total score 60 seconds after birth of the infant; changes in the score at varying intervals if they are dramatic (improvement from 0 or 1 to 8 or 9, a fall from score of 8 to 2 after a period of deep pharyngeal suction due to tight laryngospasm); type of oxygen therapy used (none, face mask, positive pressure mask; endotracheal tube, short, sharp high pressures, preferably with height of pressure recorded); the fact that the stomach was aspirated, and the volume and the description of the contents in every case. At admission to the newborn recovery room, a retraction score is noted and charted, and is observed at intervals of 3 or 4 hours if respiratory status was deficient upon admission or deteriorated from a previously satisfactory condition. Only by accurate, impersonal recording of such data in every case can clinical impressions as to therapy during the perinatal period be evaluated. Such records also are invaluable for the study of later mental, emotional, physical and psychological development.

No mention has been made of the use of drugs administered intramuscularly or into the umbilical vein. All central nervous system stimulants increase oxygen consumption, some for unpredictable lengths of time. Since a depressed infant's chief problem is to get enough oxygen for normal metabolism, it is illogical to administer drugs that demand more oxygen. The other approach, lowering metabolism to meet the lower oxygen tensions present, is more reasonable. At present, moderate hypothermia by physical means is the safest method. The status of drugs that lower body temperature remains to be determined.

N-Allylnormorphine, a pure opiate, will reverse respiratory depression caused by morphine or Demerol but not by barbiturates or physiologic abnormalities. In 2 years we found only 30 infants in whom the use of the drug seemed to be indicated. Intravenous injection of 0.25 mg. into the umbilical vein was successful in improving respiration in about 75 per cent, but it was hard to decide to what to attribute the results — the use of the drug or other treatment, such as oxygen therapy. The several neonatal deaths that occurred did not seem to be related to the use of the drug. A much better rationale is to avoid the use of undue doses of opiates, so that no antidote is necessary. Because of the many ways in which direct laryngoscopy is practiced in the depressed newborn infant, a short description of a simple technic seems to be in order.

The infant is placed in the supine position, at the end of the bassinet nearest the operator, with a small folded towel beneath his shoulders. It is *not* necessary to extend his head over the end or to have anyone else hold the head. The infant laryngoscope is held in the *left* hand at all times. The right thumb and the index finger separate the lips while the scope is introduced between the tongue and the palate (not beneath the tongue!), starting at the right angle of the mouth. The purpose of this is to push the tongue to the left and out of sight as the blade is introduced more deeply. The blade is advanced gently until the posterior pharynx is reached. Visually, any obstruction material present is aspirated. Then the scope is lifted toward the ceiling and advanced a few millimeters farther, whereupon the epiglottis or the glottis itself comes into view. The feeling in the left hand is that of lifting up the child's mandible with the tip of the scope. Force never is necessary. The glottis appears as a vertical chink in the most anterior part of the exposure thus produced. If no obstructing material is present, an endotracheal tube, held in the right hand, is advanced from the right corner of the mouth downward and through the vocal cords. The "slot" in the laryngoscope is meant for vision, not for passage of the tube. More room for vision (and the tube) is obtained if, as the scope is advanced, it is swung over to a *medial* position, although the original insertion was on the right side. The tongue should be conspicuous by its absence. The commonest error in laryngoscopy is to pass the instrument too deeply and visualize a round, dark opening, which is the esophagus, with the cricopharyngeus muscle simulating the glottic ring. Treatment is to withdraw the scope a few millimeters, the tip always being lifted upward, when the glottis will fall into view. At this point, both openings will be seen; the anterior one, vertical and smaller than the posterior one, which is round. If the tube is advanced too deeply, endobronchial intubation will take place, which is highly undesirable. After the tube has been seen to pass through the cords for about 1 cm., the scope is removed, and the left hand grasps firmly the point of the chin and the tube so that their relationship will not change. A short, sharp puff while the operator watches the chest will assure him that the tube is in the trachea. If the chest does not move and a pharyngeal gurgle is heard, the tube is in the esophagus and should be withdrawn promptly for proper insertion. Auscultation of the chest also will check the position of the tube.

The following equipment is recommended as minimal for each delivery room:

A bassinet with shallow sides, which can be kept in a head-down position to receive the infant immediately after birth.

Suction equipment: rubber bulb, approximately 30 cc. capacity, for use in clinics that practice delayed clamping of cord, or No. 12 French rubber suction catheter, with 2 orifices near tip connected to glass trap, whose volume has been measured, and rubber connecting tubing. The source of suction can be electrical, mechanical from a piped-in system, or the operator's mouth. Convenience, reliability and simplicity should guide the decision as to which should be selected.

Source of oxygen: piped-in systems very advantageous; present "keyed" tanks prevent possibility of putting wrong gas on oxygen yoke; D or E tanks if oxygen must be transported from one room to another; G tanks if source remains in one room; the operator's mouth contains about 14 per cent, better than none. Melco O_2 Reducing Valves to 40 per cent.

Airways: Berman plastic airway, infant type, satisfactory except in very large infants.

Laryngoscope that works. Pencil handle, batteries, "premature" blade and bulbs; should be tested before each case.

Endotracheal tubes: none wholly satisfactory; for short, high pressures; Kreiselman, Cole and No. 0 portex all in use; No. 00 portex with glottic stop being developed.

Malleable wire stylet of copper or brass very useful if tube has not enough curve; potentially dangerous, as is all resuscitation equipment.

Plastic catheter for suction of endotracheal tube (No. 444T BD) with Luer hub; 2 cc. Luer-Lok syringe used if tracheal suction is necessary.

Ventilating equipment: This item is left to the last intentionally, for there is none that can be recommended unqualifiedly as to safety and efficiency. With one exception, none has an automatic timing device to limit application of pressure or volume. None is available commercially. An intelligent operator is still the best "timer," whether gas is delivered from a bag and mask, from a manually operated device, such as the Mann or the Kreiselman, or from the mouth. There is no convincing evidence in favor of a negative suction phase or automatic cycling. Very few infants (0.1-0.5%) are truly apneic (*no* respiration). It is desirable to have a machine that can be controlled with electrical cycling and also fit the infant's respiration immediately when it becomes initiated. Such is not available commercially in this country; one such device is under investigation in Great Britain. Stimulation of the phrenic nerve electrically is logical if the airway has been cleared, but the adult stimulators do not seem to be efficient enough in newborn infants. Apparently, a stronger current is needed. Rocking beds assist circulation more than respiration. Some infants and experimental animals with weak respiration will change to a rhythm similar to that of the machine, but others show further reduction in ventilation. Further investigation on this point is under way. Co-operation between respiratory physiologists and manufacturers is gratifying.

Gastric insufflation of oxygen has been shown in newborn and adult animals to be wholly ineffective in relieving anoxia during apnea. Human clinical results, which on the whole, have been good, result from increased pharyngeal oxygen and diffusion respiration or occasional gasps by the infant. Oxygen delivered into the pharynx by nasal catheter accomplished the same result without the accompanying gastric and intestinal distention.

BIBLIOGRAPHY

Maternal Safeguards

Barach, A. L.: Physiologic Therapy in Respiratory Diseases, pp. 356-358, Philadelphia, Lippincott, 1948.

Hale, D. E., *Ed.*: Anesthesiology, chap. 27, Anesthetic Emergencies, pp. 557-578, Philadelphia, Davis, 1954.

McRoberts, W. A., Jr.: Postural shock in pregnancy, Am. J. Obst. & Gynec. **62:** 627-632, 1951.

Pillar, S.: Re-emphasis on bone marrow as a medium for administration of fluid, New England J. Med. **251:**846-851, 1954.

Tocantins, L. M.: Rapid absorption of substances injected into bone marrow, Proc. Soc. Exper. Biol. & Med. **45**:292-296, 1940.

INFANT SAFEGUARDS

Apgar, V. A.: Proposal for a new method of evaluation of the newborn infant, Anesth. & Analg. **32**:260-267, 1953.

Gibberd, G. F.: Mechanism, Prevention and Treatment of Asphyxia in the Newborn Infant, pp. 26-42, *in* Council for International Organizations of Medical Sciences: Anoxia of the Newborn, Oxford, Blackwell, 1953.

McCall, J. O., Jr., and Fulsher, R. W.: A study of fetal distress; its interpretations and significance, Am. J. Obst. & Gynec. **65**:1006-1019, 1953.

Silverman, W. A., and Anderson, D. A.: Controlled clinical trial of effects of Alevaire mist on premature infants, J.A.M.A. **157**: 1093-1096, 1955.

Wilson, J. A., *et al.*: Anaerobic metabolism in the newborn infant: 1. On the resistance of the fetus and newborn to oxygen lack, Pediatrics **6**:581-592, 1948.

10 Organization of Obstetric Anesthesia Service on a 24-Hour Basis

SPECIAL CONSIDERATIONS

Of the 12 million anesthesias administered each year in the United States, more than 4 million are obstetric. Even though the vast majority of obstetric anesthesias are of short duration and are administered to patients in good health without complication, at least 75,000, or approximately 2 per cent of the total, are for cesarean section. This operation carries a recognized mortality, both in the United States and in Great Britain, of 1 per cent throughout the last decade. One half of the maternal deaths in these patients delivered by cesarean section are related in whole or in part to anesthesia.

More than 10 per cent of the 3 million obstetric anesthesias are administered to patients with toxemia, hemorrhage or major complications of the circulatory, metabolic or respiratory systems. At least 5 per cent, or 180,000, of these anesthesias are administered to patients delivering premature babies in which the infant mortality ranges from 50 per cent in the 1,500-Gm. and smaller babies to 6 per cent in the 2,000-Gm. and larger babies.

Obstetrics has been declared the specialty of nocturnal practice superimposed upon an 8-hour day. At least as many babies are born by night as by day, requiring in contradistinction to a surgical anesthesia staff on 8-hour duty 3 separate staffs of physicians, nurses and anesthetists for day and night duty.

The following conditions require that obstetric anesthesia and its departmental management be given the combined special consideration of anesthetists and obstetricians and hospital administrators:

1. Each single anesthesia involves the safety of 2 persons: the mother and the baby.

2. Frequently, many hours of analgesia and seminarcosis precede anesthesia in obstetrics to provide for control of pain in labor.

3. All drugs used to control pain in labor and in delivery in sufficient quantities exert effect upon and may stop uterine contractions. Thus, there must be a blend of pain relief compatible with progress in labor.

4. Obstetric patients, unlike surgical patients for planned operations, frequently present themselves near delivery in precipitous labor after having eaten a full meal. Thus, anesthesia is called for in the unpremedicated and the unprepared patient.

5. The obstetric anesthesia staff must be relatively larger than the surgical anesthesia staff to provide adequate coverage throughout both day and night practice.

At present there are several systems of obstetric anesthesia organization employed in hospitals of various sizes throughout the United States and Canada. These are:

1. Anesthesia service provided by physician anesthesiologists on a 24-hour rotation basis, directed by a physician anesthesiologist who devotes full time to this specialty. Until recently this type of service was available in only a minority of large hospitals of the major cities of

the United States. In 1950, this type of service was available in only 5 per cent of the 107 maternity hospitals in Greater New York. Today in New York and in several other large cities it is available in more than one quarter of them.

2. Services comprised of a combination of nurse anesthetists or, indeed, obstetric nurses with little or no formal training in anesthesia, on routine rotation duty working with obstetricians capable of giving their own conduction anesthesia. Probably this is the most common type of anesthesia service available in the majority of hospitals today.

3. Anesthesia services in which nurse anesthetists on call are available in emergencies only to supplement the work of the obstetrician who frequently administers his own anesthesia.

4. Services in which the obstetrician alone is responsible for the conduction of his obstetric anesthesia and is compelled to use routine obstetric nurses and/or medical students as assistants. This type of service in hundreds of small hospitals is compelled to provide a vast number of anesthesias for obstetric delivery.

From the problems enumerated at the beginning of this text, it is obvious that special training not only in anesthesia but in obstetrics is necessary to qualify the obstetric anesthetist. The processes of natural labor must not be jeopardized by too deep or too early administration of analgesia and anesthesia. It is imperative that certain respiratory depressing agents be not used in terminal labor and in the delivery of the premature baby. Many anesthetists who have daytime responsibilities beginning at 6 A.M. are not able to render long hours of night duty regularly. For these reasons the authors feel that the following basic requirements are necessary to provide safe anesthesia on a 24-hour service:

All obstetric interns and residents and nurses must be taught fundamentals of sedation, anesthesia and resuscitation as a part of their responsibilities in obstetrics. They must know standard routines for proper oxygenation of the patient with anesthetic gas machines, especially in situations of intra-uterine fetal distress, maternal hemorrhage, overt or concealed, and in premature labors. They must be taught the management of patients under at least one simple conduction anesthesia, such as local and pudendal, saddle block spinal or caudal analgesia; the conduct of labor and delivery from the psychological standpoint in those cases in which all types of analgesia and anesthesia are contraindicated or not required or not available; they must know at least one basic systemic anesthesia technic, such as nitrous oxide-oxygen, gas-ether-oxygen anesthesia or open drop ether anesthesia. They must understand the principles of replacement fluid therapy, vasopressors and transfusions in dehydration, toxemia, anemia, hemorrhage and prematurity. So far as the house staff goes, we have found that it is easier to teach basic anesthesia to obstetricians than to teach obstetrics to anesthetists.

John J. Bonica and George H. Mix, of Tacoma, have written recently:*

> It is generally conceded that the contribution made by the rapidly developing science of anesthesiology constitutes one of the most important factors that has made possible the great advances in surgery during the past quarter of a century. Unfortunately, the same cannot be said in regard to obstetrics. While it should be readily admitted that many of the improvements in anesthetic practice have been applied to obstetrics, the contributions in this field have not been commensurate with the progress made in anesthesiology. This is especially true in regard to the administrator, a factor that, in the final analysis, is the most important to be considered. Most of the interest in obstetric anesthesia has been

* Twenty-four hour medical anesthesia coverage for obstetric patients, J.A.M.A. **159**:551-554, 1955.

focused on refinement in technics and producing better agents, but relatively little has been written or done to encourage the development of expert administrators. It serves little purpose to discuss the selection of methods of anesthesia unless there is a corresponding effort to encourage the application of these methods with the best judgment and greatest skill. A further reduction in the mortality and morbidity in obstetric anesthesia will depend to an increasing extent on the ability of the anesthesiologist and his active participation on the obstetric team to the same extent that he participates on the surgical team. Both the anesthesiologist and the obstetrician must share the blame for the fact that this is not the case at the present time.

The obstetrician has been at fault for accepting, in many instances, the barest minimum of anesthetic service at the hands of the most uninformed and the least useful person in the delivery room, whereas in his gynecologic practice he would be satisfied only with the services of an expert anesthesiologist. The obstetrician should encourage, and even demand, that the department of anesthesiology be organized to give the obstetric service expert administration of any type of analgesia or anesthesia any time it is desired. If anesthesiologists cannot offer such technics as caudal, peridural or subarachnoid blocks as a regular service, it is inevitable that they will be unavailable when most needed. The obstetrician deserves the benefit of the anesthesiologist's skill in the management of patients whose lives are threatened by hemorrhage, toxemia or other complications, as well as in those abnormal conditions that might interfere with the lifeline of the fetus, such as prolapsed cord, prolonged labor, eclampsia, dystocia and premature separation of the placenta. Moreover, he should derive the benefit of the anesthesiologist's skill in the management of asphyxia neonatorum and expert knowledge of depressant drugs and be able to rely on the latter to observe and evaluate the many and varied regimens of sedatives, narcotics and amnestic drugs recommended for the first stage of labor. The obstetrician should have the interested and informed co-operation of the anesthesiologist so that he may avoid the many occasions for hazardous synergistic combinations that exist between obstetric drugs and anesthetic agents.

The provision of such services is a responsibility of the specialty of anesthesiology. Anesthesiologists must devise ways and means of solving satisfactorily the problem of providing round-the-clock anesthesia service to the obstetric department.

The patient must be provided with expert anesthesia at reasonable fees while the obstetrician may expect more efficient and more capable service and patient care. The availability of such expert services on a 24-hour basis facilitates the hospital administration and enhances the reputation of the hospital, thus greatly improving its over-all care.

It is true, of course, that there is still a shortage of anesthesiologists and such an arrangement as herein described is obtained by an evolutionary process that requires the concerted effort and co-operation of anesthesiologists, obstetricians, hospital administrators and the nursing staff.

Anesthesia services should be organized along the following principles:

1. The prevention of maternal and fetal mortality through competent administration and proper choice of anesthesia
2. The maintenance of prolonged comfort of patients compatible with physiologic progress in labor
3. The thorough understanding of the major causes of maternal and fetal anesthetic mortality and morbidity
4. Equitable budgetary provisions for standard anesthesia, whether administered by anesthesiologist, obstetrician or nurse anesthetist

STAFF ORGANIZATION

With these principles in mind, we submit the following organization with a division of responsibility for all categories of obstetrics and anesthesia staff in the delivery room. The types of anesthesia to be administered by all personnel are listed for spontaneous delivery, for operative delivery and for cesarean section. We believe that only the simplest types of anesthesia should be administered by student nurse anesthetists and by medical student clerks. Xylocaine, a rapidly acting and spreading anesthesia in 1 per cent concentration, is a safe agent for medical students and interns to use in local injections to the perineum and as pudendal block. In those hospital services fortunate enough to have obstetric and anesthesia interns

Director Physician Anesthesiologist

Obstetrician Director — Chief Nurse Anesthetist

		Nurse Anesthetists	Obstetric Residents		Anesthesia Residents		Private Anesthetist
		Student Nurse Anesthetist	Medical Student Clerks	Staff Obstetric Interns	Obstetric Interns Assigned to Anesthesia	Anesthesia Interns	Private Obstetrician
Analgesia for labor		Trained to administer on doctor's order intravenous analgesics and intramuscular and oral sedation	None; observation only	Demerol Barbiturates Scopolamine Opiates and magnesium sulfate with resident's consultation	Systemic analgesia only in consultation, with obstetricians	Systemic analgesia only in consultation, with obstetricians	1. Demerol 2. Scopolamine 3. Barbiturates 4. Rectal ether 5. Continuous caudal
Anesthesia for spontaneous delivery	Multipara	1. Nitrous oxide 2. Vinethene 3. Drop ether 4. Trichlorethylene	Local and pudendal block	Local and pudendal saddle block Trichlorethylene Analgesia	1. Gas-oxygen 2. Saddle block 3. Caudal 4. Pentothal	1. Trilene 2. Gas-oxygen 3. Vinethene 4. Saddle block 5. Caudal 6. Pentothal	1. Caudal 2. Saddle block 3. Pudendal and local 4. Nitrous oxide 5. Trilene
	Primapara	1. Nitrous oxide 2. Vinethene 3. Drop ether 4. Trichlorethylene	Local and pudendal block	Local and pudendal block Trichlorethylene Analgesia	1. Gas-oxygen 2. Drop ether	1. Gas-oxygen 2. Trilene 3. Vinethene	1. Nitrous oxide 2. Trilene 3. Pudendal block 4. Local
Anesthesia for forceps or operative vaginal delivery	Multipara	1. Gas-oxygen-ether 2. Vinethene 3. Pentothal Sodium	None	Local and pudendal block, saddle block	1. Spinal, saddle and caudal 2. Gas-oxygen-ether	1. Spinal, saddle and caudal 2. Gas-oxygen-ether 3. Cyclopropane	All indicated systemic and conduction anesthesias
	Primapara	1. Gas-oxygen-ether 2. Vinethene 3. Pentothal Sodium	None	Local and pudendal block	None	1. Curare-supplement on indication	All indicated systemic and conduction anesthesias
Anesthesia for cesarean section		1. Pentothal Sodium* 2. Cyclopropane* 3. Gas-oxygen 4. Ether * Under experienced supervision.	None	None	1. Continuous spinal 2. Continuous caudal 3. Continuous peridural 4. Pentothal Sodium 5. Local	1. Continuous spinal 2. Continuous caudal 3. Continuous peridural 4. Pentothal Sodium 5. Cyclopropane 6. Local and Pentothal Sodium	1. Continuous spinal 2. Pentothal Sodium 3. Cyclopropane 4. Caudal and extradural 5. Local
Infant resuscitation, staff obstetric nurse and pediatrician		None	Suction and aspiration	Suction, oxygen Positive pressure resuscitation	Suction, oxygen Positive pressure resuscitation Direct vision intratracheal intubation and aspiration Blind palpation intubation Intravenous stimulants	Suction, oxygen Positive pressure resuscitation Direct vision intratracheal intubation and aspiration Blind palpation intubation Intravenous stimulants	Suction, oxygen Positive pressure resuscitation Direct vision intratracheal intubation and aspiration Blind palpation intubation Intravenous stimulants

FIG. 120. THE ORGANIZATION OF A 24-HOUR ANESTHESIA SERVICE WITH DELEGATION OF RESPONSIBILITY.

under the direct supervision of obstetric and anesthesia residents, a much wider choice of anesthesia and analgesia is permissible. However, it is our belief that the use of amnesia and analgesia should be kept primarily in the hands of the obstetrician managing the patient. The anesthesia staff serves only as consultants in this situation.

In those clinics in which the private qualified anesthetist and private obstetrician manage their own cases or in which anesthesia interns and residents are under the direct supervision of a physician anesthesiologist, a much wider range of anesthetic technics is possible, as indicated on the accompanying chart (Fig. 120).

It is significant that even today only a very few hospitals in the United States have facilities for rendering anesthesia round the clock with a specially trained staff. The usual organization, which borrows in times of emergency from the surgical anesthesia staff, is to be condemned. In many hospitals the income from obstetric anesthesia is diverted in large measure to other spheres of hospital activity. It is dangerous for obstetric anesthesia and patients to be so neglected. We recommend that anesthesiologists, obstetricians and hospital administrators reconsider immediately an improvement of this important activity.

The timeliness of this subject of organization of obstetric anesthesia service and the indications of intense interest on the part of anesthesiologists are illustrated by the two editorials which follow:

OBSTETRIC ANESTHESIA*

It is unfortunately true that anaesthesia for the obstetric patient has received too little attention from anaesthetists. There have been several reasons for this neglect. Many anaesthetists, being otherwise adequately employed, have shunned obstetric anaesthesia because of its demands on their time, particularly at night, and because of the numerous rush calls of an emergency nature which it entails. Others have considered it minor anaesthesia, taking little real interest in the unique problems involved. Many members of the profession have undoubtedly believed that the obstetric patient requires so little anaesthesia in most cases that the services of an anaesthetist are not warranted, and this attitude has been prevalent enough to make it possible in the recent past for a medically sponsored plan for prepaid medical care to make no provision for obstetric anaesthesia.

The serious need for expert attention to the problems of obstetric anaesthesia must be apparent to all when it is considered that aspiration of vomitus during delivery remains an important cause of maternal morbidity and mortality, that the part played by anaesthesia in neonatal death is yet far from being defined, and that many infants still succumb to asphyxial incidents at birth who might be salvaged by the expert care which a qualified anaesthetist can provide.

Fortunately, a number of well-qualified anaesthetists have in recent years turned their attention to the problems involved in providing analgesia and anaesthesia for the obstetric patient during labor and delivery. Their studies and experience have resulted in greater understanding of the problems involved and in the introduction of many new technics for dealing with these problems. There has also developed an ever-increasing awareness of the benefits to be derived by the patient from intelligent co-operation between the obstetrician and the anaesthetist throughout the labor. More thought has been given alike to the factors which produce pain in labor and to the effect of conventional methods of pain relief on the course of labor.

It becomes increasingly apparent that routine treatment of all obstetric patients by one method of pain relief is unsatisfactory, if not, in fact, dangerous practice. Yet publications on the subject continue to appear suggesting that all obstetric anaesthesia should be managed by one technic to the exclusion of all others. We believe that however satisfactory the results may appear, such an attitude will lead to application of the method blindly and to the detriment of some mothers and infants.

* Canad. Anaesthetists' Soc. J. 1:57, 1954.

NEGLECT OF OBSTETRIC ANESTHESIA CAN HARM OUR RELATIONS WITH PATIENTS, HOSPITALS*

Leading anesthesiologists have emphasized the important added margin of safety possible in childbirth through professional anesthesia serv-

* Report by The American Society of Anesthesiologists, February, 1955.

ices. On the other hand, this phase of anesthesiology often is neglected in the rush of more complicated procedures, and administration of obstetric anesthesia is left to technicians. Failure to develop this phase of our specialty in more and more institutions may be a serious disservice to the patient and to the hospital, from both a medical and human relations standpoint.

WHAT THE PATIENT EXPECTS

Newspapers from time to time publish articles on deaths occurring under anesthesia during the simplest operations. It is possible that many of these could not be avoided. It is equally true that a qualified anesthesiologist often can prevent shock or other conditions responsible for death under anesthesia. *The importance of having a trained physician at the head of the operating table during any surgical procedure, no matter how large or how small, is constantly emphasized by the Society.* More and more patients realize the importance of professional anesthesia. Death for any reason during elective surgery simply cannot be tolerated. The patient knows that better anesthesia care is available than ever before, and expects it.

OPPORTUNITY FOR CONFUSION

Probably no one is more confused about anesthesia than an expectant mother going to the hospital for the first time. For weeks she has been reading popular articles about new drugs, hypnosis, natural childbirth, spinals, saddle block and similar subjects. She has discussed the subject of anesthesia with her friends. And she is hopelessly confused on the subject. *Then she arrives at the hospital in pain, usually at a time when her obstetrician is not present. She may get too much analgesic, not enough analgesic, or the wrong kind of anesthetic for her condition.*

A mother having her third child recently had her baby held back until the obstetrician arrived, then had it without benefit of anesthesia whatsoever. The baby suffered a brain injury in childbirth. And this happened at a maternity hospital that supposedly is one of the finest in America.

24-HOUR SERVICE ESSENTIAL

It is worth pointing out that if professional anesthesia is desirable at 8 o'clock in the morning, it is equally desirable at midnight. A hospital with a qualified anesthesia staff has the right to expect service on a round-the-clock basis for its patients. *More and more hospitals are certain to demand such service and to take steps to obtain it if their staff physicians do not meet the challenge.* A great many anesthesiologists are recognizing this problem and meeting the need, one result being that a qualified physician usually is on hand. This can be particularly important to obstetric patients, who obviously cannot schedule their exact hour of arrival at the hospital in advance.

THE MEASURING STICK

Most obstetric patients recall the anesthesia care they receive or the lack of it as the most vivid impression of the type of medical care accorded them. *A mother who has an unpleasant experience in childbirth is going to have a sorry opinion of the quality of anesthesia care at your hospital for the rest of her life, no matter whether you had anything to do with her care or not.* How much better would it be if she received some information about anesthesia from you in advance of her confinement and knew that a physician anesthesiologist would be on hand to greet her and provide her with the finest care available before her obstetrician arrived and during the period of childbirth.

PRACTICAL PROBLEMS

Naturally, there are practical problems in many institutions where the supply of physician anesthesiologists is small and the number of maternity cases is substantial. On the other hand, who is to tell the public that professional anesthesia is vital in every surgical procedure, yet is not to be provided in obstetric cases where the well-being of both mother and child is at stake?

It may be a long time before practical problems can be removed and professional anesthesia services can be provided to every obstetric patient in your hospital. But planning towards this end is essential in our specialty. It is important from a sound medical viewpoint. And it is equally vital in terms of the sound human relationships needed for the orderly growth and development of our specialty.

In no branch of medicine is the relationship between patient and physician as close as that between a prospective mother and her obstetrician. This has led to an accentuated feeling of responsibility and possessiveness on the part of good obstetricians that make them somewhat reluctant to share that responsibility developed through the months of prenatal care. This attitude is summarized in an editorial by Keith Folger entitled, "A Quarter's Worth of Chloroform, Doctor, Please," which is quoted in part below:*

The obstetrician has experienced a change in the responsibility for the anesthesia and has been tremendously relieved to know that he could put all his thoughts on the operation at hand and not worry about the condition of the patient. This approachable Utopian goal has not been reached easily or quickly. Long years of effort in teaching and training anesthetists has started to change the anesthesia picture for medicine in the present era. Why, then, should a few dark clouds appear on the horizon for the obstetrician?

These clouds first appear when the obstetrician contemplates the matter of responsibility to the patient. This responsibility has been built up over a period of months, and in some cases years. Every time a patient is delivered each of us learns the peculiarities and tendencies of that patient to a greater degree. In the light of her experience the patient has made us promise that certain things will or will not happen the next time.

This does not refer to the legal responsibility of an anesthetic where administered by a paid medical anesthetist. A California court has ruled on that point, stating that the anesthetist is responsible for the anesthesia. Rather, this refers to pleasant or unpleasant highlights of the labor. The second labor was more painful than the first. The headache after a spinal anesthesia was unbearable. The nurse left the patient on the bed pan so long after her initial enema that phlebitis developed. "Could the loss of the baby be due to countless different 'thises' or 'thats'? Did my obstetrician arrive in time to deliver my baby?" These and a million other questions, many legitimate, must be answered to the satisfaction of the patient.

What is the picture today from our point of view? We are seeing the nurse anesthetist disappear before sufficient numbers of trained medical anesthetists are available. Even in departments headed by a well-qualified physician, the nurse anesthetist still is depended upon to give many of the anesthetics, although her status is relegated to that below the residents in training. In some instances, the young doctor, just out in practice, is making a living as a part-time anesthetist, under the direction of the head of the department. This is good, but it does not qualify him as a well-trained man in anesthesia although he may be eligible for certification by the Board in his own specialty.

Obstetrics makes far greater demands in hours on duty than any other specialty. There is no specialty in which periods of peaceful inactivity occur, alternating with jam sessions in which everyone wants to have a baby at the same moment. Crisis after crisis occurs with accidents of pregnancy and labor. The apprehension and excitability of the patient in labor is also added to the problem.

Therefore, it is essential that the anesthetist interested in obstetrics know and appreciate these attitudes and their background. He must be thoroughly familiar with good obstetrics and the milieu of the delivery floor. Also, he must recognize that not only is he required to be a patient's doctor but also to take his part in the team as the doctor's doctor.

It is impossible for the director of a surgical anesthesia service who is completely involved in the problems and the time schedule of many surgeons to render an efficient service to the obstetric patients and to the obstetricians who must, of necessity, dictate their own schedule. The solution lies in the procurement and the education of anesthesiologists within the field of obstetrics. Only then, under this type of direction, can residency training in obstetric anesthesia be meaningful.

Hospital administrators and obstetricians should recognize that the shortage of physician anesthesiologists is more apparent than real. As soon as conditions are developed in which he is invited to practice his specialty in a standard manner similar to that of any other specialist, with opportunities for both private and service practice, will personnel be found ready to share full 24-hour responsibility.

ENVIRONMENT

The advent of physician anesthesia, augmenting existing anesthesia staffs, and the application of the principles of obstetric pain relief enunciated in this volume require the renovation of both labor and delivery areas as follows:

* Obst. & Gynec. 4:588-590, 1954.

1. The noisy labor room and the rooms in which patients are managed under profound sedation and amnesia should be separated physically from the quiet labor rooms in which patients have total elimination of their pain produced through the methods of conduction anesthesia by the anatomic approach or through the nerve conditioning of psychological childbirth. It is recommended that facilities providing air-conditioning and soundproofing be instituted wherever possible. Furthermore, the construction of inlets for pure oxygen and vacuum for suction is a recommended safeguard.

2. Facilities must be developed for the normal mental activity of patients during labor managed by methods of conduction and physiologic childbirth technics. The following are suggested:

A. Attractive interior decorating of the labor room with indirect lighting and controlled reception of sunlight

B. Carefully chosen restful paintings of flowers, landscape or water scenes placed artfully round the walls

C. A small, attractive bedside library supplied with recent periodicals and short stories

D. A bedside radio or other facilities for music

E. A small bedside table from which a patient may enjoy fluids and timely and appropriately selected nourishment

F. An attractive bed with a hard sponge-rubber mattress

G. An attractive wall mirror conveniently located so that the patient may keep herself physically tidy and, thus, boost her own morale in maintaining her self-respect

H. Since many women in labor, because of endocrine disturbances, develop a nasal congestion, Benzedrine inhalers or ephedrine nose drops should be provided as part of the routine management.

I. A bedside bell or an intercommunicating system to the head nurse's desk

J. In some instances we have found that a psychological advantage ensues from having some labor rooms constructed so that 2 women may labor in the same room as companions.

K. The training of special nurse anesthesia assistants who understand the principles of blood pressure and fetal heart determinations, analgesia charting and intramuscular medication, as well as the psychological principles involved in the management of patients under the regimen of sedation in the encephalic approach, conduction anesthesia in the anatomic approach and physiologic childbirth through relaxation and the development of a conditioned blockade against labor stimulus

The patient of high intelligence who has absolute confidence in her obstetrician and goes through labor relieved of pain but conscious of her surroundings and what is being done for her has in her mind an indelible impression of what actually is the concept of modern obstetrics. In the management of a patient who is conscious, much can be and should be done to give her mental tranquility without fear of the outcome of her labor. This is accomplished by a cheerful atmosphere in the labor room, which should be furnished much like the patient's own comfortable room at home. The conversation should be along lines that have nothing to do with her present ordeal. Her interest in reading light literature should be aroused. Her thoughts can be taken away from her present environment by the judicious use of the radio. For example, one patient became so engrossed in listening to a football game that she was reluctant to leave the labor room for the delivery of her baby; another enjoyed a full program of the Metropolitan Opera during

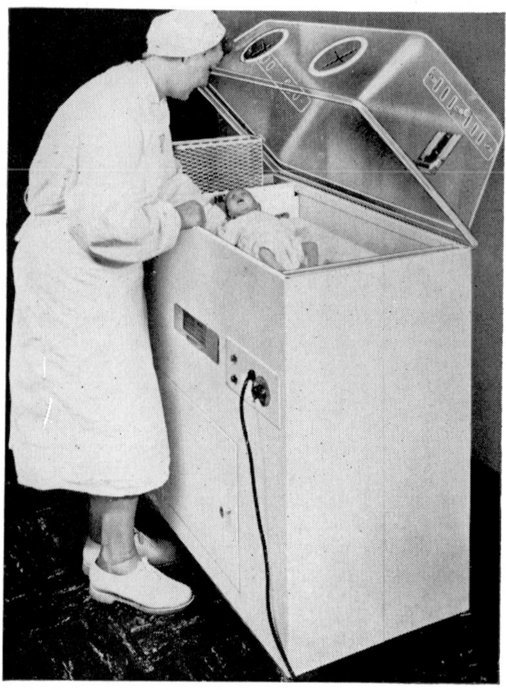

FIG. 121. The Continental Infantair is a combination of incubator, oxygen tent, surgical and isolation unit. It provides a heating element, as to temperature and humidity; is formed to satisfy the needs of the infant. Oxygen can also be administered, if so desired, with or without cooling. The built-in Ice Chamber, holding up to 10 pounds of ice, provides efficient cooling, and is easily accessible through a rustless chute in the hood.

The Plexi-glass hood with entry ports, offers complete visibility at all times, and provides easy access to the patient for both doctor and nurse at the same time without disturbing the heat, humidity or oxygen concentration, also the facility for removal of soiled linen without danger of contamination of entry ports for feeding, etc. (Continental Hospital Service)

her labor. These two incidents indicate that a suitable type of entertainment for the patient is not incompatible with good scientific management of the case. A favorite form of occupation of our patients under caudal anesthesia is a soft drink or a tea party. The hot fluids, glucose, caffeine and relaxation afforded by this repast are welcomed by both nurses and patients. When a patient is given continuous caudal analgesia, the psychology of the patient and attendants in the labor room is entirely different from the management of a patient under the sleep-producing methods.

If the labor is managed by the use of amnesic or sedative drugs, the following conditions should be instituted: (1) absolute quiet and (2) a partially darkened room conducive to sleep and rest. Particular emphasis should be placed on the conversation between those in attendance, because although the patient may seem to be entirely unconscious, often under the influence of these drugs statements are confused and are remembered after the drugs have been eliminated. Instances have been cited in which patients have been emotionally upset following their labor because they thought statements detrimental to themselves or their personality were made while they were under the influence of the drugs.

THE POSTANESTHESIA RECOVERY ROOM

On the delivery floor much attention must be given to the planning of comfortable and attractive facilities surrounding patients during their emergence from all forms of anesthesia and during the immediate postpartum period when the control of obstetric hemorrhage and postdelivery uterine relaxation is so important. All patients will remain in this area for at least 1 to 2 hours. It will contain all the safeguards of fluid therapy, stimulant and analeptic drugs, and postdelivery sedatives. Bedside wall oxifiers for the administration of humidified oxygen by nasal catheter mask or by intermittent positive pressure resuscitation, wall suction for removal of respiratory mucus and vomitus, and

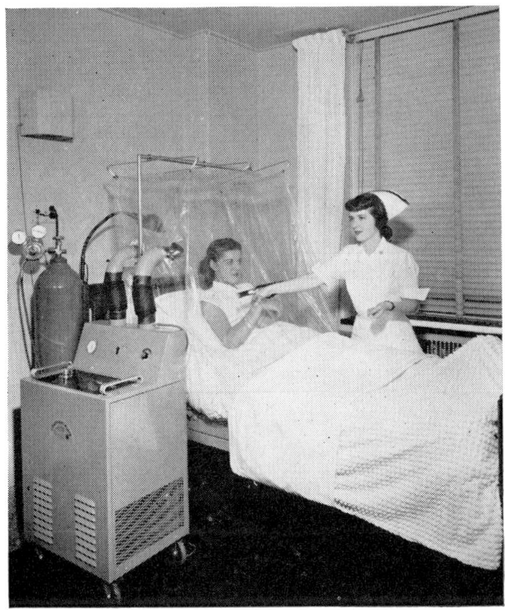

FIG. 122. Continentalair Iceless Oxygen Tent with automatic temperature control, the purpose of which is to draw the vitiated air from within the canopy, where it is cooled through variable temperature adjustments by automatic refrigeration; excess humidity is removed, and the air is changed 3 times per minute, as the ideal for air therapy.

As the condensate is accumulated in the cleaning chamber, through which the air is forced, it effects a water screening for automatic removal of airborne irritants. This expedites comfort by aerating patients following anesthesia, and is of comfort, especially during the pollen season, to asthmatic, hay-fever and cardiac patients, etc.

Oxygen concentration and increased humidity can be effected as indicated by the attending physician. (Continental Hospital Service)

beds with facilities for providing both the Trendelenburg and the Fowler positions—all are essential.

It is imperative that this area have good lighting to reveal any evidence of suboxygenation. There are many occasions on which several patients can be cared for properly in a single large room, but others on which it is necessary to provide transfusions and other types of therapy which may appear alarming to normal patients emerging from a general anesthesia or patients in full control of their mental faculties who were delivered without general anesthesia. For these reasons, and for the reasons of maintaining special equipment in the study and the protection of the patients during emergence from general anesthesia, at least one room should be separated from the larger area. We recommend that this recovery area be placed conveniently close to the office of the anesthetist and separated from the labor suite. It is a matter of practical consideration to have this room close to the elevators for transporting the patients back to their rooms and divisions and for receiving in indicated cases members of the family.

Index